Nephrology and Hypertension Board Review

Nephrology and Hypertension Board Review

Phuong-Chi T. Pham, MD, FASN

Chief
Division of Nephrology and Hypertension
Program Director
Nephrology Fellowship Program
Olive View-UCLA Medical Center
Sylmar, California
Clinical Professor of Medicine
David Geffen School of Medicine
University of California
Los Angeles, California

Phuong-Thu T. Pham, MD, FASN

Director
Outpatient Services
Kidney Transplant Program
Ronald Reagan UCLA Medical Center
Clinical Professor of Medicine
David Geffen School of Medicine
University of California
Los Angeles, California

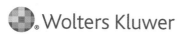
. Wolters Kluwer

Philadelphia • Baltimore • New York • London
Buenos Aires • Hong Kong • Sydney • Tokyo

Acquisitions Editor: Kel McGowan
Product Development Editor: Leanne Vandetty
Production Project Manager: Bridgett Dougherty
Design Coordinator: Joan Wendt
Manufacturing Coordinator: Beth Welsh
Marketing Manager: Rachel Mante Leung
Prepress Vendor: S4Carlisle Publishing Services

9 8 7 6 5 4 3 2 1

Printed in China

Library of Congress Cataloging-in-Publication Data

Names: Pham, Phuong-Chi T., author. | Pham, Phuong-Thu T., author.
Title: Nephrology and hypertension board review / Phuong-Chi T. Pham, Phuong-Thu T. Pham.
Description: First edition. | Philadelphia: Wolters Kluwer Heath, [2017]
Identifiers: LCCN 2016015989 | ISBN 9781496328076
Subjects: | MESH: Kidney Diseases | Hypertension, Renal | Outlines
Classification: LCC RC903 | NLM WJ 18.2 | DDC 616.6/10076--dc23 LC record available at https://lccn .loc.gov/2016015989

LWW.com

Contributing Authors

Monica S. Deshmukh, MD
Assistant Clinical Professor
David Geffen School of Medicine
University of California
Los Angeles, California
Department of Radiology
Olive View-UCLA Medical Center
Sylmar, California

Golriz Jafari, MD
Associate Program Director
Nephrology Fellowship Program
Division of Nephrology and Hypertension
Olive View-UCLA Medical Center
Sylmar, California
Assistant Clinical Professor of Medicine
David Geffen School of Medicine
University of California
Los Angeles, California

Anita Kamarzarian, MD
Assistant Clinical Professor of Medicine
David Geffen School of Medicine
University of California
Los Angeles, California
Division of Nephrology and Hypertension
Olive View-UCLA Medical Center
Sylmar, California

Jeffrey M. Miller, MD
Associate Clinical Professor of Medicine
David Geffen School of Medicine
University of California
Los Angeles, California
Division of Hematology and Oncology
Olive View-UCLA Medical Center
Sylmar, California

Cynthia C. Nast, MD
Director
Division of Renal Pathology
Cedars-Sinai Medical Center
Professor of Pathology
Cedars-Sinai Medical Center and David
  Geffen School of Medicine
University of California
Los Angeles, California

Phuong-Anh T. Pham, MD, FACC
Interventional Cardiologist
Division of Cardiology
West Palm Beach VA Medical Center
West Palm Beach, Florida

Phuong-Chi T. Pham, MD, FASN
Chief
Division of Nephrology and Hypertension
Program Director
Nephrology Fellowship Program
Olive View-UCLA Medical Center
Sylmar, California
Clinical Professor of Medicine
David Geffen School of Medicine
University of California
Los Angeles, California

Phuong-Mai T. Pham, MD
Associate Clinical Professor of Medicine
David Geffen School of Medicine
University of California
Sepulveda Ambulatory Care Center
Greater Los Angeles Veterans Administration
Los Angeles, California

Phuong-Thu T. Pham, MD, FASN
Director
Outpatient Services
Kidney Transplant Program
Ronald Reagan UCLA Medical
  Center
Clinical Professor of Medicine
David Geffen School of Medicine
University of California
Los Angeles, California

Phuong-Truc T. Pham, PhD
Associate Professor
Department of Chemistry
Penn State Worthington Scranton
Dunmore, Pennsylvania

Son V. Pham, MD, FACC
Chief
Division of Cardiology
Audie L. Murphy VA Hospital
Assistant Clinical Professor of Medicine
University of Texas Health Science Center
San Antonio, Texas

Jennifer Q. Zhang, PhD
Associate Professor
David Geffen School of Medicine
University of California
Associate Director
UCLA Immunogenetics Center
Department of Pathology and Laboratory
Medicine
Los Angeles, California

Preface

A practicing nephrologist is expected to have a firm grasp of a large array of potentially life-threatening electrolyte and acid–base disturbances, a multitude of acquired and inherited kidney diseases, acute kidney injuries, complex chronic kidney disease–related metabolic, endocrinologic, skeletal/mineral, and cardiovascular complications, difficult-to-treat hypertension, kidney stones, all forms of renal replacement therapy including kidney transplantation, among many other topics.

Mastering the wide knowledge base and current literature required for the routine practice of nephrology can be a difficult task, particularly for those working in hectic private settings.

We intended to write this book as an abbreviated review for renal fellows and general nephrologists who have limited time to study for the nephrology board certifying examination or who simply wish to review and update their nephrology knowledge. The content presented herein closely reflects the American Board of Internal Medicine blueprint outlined for the Nephrology Certifying Examination.

In honor of our most loving and supportive parents, we direct all proceeds from this book to the Pham Family Patient Assistance Fund, created in September 2015, to help financially challenged patients pay for basic fees while seeking medical care.

Phuong-Chi T. Pham and Phuong-Thu T. Pham

Abbreviations

Na^+_e; K^+_e: exchangeable Na$^+$; exchangeable K$^+$
[HCO$_3^-$]: serum bicarbonate concentration
a.k.a.: also known as
Ab–Ag: antibody–antigen complex
ACC/AHA: American College of Cardiology/American Heart Association
ACEI: angiotensin-converting-enzyme inhibitor
ACKD: acquired cystic kidney disease
ACR: acute cellular rejection
ACS: acute compartment syndrome
ACTH: adrenocorticotropic hormone
AD: autosomal dominant
ADAMST13: a disintegrin and metalloproteinase with a thrombospondin type 1 motif
ADH: antidiuretic hormone
ADHF: acute decompensated heart failure
AE-1: anion exchanger I
AER: albumin excretion ratio
AFLP: acute fatty liver of pregnancy
AG: anion gap
AGE: advanced glycosylated end product
AGE:RAGE: advanced glycosylated end-product interaction with AGE receptor
aHUS: atypical hemolytic uremic syndrome
AII: angiotensin II
AKI: acute kidney injury
AKIN: Acute Kidney Injury Network
ALT: alanine aminotransferase
AME: apparent mineralocorticoid excess
AMR: acute antibody-mediated rejection
ANCA: antineutrophil cytoplasmic antibody
ANP: atrial natriuretic peptide
APP: abdominal perfusion pressure
APS: antiphospholipid syndrome
AQP: aquaporin
AR: autosomal recessive
ARB: angiotensin-receptor blocker
ARDS: acute respiratory distress syndrome
ARR: aldosterone–renin ratio
AST: aspartate aminotransferase

ATIN: acute tubulointerstitial nephritis
ATN: acute tubular necrosis
ATP: adenosine triphosphate
AV: atrioventricular
AVF: arteriovenous fistula
AVG: arteriovenous graft
AVN: avascular necrosis
AVP: vasopressin
AVR: vasopressin receptor
AVS: adrenal venous sampling
AZA: azathioprine
BKN: BK nephropathy
BMI: body mass index
BP: blood pressure
BUN: blood urea nitrogen
CA: cancer
CABG: coronary artery bypass grafting
CAD: coronary artery disease
CAII: carbonic anhydrase II
CAIV: carbonic anhydrase IV
CAPD: continuous ambulatory peritoneal dialysis
CaSR: calcium-sensing receptor
CCB: calcium channel blocker
CCT: cortical collecting tubule
CDC: complement-dependent cytotoxicity
cDI: central diabetes insipidus
CHF: congestive heart failure
CI-AKI: contrast-induced acute kidney injury
CKD: chronic kidney disease
CKD-EPI: chronic kidney disease epidemiology collaboration
CMV: cytomegalovirus
CNI: calcineurin inhibitor
CNS: central nervous system
CO: cardiac output
COPD: chronic obstructive pulmonary disease
C$_{OSM}$: osmolar clearance
CPK: creatine phosphokinase

cPRA: calculated cytotoxicity panel of reactive antibodies
CR: complete remission
CrCl: creatinine clearance
CRRT: continuous renal-replacement therapy
CRS: cardiorenal syndrome
CSA: cyclosporine
CSW: cerebral salt wasting
CT: computed tomogram
CTG: chronic transplant glomerulopathy
CTIN: chronic tubulointerstitial nephritis
CTLA-4: cytotoxic T-lymphocyte–associated antigen-4
CVD: cardiovascular disease
CVP: central venous pressure
CVVH or CAVH: continuous venovenous (or arteriovenous) hemofiltration
CVVHDF: continuous venovenous hemodiafiltration
CYC: cyclophosphamide
D5: 5% dextrose solution
DBP: diastolic blood pressure
DCT: distal convoluted tubule
DDAVP: desmopressin acetate
DDD: dense deposit disease
DEXA: dual energy X-ray absorptiometry
DGF: delayed graft function
DHP: dihydropyridine
DI: diabetes insipidus
DIC: disseminated intravascular coagulation
DKD: diabetic kidney disease
DM: diabetes mellitus
DOPPS: dialysis outcomes and practice patterns study
DR: diabetic retinopathy
dRTA: distal renal tubular acidosis
DSA: donor-specific antibodies
DVT: deep vein thrombosis
EBV: Epstein–Barr virus
ECG: electrocardiogram
EF: ejection fraction
EFWC: electrolyte-free water clearance
EGF: epithelial growth factor
eGFR: estimated glomerular filtration rate
eKT/V: equilibrated KT/V
EM: electron microscopy
ENaC: sodium epithelial channel
EPO: erythropoietin
ESA: erythropoiesis-stimulating agent
ESRD: end-stage renal disease
ESWL: extracorporeal shock-wave lithotripsy
ET: endothelin
EVAR: endovascular aortic aneurysm repair
FBS: fasting blood sugar

FeHCO$_3$: fractional excretion of bicarbonate
FeMg: fractional excretion of magnesium
FeNa: fractional excretion of sodium
FePO$_4$: fractional excretion of phosphate
FeUrea: fractional excretion of urea
FGF-23: fibroblast growth factor 23
FHH: familial hyperkalemic hypertension (Gordon) or familial hypocalciuric hypercalcemia
F$_{IO_2}$: fraction of inspired oxygen
FLC: free light chain
FMD: fibromuscular dysplasia
FSGS: focal segmental glomerulosclerosis
FWC: free water clearance
GBM: glomerular basement membrane
GFR: glomerular filtration rate
GI: gastrointestinal
GN: glomerulonephropathy
GRA: glucocorticoid remediable aldosteronism
GU: genitourologic
HAART: highly active antiretroviral therapy
hANP: human atrial natriuretic peptide
Hb: hemoglobin
HbA1C: hemoglobin A1C
HBV: hepatitis B virus
HCTZ: hydrochlorothiazide
HCV: hepatitis C virus
HD: hemodialysis
HDL: high-density lipoproteins
HELLP: hemolysis, elevated liver enzymes, low platelets syndrome of pregnancy
HF: heart failure
HIT: heparin-induced thrombocytopenia
HIV: human immunodeficiency virus
HLA: human leukocyte antigen
HMGCoA: hydroxymethylglutaryl-CoA
HPF: high power field
hPTH: hyperparathyroidism
HR: hazard ratio
HRS: hepatorenal syndrome
HSP: Henoch–Scholein purpura
HSS: hypertonic saline
HTN: hypertension
HUS: hemolytic uremic syndrome
IAH: intra-abdominal hypertension
IAP: intra-abdominal pressure
IC: immune-complex
ICP: intracranial pressure
ICU: intensive care unit
IDH: isolated diastolic hypertension
IDWG: interdialytic weight gain
IF: immunofluorescent microscopy
IgAN: IgA nephropathy
IGIV: intravenous immunoglobulin

iMGN: idiopathic membranous glomerulonephropathy
INR: prothrombin time/international normalized ratio.
IRRT: intermittent renal-replacement therapy
ISH: isolated systolic hypertension
IV: intravenous
IVC: inferior vena cava
KDIGO: kidney disease: improving global outcomes organization
KDOQI: kidney disease outcomes quality initiative
LDH: lactate dehydrogenase
LDL: low-density lipoproteins
LM: light microscopy
LN: lupus nephritis
LVEAD: left ventricular end diastolic area
MAG3: mercaptoacetyltriglycine (used in nuclear renal scanning)
MAHA: microangiopathy ad hemolytic anemia
MAP: mean arterial pressure
MARS: molecular adsorbent recycling system
MBD: mineral bone disease
MCD: minimal change disease
MDRD: modification of diet in renal disease study
MELD: model for end-stage liver disease
MFI: mean fluorescence intensity
MGN: membranous glomerulonephropathy
MHC: major histocompatibility complex
MM: multiple myeloma
MMF: mycophenolate mofetil
MPA: mycophenolic acid
MPGN: membranoproliferative glomerulonephropathy
MPO: myeloperoxidase
MRA: mineralocorticoid-receptor antagonist
MRI: magnetic resonance imaging
mTOR: mammalian target of rapamycin
NBC: sodium bicarbonate cotransporter
NCC: sodium chloride cotransporter
nDI: nephrogenic diabetes insipidus
NE: norepinephrine
NFAT: nuclear factor of activated T cells
NHE3: sodium–hydrogen exchanger 3
NODAT: new-onset diabetes mellitus after transplant
NOS: not otherwise specified
NPT: sodium–phosphate transporter
NS: normal saline
NSAIDS: nonsteroidal anti-inflammatory drugs

NSF: nephrogenic systemic fibrosis
NSIAD: Nephrogenic syndrome of inappropriate antidiuresis
NT-proBNP: N-terminal of the prohormone brain natriuretic peptide
ODS: osmotic demyelinating syndrome
OGTT: oral glucose tolerance test
OPTN/UNOS: Organ Procurement and Transplantation Network/United Network of Organ Sharing
P[K⁺]: plasma potassium
P[Na⁺]: plasma sodium concentration
PA: pulmonary artery
PAI-I: plasminogen-activating-factor inhibitor
PAN: polyarteritis nodosa
PAoP: pulmonary arterial occlusion pressure
PaO₂: arterial partial pressure
PCR: polymerase chain reaction
PCR: protein-to-creatinine ratio
PD: peritoneal dialysis
PDG: phosphate-dependent glutaminase
PEEP: positive end–expiration pressure
PEPCK: phosphoenolpyruvate carboxykinase
PGL: paraganglioma
PGNMID: proliferative glomerulonephropathy with monoclonal Ig deposits
PH: primary hyperoxaluria
PHA: pseudohypoaldosteronism
PHEO: pheochromocytoma
PMN: polymorphonuclear leukocytes
POSEIDON trial: left ventricular end-diastolic pressure–guided fluid administration among patients undergoing cardiac catheterization trial
PPAR: peroxisome proliferator-activated receptor
PPV: pulse pressure variation
PR: partial remission
PR3: proteinase 3
PRA: cytotoxicity panel-reactive antibodies
PRA: plasma renin activity
PRCA: pure red cell aplasia
PRES: reversible posterior leukoencephalopathy syndrome
pRTA: proximal renal tubular acidosis
PTF: pentoxifylline
PTH: parathyroid
PTHrp: parathyroid hormone–related peptide
PTLD: posttransplant lymphoproliferative disease
PTRA: percutaneous transluminal renal angioplasty

PTT: activated prothrombin time
PVR: peripheral vascular resistance
RAAS: renin–angiotensin–aldosterone system
RBC: red blood cells
RCC: renal cell carcinoma
RIFLE: risk, injury, failure, loss of kidney function classification of acute kidney injury, and end-stage renal disease
ROMK: renal outer medullary kidney channel
RRT: renal-replacement therapy
RTA: renal tubular acidosis
RUA: routine urinalysis
S[K$^+$]: serum potassium
S[Na$^+$]: serum sodium concentration
SAG: serum anion gap
SBP: systolic blood pressure
SCa: total serum calcium
SCD: sickle cell disease
SCr: serum creatinine
SCUF: slow continuous ultrafiltration
SCvo$_2$: central venous oxygen saturation
sFLt1: soluble fms-like tyrosine kinase 1
SGLT2: sodium–glucose cotransporter 2
SIADH: syndrome of inappropriate secretion of antidiuretic hormone
SLE: systemic lupus erythematosus
SLEDD: sustained low-efficiency daily dialysis
SNAT3: sodium-dependent amino acid transporter
SNS: sympathetic nervous system
SOG: serum osmolality gap
S$_{OSM}$: serum osmolality
SPEP: serum protein electrophoresis
S$_{PO_4}$: serum phosphate concentration
SRC: scleroderma renal crisis
SSRI: serotonin reuptake inhibitors
SVR: systemic vascular resistance
SV: stroke volume
SVV: stroke volume variation

t$^{1\!/\!2}$: half-life
TAC: tacrolimus
TB: tuberculosis
TBM: tubular basement membrane
TBMN: thin basement membrane nephropathy
TEB: thoracic electrical bioimpedance
TG: triglycerides
TGF: tumor growth factor
TIPS: transjugular intrahepatic portosystemic shunt
TLS: tumor lysis syndrome
TMP: transmembrane pressure
TRALI: transfusion-related acute lung injury
TRIM: transfusion-related immunomodulation
TRPV5: transient receptor potential cation channel, subfamily V, member 5
TSAT: serum transferrin saturation
TTP: thrombotic thrombocytopenic purpura
TZD: thiazolidinedione
U[K$^+$]: urine potassium concentration
U[Na$^+$]: urine sodium concentration
UCreat: urine creatinine concentration
UF: ultrafiltration
U$_{GLUCOSE}$: urine glucose concentration
U$_{OSM}$: urine osmolality
uPCR: urine protein-to-creatinine ratio
UPEP: urine protein electrophoresis
U$_{PO_4}$: urine phosphate concentration
URR: urea-reduction ratio
UT: urea transporter
U$_{UREA}$: urine urea concentration
Vd: volume of distribution
VDRA: vitamin D-receptor agonist
VEGF: vascular endothelial growth factor
VZV: varicella zoster
WBC: white blood cells
WCH: white coat hypertension
WNK: with-no-lysine kinase
WRN: warfarin-related nephropathy
XO: xanthine oxidase

Acknowledgments

We thank all our mentors for their guidance through the exciting field of nephrology and hypertension.

We thank our parents for their guidance and unconditional love and support.

Contents

Sodium/Water

Phuong-Chi T. Pham and Phuong-Thu T. Pham

HYPONATREMIA

Background

- Plasma sodium concentration ($P[Na^+]$) refers to [Na+] in the plasma in vivo or in the plasma of anticoagulated blood ex vivo. Serum sodium concentration ($S[Na^+]$) refers to [Na+] measured in the serum of coagulated blood ex vivo. P[Na+] and $S[Na^+]$ are often used interchangeably. Hyponatremia is typically defined as having $S[Na^+] < 136$ mEq/L.
- Clinical significance of hyponatremia:
  - Increased mortality
  - Impaired attention, mentation slowing even with mild hyponatremia
  - Predictor of hepatorenal syndrome (HRS), hepatic encephalopathy, and death in patients with liver disease
  - Increased risks for osteoporosis, gait instability, fall, and fracture
  - Associated with marked bone loss, myocardial fibrosis, and evidence of early senescence in rats
- The early Edelman equation predicts $P[Na^+]$ as follows:

$$P[Na^+] = 1.11 \times (Na^+_e + K^+_e)/(\text{total body water}) - 25.6,$$

  where ($Na^+_e + K^+_e$) represents the sum of total body *exchangeable* Na^+ and K^+ and the *constant 25.6* represents the pool of *osmotically inactive* Na^+ and K^+ (e.g., *"inexchangeable" Na^+ and K^+ sequestered in bones, nonfluid phase*).
- The Edelman equation indicates that disorders of water balance can cause changes in $P[Na^+]$. Indeed, "sodium disorders" typically reflect disorders of water balance.
- Note that body fluid tonicity = plasma tonicity = cell tonicity. Cell tonicity reflects plasma tonicity. Any change in plasma tonicity leads to a matching change in cell tonicity via free water shift, thus cell volume. Essentially, plasma tonicity determines cell volume.
- In acute hyponatremia, free water shifts into brain cells causing brain swelling. Severe neurologic complications and death can ensue due to the confinement of the brain within the skull.
- Two major determinants of body tonicity: antidiuretic hormone (ADH), a.k.a. arginine vasopressin and thirst
- Arginine vasopressin (AVP):
  - Synthesized in the paraventricular neurons of hypothalamus as pre-pro-AVP and proteolytically cleaved into vasopressin (a.k.a. ADH), neurophysin II, and *copeptin.* These molecules are stored in secretory granules in the posterior

pituitary and released upon osmotic (e.g., hyperosmolality) and nonosmotic stimuli (e.g., volume depletion, stress, drug-induced, nausea, etc.).
  - ADH may be seen as a "pituitary bright spot" or hyperintense T1 signal within the posterior pituitary on brain MRI. The loss of this "pituitary bright spot" is consistent with the lack of ADH, thus central diabetes insipidus (cDI).
- *Copeptin* as a surrogate for ADH:
  - Blood levels of copeptin are more easily measured than ADH (greater stability than ADH) and have been suggested to be a good ADH surrogate.
  - Copeptin levels have been shown parallel to ADH levels in various clinical settings, including increased levels in heart failure (HF), syndrome of inappropriate ADH secretion (SIADH), and sepsis, and reduced levels in cDI.
  - Copeptin level has been shown to increase earlier than troponin in acute myocardial infarction and has been suggested to be used as an early marker for its diagnosis.
  - Copeptin measurement is not yet commercially available in the United States.

Clinical Manifestations
- Risk and severity of neurologic effects depend on the degree and rate of change of $S[Na^+]$.
- Mild: $S[Na^+] \geq 125$ mEq/L: usually asymptomatic to minimally symptomatic
- Moderate: lethargy, headaches, nausea/vomiting, disorientation, muscle cramps, reduced reflexes
- Severe: hyponatremic encephalopathy, seizures, coma, respiratory arrest, brain stem herniation, death

Broad Categorization of Hyponatremia
- Pseudohyponatremia:
  - Refers to falsely low-measured $S[Na^+]$. Flame photometric assay is an old method used to detect sodium content via intensity of flame color divided by serum volume. In patients with falsely elevated serum volume due to space-occupying paraproteins or lipids, the $S[Na^+]$, defined as sodium content ÷ serum volume, will be falsely low. Newer methods of measuring $S[Na^+]$ are now widely used to avoid pseudohyponatremia:
    - Ion-specific electrodes which measure $S[Na^+]$ directly from the serum
    - Supracentrifugation of serum to remove paraproteins/lipids prior to measuring $S[Na^+]$
  - Conditions with falsely high plasma volume leading to "pseudohyponatremia":
    - Severe hyperlipidemia
    - Hyperparaproteinemia (multiple myeloma, Waldenstrom macroglobulinemia)
- Hyponatremia due to extracellular free H_2O shift with osmotically active agents:
  - Hyperglycemia
  - Hypertonic mannitol
  - Sucrose, maltose (mixed in intravenous IgG solutions)
- True hyponatremia: truly low Na^+ content per unit volume, due to increased free water retention, excessive Na^+ loss, or both leading to a hypoosmolar state

Differential Diagnoses of True Hyponatremia
Hypovolemic hyponatremia:
- Appropriate increase in ADH secretion + high H_2O intake + increase renal salt reabsorption (Table 1.1):
  - Bodily fluid loss, chronic diuretics (thiazides), third-spacing

- Typical presentation: hypovolemia, urine Na^+ concentration ($U[Na^+]$) < 20 mEq/L (unless poor kidney function with inability to maximally reabsorb Na^+), urine osmolality (U_{OSM}) typically >300 mOsm/kg
- Renal salt wasting $\rightarrow$ volume depletion $\rightarrow$ appropriate increase in ADH secretion + high H_2O intake:
  - Acute, recent diuretic use
  - Mineralocorticoid insufficiency
  - Cerebral salt wasting (CSW)
  - Typical presentation: hypovolemia, $U[Na^+] > 20$ to 30 mEq/L, U_{OSM} typically >300 mOsm/kg

Euvolemic hyponatremia:

- ADH-dependent, but ADH secretion is inappropriate (i.e., ADH is not secreted in response to volume loss or hyperosmolar state):
  - SIADH: central nervous system (CNS) or pulmonary pathology, drugs affecting CNS, antipsychotics, antiepileptics, antidepressants, nonsteroidal anti-inflammatory drugs (NSAIDS), cyclophosphamide, acute pain, nausea/vomiting, symptomatic HIV
  - Severe hypothyroidism (myxedema coma or thyroid-stimulating hormone > 50 mIU/mL) $\rightarrow$ reduced cardiac output, peripheral vascular resistance, and renal perfusion $\rightarrow \uparrow$ADH secretion

Table 1.1	Differential diagnoses of true hyponatremia			
	ADH-Dependent $U_{OSM} > 100\text{--}150$ mOsm/kg		**ADH-Independent** Variable U_{OSM}	
	Appropriate ADH secretion	Inappropriate or dysregulated ADH secretion	$U_{OSM} < 100$ mOsm/kg	$U_{OSM} > 100$ mOsm/kg
Sodium retention $U[Na+] < 20$ mEq/L	Chronic thiazides Bodily fluid losses Third-spacing Mineralocorticoid deficiency	SIADH + low salt intake Congestive heart failure Cirrhosis Nephrotic syndrome		Nephrogenic SIAD + low salt intake
No sodium retention $U[Na+] > 30$ to 40 mEq/L	Mineralocorticoid deficiency Renal salt wasting Recent diuretic use Bodily fluid loss + poor kidney function Cerebral salt wasting	SIADH + normal salt intake Hypocortisolism Severe hypothyroidism		Kidney failure (U_{OSM} is typically ~300 mOsm/kg) Nephrogenic SIAD + normal salt intake
Variable sodium excretion: Diet-dependent	Pregnancy (physiologically appropriate—see text)		Polydipsia Low solute intake Hypotonic fluids	
				Reset osmostat

- Hypocortisolism → ↑synthesis of corticotropin-releasing hormone, which is co-expressed with ADH, hence ↑ADH
- Pregnancy: reduced threshold for ADH secretion + increased thirst
- Typical presentation for all conditions associated with "inappropriate" ADH secretion above: euvolemia, U[Na$^+$] > 30 to 40 mEq/L (on normal dietary water and sodium intake), U$_{OSM}$ > 100 mOsm/kg, low serum uric acid. NOTE: In the presence of hyponatremia, the kidneys are expected to maximally dilute the urine to <100 mOsm/kg. Any urine osmolality > 100 mOsm/kg indicates sub-optimal urine dilution, which implies either presence of ADH or poor kidney function.
- For the diagnosis of SIADH: In addition to typical presentation above, hypo-thyroidism, hypocortisolism, diuretic use (particularly thiazides), and renal in-sufficiency must also be ruled out.
- ADH-independent:
  - Reset osmostat: normal variant (lower osmotic threshold for ADH release), hy-pothalamic injury, malnutrition. Urine sodium and osmolality vary according to volume status and serum osmolality (S$_{OSM}$).
  - Primary polydipsia (psychogenic polydipsia – psychiatric patients +/− pheno-thiazines with associated dry mouth, hypothalamic infiltrative disease such as sarcoidosis affecting thirst center)
  - Tea and toast syndrome, beer potomania: insufficient solute intake to provide the necessary solute load required by kidneys to excrete water. Kidneys cannot excrete pure free water. Kidneys need a minimum of 50 to 100 mOsm of solute to excrete every 1 L of water (i.e., maximal diluting capacity of healthy kidneys is typically 50 to 100 mOsm/kg).
  - Increase H$_2$O absorption from the use of irrigation fluids with various proce-dures (transurethral resection, hysteroscopy, nephrolithotomy):
    - Hypoosmotic 1.5% glycine solution, osmolality = 200 mOsm/kg. Of interest, the use of >1.5 to 2.0 L of 1.5% glycine solution may also directly stimulate ADH.
    - Hypoosmotic 3% sorbitol, osmolality = 165 mOsm/kg. Sorbitol is metabo-lized to glucose + fructose in liver, then to CO$_2$ and H$_2$O.
    - Isoosmotic 5% mannitol, osmolality = 275 mOsm/kg. 5% mannitol solution usually does not cause hyponatremia because it is isotonic to plasma.
  - Typical presentation for all ADH-independent conditions above: euvolemia, U[Na$^+$] variable depending on sodium intake; U$_{OSM}$ < 100 to 150 mOsm/kg.
  - Constitutively activated ADH-receptor without presence of ADH: Nephrogenic syndrome of inappropriate antidiuresis (NSIAD). Not to be confused with SIADH
    - X-linked gain of function mutation of vasopressin 2 (AVP2) receptor
    - Clinically, patients resemble those with SIADH, but no stimulus for the ADH secretion is found and plasma ADH level is undetectable (in contrast to SIADH where ADH levels are high). In SIAD, the ADH receptor is activated without actual ADH binding. Diagnosis of SIAD is possible in older age (e.g. 70's).
    - Typical presentation: similar to SIADH, except ADH level is undetectable
    - Diagnosis requires sequencing of the *AVP2* receptor gene.
    - Carriers of the mutation have abnormal response to water-loading test.

Hypervolemic hyponatremia:

- ADH-dependent: dysregulated continuing ADH secretion due to conditions as-sociated with reduced effective circulating volume (e.g. heart failure, cirrhosis, nephrotic syndrome)
- ADH-independent: kidney failure with poor diluting capacity.

Drugs Associated with Hyponatremia

- Drugs affecting both sodium and H_2O homeostasis: diuretics (most common: thiazides, others less common: indapamide, amiloride, furosemide)
- Drugs affecting H_2O homeostasis:
  - Increase hypothalamic ADH production: antidepressants (amitriptyline, protriptyline desipramine, selective serotonin reuptake inhibitors, monoamine oxidase inhibitors), antipsychotics (thioridazine, trifluoperazine, haloperidol), antiepileptics (carbamazepine, oxcarbazepine, sodium valproate), chemotherapeutic agents (vincristine, vinblastine, IV cyclophosphamide, melphalan, ifosfamide, methotrexate, interferon α and γ, levamisole, pentostatin, monoclonal antibodies), opiates
  - Potentiate ADH effect: antiepileptics (carbamazepine, lamotrigine), antidiabetics (chlorpropamide, tolbutamide), anticancer agents (IV cyclophosphamide), NSAIDS
- Drugs that reset osmostat: antidepressants (venlafaxine), antiepileptics (carbamazepine)

Other Noteworthy Causes of Drug-Induced Hyponatremia

- Angiotensin-converting enzyme inhibitors (ACEI) , although likely rarely observed: ACEI inhibits conversion of angiotensin I (AI) to II (AII) in peripheral tissue, but not in brain. In the brain, AI is converted to AII, which can stimulate thirst and ADH release. Use of ACEI increases AI levels, hence increased brain AII. ACEI may also induce increase ADH secretion by delaying bradykinin degradation.
- Intravenous immune globulins mixed in maltose or sucrose: Hyponatremia may occur via (1) pseudohyponatremia if measured by flame photometric assay due to large amount of space-occupying globulins and (2) dilutional hyponatremia due to extracellular free water shift with accumulation of maltose or sucrose (important if poor kidney function and reduced excretion of maltose or sucrose)
- Amphetamines, 3,4-methylenedioxymethylamphetamine a.k.a. "ecstasy": increased hypothalamic ADH secretion and excessive water intake due to associated hyperthermia.
- Less-common causes: nicotine patch, colchicine poisoning, dopaminergic agents, unfractionated heparin, hydroxyurea, azithromycin, clonidine, glipizide, tacrolimus, co-trimoxazole, theophylline, proton pump inhibitors

Management of Hyponatremia

- General considerations:
  - Provide adequate *oxygenation*, mechanical ventilation support, if necessary. Hypoxemia may exacerbate hyponatremic encephalopathy.
  - *Potassium and sodium are equivalent effective, exchangeable* osmoles. Any K^+ given during the treatment of hyponatremia will correct $S[Na^+]$ *exactly* as if the same amount of Na^+ was given.

Example: If a patient needs 200 mEq of Na^+ to raise his hyponatremia to goal, but also needs 75 mEq K^+ for concurrent hypokalemia, the clinician should give
  - 125 mEq of Na^+ + 75 mEq of K^+ = 200 mEq total of Na^+ + K^+ *instead of*
  - 200 mEq of Na^+ + 75 mEq K^+ = 275 mEq total of Na^+ + K^+. The latter combination would overshoot the goal $S[Na^+]$.

  - *Monitor urine output*: Hypotonic polyuria can easily overcorrect hyponatremia if not recognized. Hypotonic polyuria may be seen during the management of hyponatremia with the following conditions: post-pituitary infarction, glucocorticoid replacement in patient with cortisol insufficiency, discontinuation of desmopressin (DDAVP) in patients with chronic use (e.g., cDI), excessive

gastrointestinal or skin hypotonic fluid loss, recovery from acute respiratory failure, withdrawal of thiazides, water deprivation in primary polydipsia, rapid volume expansion with intravenous saline
- Cases of osmotic demyelination syndrome (ODS) have been reported in patients with concurrent hypokalemia, hypomagnesemia, hypophosphatemia, thiamine deficiencies, or any combination of these deficiencies *INDEPENDENT* of the rate of Na^+ correction. Monitor and correct these deficiencies during the management of hyponatremia.
- Rate of correction:
  - A 5% increase in $S[Na^+]$ should substantially reduce cerebral edema.
  - Rapid correction can lead to ODS previously known as central pontine myelinolysis (CPM) due to insufficient time allowed for brain synthesis of organic osmolytes or "idiogenic osmoles" to counteract the acute rise in extracellular osmolality. Major brain organic osmolytes include glutamine, glutamate, taurine, myo-inositol, among others.
    - *High risks for ODS*: $S[Na+] < 105$ mEq/L, alcoholism, malnutrition, advanced liver disease, hypokalemia
    - Clinical manifestations of ODS:
      - 1 to 2 days: generalized encephalopathy
      - 2 to 3 days: behavioral changes, cranial nerve palsies, progressive weakness, quadriplegia with "locked-in" syndrome; death possible. Partial to complete resolution of mild to moderate neurological complications may be possible.
  - Reversal of overcorrection with hypotonic fluids and DDAVP has been shown to be beneficial in rats and human case reports.
- Correction rate for acute symptomatic hyponatremia (onset < 48 hours):
  - 2 mEq/L/h $\times$ 2 to 3 hours (4 to 6 mEq/L) or until neurologic symptoms resolve
  - Do not exceed 6 to 8 mEq/L/d.
- Correction rate for chronic (onset $\geq$ 48 hours):
  - 4 to 8 mEq/L/d
  - Use lower target for high ODS risk patients (4 to 6 mEq/L/d).
  - Normal risk for ODS: may correct 10 to 12 mEq/L in any 24-hour period, but not to exceed 18 mEq/L in any 48-hour period

Specific Treatment Options

- Fluid restriction: consider for euvolemic or hypervolemic patients.
  - "Fluid" implies all fluid consumed by drinking, not just water.
  - Restriction volume should be aimed at 500 mL below the patient's average daily urine volume.
  - Predictors of likely failure with fluid restriction alone:
    - High U_{OSM} (>500 mOsm/kg)
    - $(U[Na^+] + U[K^+])/(S[Na^+]) > 1$
    - Baseline urine volume < 1500 mL/d
- Salt supplement:
  - Normal saline (NS): recommended for hypovolemic patients
  - Hypertonic saline:
    - Indicated for severely symptomatic, for example, seizures, severely depressed mental status: 100 mL of 3% saline bolus every 10 minutes as needed to break seizures or up to a total of 3 boluses, whichever comes first

- May also be considered at low infusion rates for patients with severe SIADH + severe hyponatremia whose $U_{OSM} >> 300$ mOsm/kg

> **NOTE** NS can worsen hyponatremia in SIADH patients with $U_{OSM} >> 300$ mOsm/kg. This is due to a process called "*desalination*."

Example: Imagine a patient with severe SIADH, whose kidneys **always** concentrate the urine to an osmolality of 600 mOsm/kg ~600 mOsm/L of urine.

- If this patient receives 1 L of NS, he receives a solution consisting of 308 mOsm of solutes (154 mEq Na + 154 mEq Cl) plus 1 L of free water, which is approximately 300 mOsm of solutes plus 1 L of free water.
- Kidneys see: 300 mOsm of solutes plus 1 L of free water
- Kidneys' task: excrete a urine with osmolality 600 mOsm/kg ~600 mOsm/L.
- Kidneys use up all 300 mOsm of solutes but only 500 mL of water from the fluid administered to make a urine with osmolality 600 mOsm/kg.
- That means, the remaining 500 mL of water gets reabsorbed into the patient. This leads to worsening of the patient's existing hyponatremia!
- In effect, the kidneys "desalinate" or remove all NaCl from the NS to make a urine with the high osmolality dictated by the patient's degree of SIADH. The "leftover" water gets reabsorbed into the patient.
- By the same reasoning, imagine another patient with moderate SIADH with a typical U_{OSM} of 300 mOsm/kg. The use of NS would never correct the patient's hyponatremia because this patient's kidneys typically excrete a urine with the same osmolality as NS. Thus, no salt gained, no water lost, no improvement in hyponatremia.

  Bottom line: Any saline solution used in a patient with SIADH for the sole purpose of increasing $S[Na^+]$, the osmolality of the solution must be higher than that of the urine.
- Salt tablets: may be preferred over strict fluid restriction in stable euvolemic patients with SIADH and terminal conditions (i.e., metastatic malignancy for better quality of life—authors' opinion)
- Increase renal H_2O excretion:
  - Increase solute load if poor nutrition: parenteral feeding, dietary concentrated protein supplements, urea 15 to 60 g/d
  - Correct underlying disease/condition that cause SIADH.
  - ADH antagonists:
    - Demeclocycline: thought to inhibit ADH binding to its receptor. Contraindicated during pregnancy and children due to interfering with bone development, teeth discoloration. Other: photosensitive rash, nephrotoxicity
    - ADH receptor antagonists (a.k.a. vaptans, aquaretics): for euvolemic and hypervolemic hyponatremic patients
      - FDA-approved agents:
        - Conivaptan: intravenous formulation only; combined V1a and V2 receptor antagonist; limit use to 4 days due to significant drug interactions with other agents metabolized by CYP3A4.
        - Tolvaptan: oral formulation; V2 receptor antagonist

- Both agents improve free water excretion and improve $S[Na^+]$ without altering 24-hour sodium excretion.
  - Vaptans have not been shown to improve long-term outcome.
- Use of vaptans is not recommended immediately following cessation of other treatments of hyponatremia, particularly 3% saline.
- Vaptans are ineffective in patients with reduced kidney function (i.e., serum creatinine (SCr) > 3 mg/dL)
- Major side effects/risks: thirst, transaminitis, gastrointestinal bleed
- Overly rapid correction leading to ODS is possible particularly if used concurrently with diuretics or used in patients without access to free water (e.g., patients who are mechanically ventilated or debilitated, bed-bound).
- Relowering of $S[Na^+]$ should be considered in cases with overly rapid corrections.
- Data are lacking to recommend use of vaptans in severe asymptomatic hyponatremia, that is $S[Na^+] < 120$ mEq/L.
- Furosemide: may be used in patients with hypervolemia. Concurrent use with vaptan is not recommended due to risk of overly rapid free H_2O excretion and over-correction of hyponatremia.
- Correction of hyponatremia in the dialysis patient:
  - Uremic patients are thought to be protected from ODS with overly rapid correction of hyponatremia during dialysis because of the simultaneous removal of uremic solutes. However, ODS has been reported in patients with rapid sodium correction with dialysis.
  - Correction rates should therefore follow the same guidelines as nonuremic patients.
  - Minimization of sodium correction may be achieved by using the dialysate with the lowest sodium concentration appropriate for patient's $S[Na^+]$ level (lowest dialysate $[Na^+]$ is typically 130 mEq/L) and lowest blood flow rate.
    - Calculations of blood flow for intermittent hemodialysis:
      - One can assume that 100% of the $[Na^+]$ difference from the dialysate will transfer to the blood if the blood is allowed to flow very slowly against a high dialysate flow rate of 800 mL/min.
      - Consider a patient with $S[Na^+]$ of 120 mEq/L; goal correction of 6 mEq/L over a 3-hour dialysis session using a dialysate with $[Na^+]$ of 130 mEq/L.
      - Assuming 100% Na^+ transfer from the dialysate, every 1 L of blood that passes through the dialyzer will gain 10 mEq of Na^+.
      - If goal $S[Na^+]$ is 126 mEq/L and patient has total body volume of 30 L, the total amount of Na^+ needed is 6 mEq/L $\times$ 30 L = 180 mEq. Since every 1 L of blood that passes through the dialyzer picks up 10 mEq of Na^+ from the dialysate, a total blood volume of 180 mEq/10 mEq/L = 18 L would need to pass through the dialyzer over 3 hours. The blood flow rate would thus be 18 L/3 h or 100 mL/min. This may be achieved by using the pediatric mode on the dialyzer.
    - Calculations of blood flow for continuous renal replacement therapy: same as above, but the total blood volume will be run over 24 hours.
- Management of overly rapid correction of hyponatremia:
  - For acute water intoxication, relowering of sodium is not necessary.
  - For patients with presenting $S[Na^+] < 120$ mEq/L, relowering of $S[Na^+]$ should be considered (particularly in patients with high risks for ODS):
    - Replace water losses with intravenous 5% dextrose (D5) water or oral water to achieve desired goal.

- Administer DDAVP 2 to 4 µg every 8 to 12 hours parenterally (intravenous). Authors' experience: intravenous DDAVP 2 mg q18-24 h typically suffices.

> **NOTE** Do *not* give excessive water replacement while patient receives DDAVP. Rapid and excessive relowering of S[Na$^+$] can easily occur.

- If patient was given vaptan, hold the next dose if correction exceeds 8 mEq/L/24 h. In case of unsafe overcorrection, administer free water and DDAVP as above.
- Monitor S[Na$^+$] closely.
- Consider administration of high-dose glucocorticoids (e.g., dexamethasone 4 mg q6h for 24 to 48 hours) in severe overcorrection cases.
- Special notes about therapy:
  - Hyponatremia in patients with HF:
    - For mild to moderate symptoms:
      - Fluid restrict 1 L/d. Add loop diuretic as needed for volume overload.
      - Tolvaptan may be considered, but must be closely monitored to assess long-term need.
    - For severely symptomatic patients with severe hyponatremia, administer 3% NaCl plus loop diuretics. Very close monitoring is REQUIRED.
  - For primary polydipsia, consider
    - Behavioral therapy
    - Clozapine (antipsychotic, dibenzazepine derivative) has been reported to be useful in some cases of psychogenic polydipsia.
  - NSIAD: treatment is also free water restriction as in SIADH + increase solute intake (urea); hypertonic saline when severe and/or symptomatic hyponatremia. Vaptans have been reported to be *ineffective* in this syndrome presumably because they cannot deactivate the constitutively activated ADH receptor.

Sodium Correction Formulas

Adrogue–Madias Equation:

$$Na_2 = \frac{(Na_1 \times TBW) + [Vol_{inf} \times (Na+K)_{inf}]}{TBW + Vol_{inf}}$$

Barsoum–Levine Equation:

$$Na_2 = \frac{(TBW \times Na_1) + [Vol_{input} \times (Na+K)_{input} - Vol_{out} \times (Na+K)_{out}]}{TBW + \Delta Vol}$$

Nguyen–Kurtz Equation:

$$Na_2 = \frac{[(Na_1 + 23.8) \times TBW] + \left[1.03 \times [(Na+K)_{input} - (Na+K)_{out}]\right]}{TBW + \Delta Vol} - 23.8$$

TBW, Total body water, Vol, Volume Inf, Infused. For calculations involving multiple sources of input and output and estimates for both fluid tonicity and rate administration, see CurbsideConsultant.com → Nephrology and Hypertension → Calculations of expected serum sodium or Calculations for fluid tonicity and rate.

FLUID MANAGEMENT

Basic Concepts and Formulas

Osmolar Clearance (C_{OSM})

- $C_{OSM} = U_{OSM} \times V/P_{OSM}$, where U_{OSM} is the urine osmolality, V is urine volume, and P_{OSM} is the plasma osmolality.
- A typical osmolar clearance is <3 L/d.
- $C_{OSM} > 3$ L/d indicates the presence of a solute diuresis.

Urine output (V) $= C_{OSM} + C_{H_2O}$, or $C_{H_2O} = V - C_{OSM}$, where C_{H_2O} is the free water clearance (FWC). In a patient with high solute diuresis, that is $C_{OSM} >> 3$, C_{H_2O} may be negative, but this does not imply that patient holds on to water and becomes hyponatremic. The development of hyponatremia depends on the quantity of Na^+ and K^+ loss in the osmolar clearance.

(Osmolar)-Free Water Clearance

$$\text{Free water clearance (FWC)} = \text{urine volume} \times (1 - U_{OSM}/S_{OSM})$$

Essentially, FWC is the urine volume with osmolality of zero that remains after the portion of urine normalized to serum osmolality has been extracted/removed from the initial total volume. Depending on the urine and serum osmolalities, FWC may be positive or negative.

A positive FWC indicates that a patient makes urine that is hypotonic to the plasma, thereby losing free water and increasing plasma osmolality, whereas a negative FWC indicates that a patient makes urine that is hypertonic to the plasma, thereby gaining free water and lowering plasma osmolality. The change in plasma osmolality does not necessarily imply a change in serum sodium concentration. This leads to the concept of electrolyte-free water clearance (EFWC) (Fig. 1.1).

Electrolyte-Free Water Clearance

$$\text{Electrolyte-free water clearance (EFWC)} = \text{urine volume} \times$$
$$(1 - U[Na^+ + K^+]/S[Na^+ + K^+])$$

Since $S[K^+]$ is $<<S[Na^+]$, EFWC is typically simplified to

$$\text{EFWC} = \text{urine volume} \times (1 - U[Na^+ + K^+]/S[Na^+])$$

Essentially, EFWC is the electrolyte-free urine volume that remains after the portion of urine normalized to plasma sodium has been extracted/removed from the initial total volume. Depending on the urine and serum $Na^+ + K^+$, EFWC may be positive or negative.

A positive EFWC indicates that a patient makes urine that has a lower electrolyte ($Na^+ + K^+$) concentration compared to that in the plasma, which can thereby increase the plasma sodium concentration, whereas a negative EFWC indicates that a patient makes urine that has higher electrolyte concentration ($Na^+ + K^+$) compared to that of plasma, which can thereby lower the plasma sodium concentration.

Alternatively, if there is more electrolyte loss in the urine compared to plasma electrolyte per unit volume (i.e., $(U[Na^+ + K^+])/(S[Na^+]) > 1$), there is net electrolyte-free water gain, and if there is less electrolyte loss in the urine compared to plasma electrolyte per unit volume (i.e., $(U[Na^+ + K^+])/(S[Na^+]) < 1$), there is net electrolyte-free water loss.

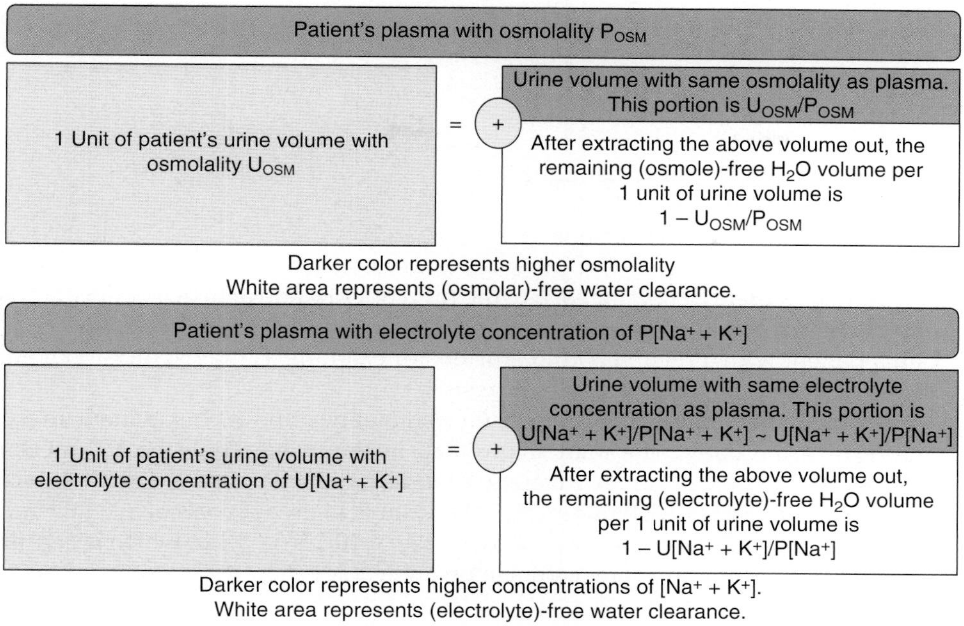

Patient's plasma with osmolality P_{OSM}		
1 Unit of patient's urine volume with osmolality U_{OSM}	$=$ $+$	Urine volume with same osmolality as plasma. This portion is U_{OSM}/P_{OSM}
		After extracting the above volume out, the remaining (osmole)-free H_2O volume per 1 unit of urine volume is $1 - U_{OSM}/P_{OSM}$

Darker color represents higher osmolality
White area represents (osmolar)-free water clearance.

Patient's plasma with electrolyte concentration of $P[Na^+ + K^+]$		
1 Unit of patient's urine volume with electrolyte concentration of $U[Na^+ + K^+]$	$=$ $+$	Urine volume with same electrolyte concentration as plasma. This portion is $U[Na^+ + K^+]/P[Na^+ + K^+] \sim U[Na^+ + K^+]/P[Na^+]$
		After extracting the above volume out, the remaining (electrolyte)-free H_2O volume per 1 unit of urine volume is $1 - U[Na^+ + K^+]/P[Na^+]$

Darker color represents higher concentrations of $[Na^+ + K^+]$.
White area represents (electrolyte)-free water clearance.

FIGURE 1.1 (Osmole)-free water clearance and (electrolyte)-free water clearance.

PROBLEMS

1. How would the $S[Na^+]$ change (increase or decrease) in a patient with current $S[Na^+]$ 132 mEq/L and making 4 L of urine with $U[Na^+]$ 38 mEq/L and $U[K^+]$ 13 mEq/L while receiving 7 L of 5% D5 half NS (77 mEq/L of NaCl)?
   - EFWC of urine $= 4 \times (1 - (38+13)/132) = 2.45$ L
   - EFWC of fluid $= 7 \times (1 - 77/132) = 2.92$ L
   - There will be a net gain of 0.47 L of electrolyte-free H_2O so $S[Na^+]$ would decrease.

2. A patient undergoing postobstructive diuresis with current $S[Na^+]$ 135 mEq/L, $P[osm]$ 297 mEq/L and urine rate of 300 mL/h with U_{OSM} 450 mOsm, $U[Na^+]$ 73 mEq/L, $U[K^+]$ 20 mEq/L. Would his $S[Na^+]$ increase or decrease with time if he continues current urine output?
   - EFWC of urine $= 0.3 \times (1 - (73+20)/135) = 0.093$ L or 93 mL/h.
   - The positive EFWC indicates that at the current rate of electrolyte-free water loss, the patient's $S[Na^+]$ will be expected to increase with time.

3. Can a patient with a urine osmolality greater than serum osmolality develop hypernatremia?
   - Yes, as long as the EFWC is positive
   - Example: patient with U_{OSM} of 500 mOsm/kg, $U[Na^+]$ of 15 mEq/L, $U[K^+]$ of 17 mEq/L, $S[Na^+]$ of 140 mEq/L
   - EFWC $= (1 - (15+17)/140) = 0.77$; for every liter of urine lost, 77% of the volume is free of Na^+ and K^+. This *electrolyte-free water loss* (EFWC) would be expected to lead to hypernatremia.

4. A patient with congestive heart failure (CHF) on continuous bumetanide infusion with $S[Na^+]$ 148 mEq/L and urine output of 125 mL/h with urine $[K^+]$ 15 mEq/L and $U[Na^+]$ 75 mEq/L. Which one of the following fluids will not worsen the fluid

overload state *and* not increase current S[Na$^+$]? Which one of the fluids will not worsen the fluid overload *and* could decrease S[Na$^+$]? Which one of the fluids will increase S[Na]?

- 125 mL/h of NS per hour
- 125 mL/h of ½ NS per hour
- 50 mL/h of 5% D5 water per hour
- 75 mL/h of D5 water per hour
- 125 mL/h of D5 ¼ NS per hour

Hint: The amount of free H_2O loss in the urine is $125 \times (1 - (15 + 75)/148) = 50$ mL/h. Calculate EFWC for each of the fluid options above to determine if there is a net electrolyte free water gain or loss.

5. Can a patient with a relatively dilute urine, for example, U_{OSM} 150 mOsm/kg and P[osm] 277 mEq/kg, have a solute diuresis?
   - Yes. Example: same urine and serum osmolalities above, but patient makes 10 L of urine daily. The total solute load in the urine would be 150 mOsm/kg $\times$ 10 L = 1,500 mOsm. An average American diet intake would give a typical urine solute load of ~800 mOsm. 1,500 mOsm is in great excess of 800 mOsm.
   - Alternatively, $C_{OSM} = U_{OSM} \times V/P_{OSM} = 150 \times 10/277 = 5.4$ L, which is $>>$ the typical <3 L/d for an average person on an average diet.

HYPERNATREMIA AND HYPEROSMOLALITY

Hypernatremia Background

- Hypernatremia is typically defined as having S[Na$^+$] > 145 mEq/L.
- Hypernatremia may be due to one or more of the following factors:
  - Inadequate free H_2O intake (e.g., limited access to free H_2O or defective thirst sensation)
  - Excessive free H_2O loss
  - Excessive sodium intake/retention
  - Transient intracellular free water uptake

> **NOTE** Hypernatremia typically does not develop unless patients (even in those with diabetes insipidus [DI]) have limited access to free water, for example, debility, surgical patients, or thirst defect.

Clinical Manifestations of Hypernatremia

Lethargy, weakness, irritability, seizures, intracerebral and subarachnoid hemorrhages due to rupture of cerebral veins with marked decrease in brain volume, coma, death

Differential Diagnoses of Hypernatremia

- Water loss/deficit:
  - Inadequate intake, poor water access
  - Increased insensible loss: skin, respiratory
  - Hypothalamic disorders:
    - Primary hypodipsia
    - Reset osmostat in primary mineralocorticoid excess:
      - Chronic sodium retention/volume expansion in this condition leads to mild chronic ADH suppression which is, in effect, a state of "reset osmostat."

- The use of diuretics corrects the volume expansion and releases the chronic suppression of ADH. Once ADH is synthesized and released, free water reabsorption can occur to correct the chronic hypernatremia.
- Presenting $S[Na^+]$ in primary mineralocorticoid excess is typically ~143 to 147 mEq/L
- Adipsic DI a.k.a. "essential hypernatremia":
  - Combined defects in osmoreceptor function and thirst. Osmolality-dependent ADH secretion is defective, but volume-regulated ADH secretion is intact.

> **NOTE** In contrast to adipsic DI, the typical central DI patient cannot stimulate ADH release with either hyperosmolar or hypovolemic state.

  - Clinical manifestations of adipsic DI:
    - Typically asymptomatic due to chronicity of condition
    - $S[Na^+]$ is typically ~155 to 190 mEq/L.
    - Patient may be hypovolemic with associated high renin/aldosterone state and hypokalemic metabolic alkalosis.
    - Adipsic DI is associated with obesity, sleep apnea, venous thrombosis during episodes of hypernatremia, thermoregulatory dysfunction, seizures, and increased mortality.
  - Causes of adipsic DI: congenital or acquired CNS lesions/sarcoidosis
  - Classic clinical scenario of adipsic DI:
    - A patient with hypernatremia not correcting with hypotonic fluid administration (patient *cannot* secrete ADH in response to hyperosmolality/hypernatremia, hence no ADH to reabsorb free H_2O from the fluid administration to correct the hypernatremia), *but*
    - Patient can concentrate the urine with fluid restriction (patient *can* secrete ADH in response to volume depletion, hence normal H_2O reabsorption with volume depletion, or ability to concentrate urine).
    - Patient with this condition may be treated with DDAVP.
- Diabetes insipidus:
  - Primary/familial cDI: rare
  - Secondary cDI: See Polyuria section for causes.
- Nephrogenic causes:
  - Hereditary nephrogenic diabetes insipidus (nDI): mutation of aquaporin 2 (AQP2) channel, ADH receptors
  - Secondary nDI: hypercalcemia, hypokalemia, pregnancy, lithium, demeclocycline, methoxyflurane, foscarnet, aminoglycosides, amphotericin B, cidofovir, vaptans
- Water *and* sodium loss:
  - Extrarenal loss: skin (burns, excessive sweating), gastrointestinal tract (nasogastric suction, viral gastroenteritis, nonelectrolyte osmotic diarrhea, e.g., lactulose, vomiting)
  - Renal loss: loop diuretics, osmotic diuresis (hyperglycemia, mannitol, high-protein diet, tissue catabolism, urea), postobstructive diuresis, postacute tubular necrosis diuresis.
- Water shift into cells (*transient*): seizures or rigorous exercise, rhabdomyolysis (increase in intracellular breakdown of larger molecules into many smaller molecules, hence increase intracellular osmolality and subsequent intracellular free H_2O shift).

- Sodium load:
  - Administration of hypertonic saline or $NaHCO_3$ (e.g., excessive $NaHCO_3$ administration during code or inadvertent mixing of 2 to 3 ampules of $NaHCO_3$ in NS instead of 5% D5 water – 1 amp of $NaHCO_3$ contains approximately 45 mEq/L of Na^+.)
  - Acute salt poisoning (e.g., accidental salt feeding in babies [salt instead of sugar or baby formula] – 1 teaspoon contains ~100 mEq Na^+); intrauterine instillation of hypertonic saline for abortion; salt water ingestion

Diagnosis

- Obtain full medical history.
- Assess volume status, urine osmolality (Table 1.2).
- Conditions that improve with DDAVP: partial and complete cDI, adipsic cDI

Management of Hypernatremia

- Estimating water deficit = total body water $\times$ {(S[Na^+]/140) – 1}, where total body water = 0.5 to 0.6 $\times$ euvolemic ideal body weight.
- Correction rates are similar to those recommended for hyponatremia.
- Fluid selection depends on hemodynamic stability and recent or ongoing salt loss.
  - Hemodynamically unstable, hypotensive: use NS for rapid intravascular expansion.
  - For recent or ongoing salt loss: 2.5% or 5% dextrose (D2.5 or D5) ¼ NS or ½ NS
  - For pure water loss or salt poisoning: D2.5 or D5 water
  - For volume overloaded patients: loop diuretics *plus* 2.5% or 5% D5 water, *never* furosemide alone as furosemide produces hypotonic urine and can worsen hypernatremia.
- Dialysis if concurrent kidney failure, anuria
- Special treatment considerations:
  - For any reversible cause, treat underlying disease/condition.

Table 1.2	Evaluation of hypernatremia and hyperosmolality		
Urine Osmolality	**Hypovolemia**	**Euvolemia**	**Hypervolemia**
<300 mOsm/kg	Complete central or nephrogenic diabetes insipidus: volume status depends on access to H_2O.		
300–600+ mOsm/kg	Partial central or nephrogenic diabetes insipidus: volume status depends on access to H_2O; Osmotic diuresis (intrinsic, e.g., poorly controlled diabetes mellitus): volume status depends on access to H_2O.		
>600–700 mOsm/kg	High insensible fluid loss Diarrheal fluid loss Primary hypodipsia Inability to access free water	Sodium, osmotic overload (iatrogenic, e.g., large volume of hypertonic saline infusion or large volume parenteral feeding): volume status depends on ability of kidneys to excrete excess solute and water load.	
Variable	Intracellular free water shift (e.g., rhabdomyolysis, seizures): volume status depends on access to H_2O. Adipsic central diabetes insipidus: urine osmolality can increase with fluid restriction.		Reset osmostat Primary mineralocorticoid excess

- Central diabetes insipidus: DDAVP (oral, nasal spray, subcutaneous, or intravenous). In the case of nasal mucosal inflammation or mechanical ventilation, avoid nasal spray due to unpredictable absorption.
- Partial cDI: Medications that potentiate ADH secretion or action may be considered *only* if safe: chlorpropamide, carbamazepine, clofibrate
- Nephrogenic diabetes insipidus: thiazides can produce a paradoxical antidiuretic effect via tubuloglomerular feedback.
- Lithium-induced nDI: If lithium must be used, add amiloride to reduce renal uptake via principal cells of collecting duct.
- Decrease solute load with low salt and protein may help (nutrition consult recommended to avoid malnutrition).
- Kidney failure, anuric: dialysis
- Adipsic DI: DDAVP
- Primary mineralocorticoid excess: mild diuretic

SALT EXCESS (EDEMATOUS STATES)

Regulation of Fluid Exchange between Plasma and Interstitium

$$\text{Starling's law: Net filtration} = \text{LpS} \times (\Delta\text{hydraulic pressure} - \Delta\text{oncotic pressure})$$
$$= \text{LpS} \times [(P_{CAP} - P_{IF}) - s(\pi_{CAP} - \pi_{IF})]$$

where Lp is the permeability or porosity of the capillary wall, S is the surface area available for filtration, P_{CAP} is the capillary hydraulic pressure, P_{IF} is the interstitial hydraulic pressure, π_{CAP} is the capillary oncotic pressure, π_{IF} is the interstitial oncotic pressure, and s is the reflection coefficient of proteins across the capillary wall (with values ranging from 0 if completely permeable to 1 if completely impermeable).

- An intravascular hydraulic pressure that is higher than that in the interstitium will favor water movement into the interstitium and vice versa.
- A higher intravascular oncotic pressure will favor water movement into the intravascular space and vice versa.
- Normally, there is a small mean gradient of ~0.3 mm Hg favoring filtration out of the vascular space; the fluid is then returned to the systemic circulation by the lymphatics so fluid accumulation in the interstitium is prevented.
- Edema formation occurs when there is alteration in ≥1 Starling's forces
  - ↑Capillary hydraulic pressure
  - ↑Capillary permeability
  - ↑Interstitial oncotic pressure
  - ↓Plasma oncotic pressure,
  or
  - Lymphatic obstruction
  - Excess renal sodium and water retention

Common Clinical Edematous Conditions, Pathophysiology of Edema Formation

Congestive Heart Failure (CHF)

- Poor cardiac output → decreased effective circulating volume
- Renin angiotensin aldosterone system (RAAS), sympathetic nervous system (SNS), ADH are stimulated → sodium and free H_2O retention → increased plasma volume. In early CHF, the increased plasma volume can enhance cardiac

contractility, hence cardiac output (Frank–Starling curve). As the disease progresses, the continuing accumulation of plasma volume will reach a point where cardiac contractility cannot be further improved to improve cardiac output. The continuing Na^+ and H_2O retention only leads to further volume expansion → edematous state, decompensated HF.

Management of Acute Decompensated Heart Failure
Diuresis and Ultrafiltration: Summary of Major Trials

Diuretic Optimization Strategies Evaluation Trial (DOSE trial):
- Evaluated various diuretic strategies (**loop diuretics**) for patients with acute decompensated heart failure (ADHF) × 72 hours:
- Low dose (1 × outpatient oral dose) given intravenously q12h
- Low dose (1 × outpatient oral dose) given as continuous intravenous infusion
- High dose (2.5 × outpatient oral dose) given intravenously q12h
- High dose (2.5 × outpatient oral dose) given as continuous intravenous infusion
- Findings:
  - There was no statistically significant difference in global symptom relief or change in renal function at 72 hours for either:
    - q 12 dosing or continuous infusion
    - Low dose or high dose
  - High intensification (2.5 × oral dose) was associated with trends toward greater improvement in multiple domains: symptom relief (global assessment and dyspnea), weight loss and net volume loss, proportion free from signs of congestion, and reduction in NT-proBNP.

Efficacy of Vasopressin Antagonism in Heart Failure Outcome Study with Tolvaptan (EVEREST trial):
- >4,000 patients studied
- Early benefit in dyspnea on day 1 and edema/weight on day 7, but no benefit on HF hospitalization or mortality. The cost for 30 days is close to $6,000.
- NO overall benefit (need subgroup analyses and more trials)

Ultrafiltration: Ultrafiltration (UF) versus intravenous (IV) diuretics for patients hospitalized for ADHF (UNLOAD):
- Aim: study the effectiveness of ultrafiltration versus aggressive loop diuretic in patients with ADHF.
- Ultrafiltration arm: ultrafiltration up to 500 mL/h, volume and rate determined per clinician, versus diuretic arm: intravenous diuretics at least two times outpatient oral dose within 48 hours of randomization
- Findings:
  - Early UF produces greater weight and fluid loss than intravenous diuretics, without adverse impact on kidney function.
  - Early UF reduces 90 day: percentage of patients requiring rehospitalization for HF, number of HF rehospitalizations, days of rehospitalization for HF, emergency department and unscheduled office visits.
  - UNLOAD suggested superiority of UF over diuretics in patients hospitalized for volume overloaded HF.

UF in decompensated HF with cardiorenal syndrome:
- 188 patients with ADHF, worsened kidney function, randomized to receive stepped pharmacologic therapy versus UF.

- Findings: The use of a stepped pharmacologic therapy algorithm was superior to a strategy of ultrafiltration for the preservation of renal function at 96 hours, with a similar amount of weight loss with two approaches. UF was associated with a higher rate of adverse events.

> **NOTE** Compared to UNLOAD trial, the medical arm in current study using the stepped pharmacologic therapy achieved greater fluid removal. This may have made the difference in outcome.

Acute Study of Clinical Effectiveness of Nesiritide in Decompensated Heart Failure (ASCEND-HF):
- Aim: To assess the safety and efficacy of nesiritide (recombinant B-type natriuretic peptide) in acute HF syndrome
- Over 7,000 patients randomized to receive nesiritide versus placebo
- Findings:
  - Nesiritide did not reduce the rate of recurrent HF hospitalization or death at 30 days.
  - Nesiritide reduced dyspnea to a modest degree, consistent with previous findings but did not meet prespecified protocol criteria for statistical significance at 6 and 24 hours.
  - Nesiritide did not affect 30-day all-cause mortality; nor did it worsen kidney function as had been suggested by prior meta-analyses of smaller studies.

Others: Vasodilators, Inotropes, Vasopressors
- Vasodilators for patients with adequate end-organ perfusion (i.e., normal or elevated blood pressure): nitroglycerin or nitroprusside
- Intravenous inotropes (e.g., dobutamine or milrinone) for patients with known systolic HF (low ejection fraction) and with signs of shock or hypotension
- Intravenous vasopressor (phenylephrine) for patients with diastolic HF with signs of shock or hypotension—do not give inotrope.
- Unknown cardiac status with signs of shock or hypotension: intravenous inotropes (e.g., dobutamine or milrinone), +/− vasopressor and mechanical support

Bottom Line for the Management of ADHF
- Diuresis:
  - Continuous furosemide infusion = bolus therapy in terms of efficacy.
  - Double home dose of furosemide results in trend for faster improvement without more adverse effects.
  - Continuous infusion has a lower risk of ototoxicity than bolus therapy.
  - Outpatient bumetanide or torsemide has better bioavailability than furosemide.
- Ultrafiltration is not superior to step-approach medical therapy.

Nephrotic Syndrome

- Underfilling theory: Hypoalbuminemia due to urinary loss and/or altered albumin metabolism reduces intracapillary oncotic pressure, thus arterial "underfilling." This leads to stimulation of the RAAS, SNS, and ADH systems to enhance renal sodium and water retention. This is likely not the sole mechanism of edema in nephrotic syndrome because edema may improve with kidney disease improvement prior to any rise serum albumin.

- Overfilling theory: Edema is due to avid renal sodium retention induced by the underlying diseased kidneys independent of hypoalbuminemia. This occurs via
  - Increased Na^+-K^+-ATPase and epithelial sodium channel (ENaC) activities in cortical collecting tubules.
  - Relative resistance to atrial natriuretic peptide and urodilatin
  - Enhanced proximal tubular reabsorption via increased sodium–hydrogen exchanger activity
- Management of nephrotic syndrome:
  - Diuretics:
    - Loop diuretics +/−
    - K-sparing diuretics (e.g., amiloride to block ENaC), thiazides
  - Salt-poor albumin infusion: Formation of diuretic-albumin complexes keep the diuretic within the vascular space, thereby increasing the rate of loop diuretic secretion into tubular lumen where the free loop diuretic works. Unfortunately, more albumin will also be available to be filtered into the tubular lumen where it binds to the secreted loop diuretic and renders it ineffective. Albumin infusion in nephrotic syndrome has also been suggested to lower thrombotic complication risks during rapid and aggressive diuresis.
  - Sodium restriction: 2 to 3 g/d
  - Angiotensin inhibition: reduce proteinuria/albuminuria, which could enhance loop diuretic action and slow progression of kidney disease.

Ascites and Hepatorenal Syndrome with Advanced Liver Disease, Cirrhosis

- Three major hemodynamic changes induced by advanced liver disease, hepatic cirrhosis:
  - *Portal hypertension* (HTN), as a result of
    - Postsinusoidal obstruction induced by hepatic fibrosis *and*
    - Increased portal venous inflow as a consequence of splanchnic arterial vasodilation
  - *Splanchnic vasodilatation*, due to
    - Local release of potent vasodilators, for example, nitric oxide (NO), thought to be driven by portal HTN and reduced clearance of bacterial products, which leads to → splanchnic blood pooling → fall in systemic effective circulating volume, *and*
  - Reduced systemic vascular resistance
- Early compensation: *HYPERdynamic* circulation (increased cardiac output)
- With disease progression, there may be cardiac dysfunction; cardiac output cannot adequately compensate the increasing splanchnic arterial vasodilation, hence *effective arterial hypovolemia*, → followed by activation of RAAS, SNS, and ADH systems to promote Na^+ and H_2O retention and vasoconstriction of liver and extra-splanchnic organs (kidneys, brain, adrenals). While the continuing Na^+ and H_2O retention leads to edema and ascites formation, the severe renal vasoconstriction leads to a precipitous fall in glomerular filtration (GFR). This state of *functional* renal dysfunction is referred to as the "hepatorenal syndrome" and may be reversed with a liver transplant.

Hepatorenal Syndrome

Definition of HRS by the Ascites International Club: *"HRS is a clinical condition that occurs in patients with chronic liver disease, advanced hepatic failure, and portal hypertension characterized by impaired renal function and marked abnormalities in the arterial circulation and activity of the endogenous vasoactive systems. In the kidney, there is marked renal vasoconstriction that results in a low GFR. In the extrarenal circulation, there is predominance of arterial vasodilation that results in reduction of total systemic vascular resistance and arterial hypotension."*

- Ascites International Club criteria for HRS:
  - Cirrhosis with ascites
  - Acute kidney injury (AKI) defined by the Acute Kidney Injury Network/Kidney Disease Outcome Quality Initiative (AKIN/KDOQI) as:
    - Increase in SCr by ≥0.3 mg/dL from stable baseline in less than 48 hours, *or*
    - ≥50% increase in stable baseline SCr within the prior 3 months
  - No improvement in SCr after at least 2 days with diuretic withdrawal and volume expansion with 20 to 25% albumin (recommended dose: 1 g/kg of body weight per day up to a maximum of 100 g/d)
  - Absence of shock
  - No current or recent treatment with nephrotoxic drugs
  - Absence of parenchymal kidney disease as indicated by proteinuria > 500 mg/d, microhematuria (>50 red blood cells per high power field), and/or abnormal renal ultrasonography
- Subtypes of HRS:
  - Type 1: ≥doubling of initial SCr to >2.5 mg/dL or a 50% reduction of the initial creatinine clearance (CrCl) to <20 mL/min within 2 weeks; type 1 may occur spontaneously, but frequently occurs in close relationship with a precipitating factor: severe bacterial infection (spontaneous bacterial peritonitis [SBP]), GI hemorrhage, major surgical procedure, or acute hepatitis superimposed on cirrhosis
  - Type 2: a moderate and stable reduction in GFR. Renal failure does not have a rapidly progressive course; type 2 is thought to represent the extreme expression of renal vasoconstriction; dominant clinical feature of type 2: severe ascites with poor or no response to diuretics.
- Incidence: 18% at 1 year; 39% at 5 years
- Prognosis: Renal function rarely spontaneously improves (<5%). Median survival without dialysis support for type I HRS: 2 weeks; type 2 HRS: 6 months
- Management of HRS:
  - Preventive measures to reduce HRS risk:
    - Prophylactic antibiotic therapy for SBP in those at risk:
      - Short-term therapy:
        - Patients hospitalized for gastrointestinal bleed (ceftriaxone 1 g/d); transition to oral quinolone or trimethoprim–sulfamethoxazole b.i.d. × 7 days after stabilization
        - Patients hospitalized for other reasons with ascitic total protein < 1 g/dL
      - Prolonged therapy: (quinolone or trimethoprim–sulfamethoxazole double-strength daily):
        - Patients with ≥1 episode of SBP
        - Patients with cirrhosis and ascitic fluid total protein < 10 g/L with Child–Pugh score > 9, serum bilirubin > 3 mg/dL, SCr > 1.2 mg/dL or blood urea nitrogen (BUN) > 20 mg/dL or S[Na$^+$] < 130 mEq/L
    - Use of tumor necrosis factor inhibitor pentoxifylline in severe alcoholic hepatitis.
    - Avoidance of nephrotoxic agents, NSAIDS, overdiuresis
  - Albumin administration:
    - Initial presentation of kidney injury as volume-expanding challenge: 1 g/kg/d up to 100 g/d for ≥48 hours
    - At diagnosis of SBP to reduce HRS risk: 1.5 g/kg at diagnosis and 1 g/kg IV 48 hours later
    - Large volume paracentesis > 4 to 5 L: albumin infusion at 6 to 8 g/L of ascitic fluid removed

- Transjugular intrahepatic portosystemic shunts (TIPS):
  - Divert portal blood flow to hepatic vein
  - Redistribute splanchnic/portal blood to central volume
  - Improve variceal bleed
  - Improve renal perfusion
  - Complications: bleeding, infections, hepatic encephalopathy, renal failure; typically not tolerable in patients with end-stage liver failure (Child–Pugh class C)
- Vasopressors:
  - Splanchnic vasoconstrictors:
    - Synthetic analogues of vasopressin with decreased antidiuretic properties: (e.g., terlipressin—not available in the United States)
    - Synthetic analog of the pancreatic hormone somatostatin octreotide is used as a splanchnic vasoconstrictor via its inhibition of glucagon. Glucagon is thought to act as a splanchnic vasodilator.
  - Systemic vasoconstrictor: midodrine

> **NOTE** Combination midodrine + octreotide ± albumin is typically used in the United States and has been reported to result in variable success in the management of HRS. If no response after 3 days, transfer to ICU for a trial of noradrenaline norepinephrine (levophed) 0.5 mg/h, to increase mean arterial pressure (MAP) by ≥10 mm Hg or increase in 4-hour urine output > 200 mL. If goals not met, increase dose every 4 hours in steps of 0.5 mg/h, up to maximum dose of 3 mg/h. Recent meta-analysis revealed equivalent reversal of HRS with terlipressin as it is with norepinephrine. Data for comparative efficacy between midodrine/octreotide combination versus norepinephrine are not available.
>
> *Midodrine: start at 7.5 mg orally t.i.d., titrate up to 12.5 mg t.i.d. to increase MAP of at least 15 mm Hg.*
> *Octreotide: start at 100 µg t.i.d. subcutaneously then, if necessary, increase to 200 µg t.i.d.*
> *Albumin: give 20 to 40 g/d, increase to 40 g daily if central venous pressure (CVP) < 12 mm Hg (or plasma renin activity (PRA) not reduced by >50% of basal value after 3 days of treatment).*

- Molecular adsorbent recycling system
  - Combination of both kidney and liver dialyses. Regular dialysis only removes water-soluble toxins. Molecular adsorbent recycling system (MARS) adds an albumin circuit mimicking normal liver removal of albumin-bound toxins.
  - Not yet widely available or approved for treatment of chronic liver disease
- Liver transplants: UNOS Model of End-stage Liver Disease (MELD) score in liver disease
  - Predict mortality risk
  - Assess disease severity to aid in organ allocation prioritization

$$\text{Risk score} = 10 \times ((0.957 \times \ln(\text{SCr})) + (0.378 \times \ln(\text{Bilirubin}) + (1.12 \times \ln(\text{INR}))) + 6.43$$

If a patient is on hemodialysis, SCr is set to 4, the maximum creatinine level allowed in the model. INR: prothrombin time/international normalized ratio. MELD score can range from 6 to 40 (anything >40 is grouped into 40 maximum), where a higher range indicates higher urgency for liver transplantation.

SALT DEPLETION

Diuretics: Loop and Thiazide Diuretics

Loop Diuretics

Diuretics	Bioavailability	IV to oral conversion	Dose equivalent	Comments
Bumetanide	75%	1:1	1	
Furosemide	50%	1:2	40	Most used
Torsemide	80%	1:1	20	
Ethacrynic acid	100%	1:1	50	No sulfa group

> **NOTE** All loop diuretics except ethacrynic acid have a sulfa group. Furosemide and especially ethacrynic acid are highly ototoxic. Ethacrynic acid should only be used if sulfa allergic.

Thiazide Diuretics

- Hydrochlorothiazide: short half-life ($t_{1/2}$) 6 to 15 hours
- Chlorthalidone: long $t_{1/2}$ 48 to 72 hours
- Both hydrochlorothiazide and chlorthalidone have poor efficacy when GFR < 30 mL/min/1.73 m².
- Metolazone:
  - Maximal effect within an hour of oral intake, lasting up to 24 hours
  - Effective even at GFR < 20 mL/min/1.73 m²
  - Often used with furosemide for synergy

Loop Diuretics versus Thiazides

Common features: Both induce volume depletion and compensatory increase in ADH secretion.
Differences:
- Diuretic effect:
  - Loop diuretics are much more potent than thiazides
  - Antidiuretic activity duration: short lived (i.e., <2 weeks) with thiazides due to upstream compensation
- Calcium: calcium wasting with loop, calcium-sparing with thiazides
- Hyponatremia:
  - Hyponatremia is commonly seen with thiazides, but not with loop diuretics
  - Mechanisms:
    - Loop diuretics inhibit Na^+-K^+-$2Cl^-$ cotransporter, hence
      - Reduction in free H_2O production (i.e., reduction of maximal urinary dilution) and consequently, less free H_2O delivery to collecting tubules for reabsorption
      - Reduction of medullary concentration gradient. Optimal H_2O reabsorption at the collecting tubules depends on a high medullary concentration gradient. The lack of a high medullary concentration gradient reduces efficiency of free H_2O reabsorption.

- The impaired free H_2O reabsorption with loop diuretics from mechanisms above "protects" patients from developing hyponatremia despite increased ADH.
  - Thiazide diuretics do not affect luminal free H_2O production nearly as much as loop diuretics and do not affect the medullary concentration gradient. A compensatory increase in ADH with thiazides, therefore, will lead to avid free H_2O reabsorption in the presence of any free H_2O intake. Consequently, hyponatremia may develop within 5 to 14 days. At-risk patients include underweight women and elderly patients (particularly elderly women).
- Of interest, potassium depletion (e.g., associated with diuretic use) may directly stimulate water intake via alterations in osmoreceptor sensitivity and increase thirst. This may play a contributory role in diuretic induced hyponatremia.

Salt-Losing Nephropathy

- Advanced kidney disease (i.e., GFR < 15 mL/min): typical labs: $U[Na^+] > 20$ mEq/L, U_{OSM} ~300 mOsm/kg
- Interstitial diseases:
  - Proximal renal tubular acidosis: obligatory Na^+ and K^+ losses due to bicarbonaturia (see Renal Tubular Acidosis , in Acid-Base/Potassium chapter)
  - Medullary cystic kidney disease, a.k.a. autosomal dominant interstitial kidney disease, familial juvenile hyperuricemic nephropathy, uromodulin-associated kidney disease (see Renal Cystic Diseases, in Tubular, Interstitial, and Cystic Disorders chapter)

Mineralocorticoid Deficiency

- Aldosterone deficiency:
  - Primary adrenal insufficiency:
    - Reduced Na^+ reabsorption and reduced distal K^+ secretion at aldosterone-sensitive distal nephron (i.e., late distal convoluted tubules (DCT), connecting segment, and cortical collecting tubules)
    - Laboratory findings: hyperkalemia due to aldosterone deficiency, hyponatremia due to concurrent hypocortisolism-induced ADH secretion.

> **NOTE** Secondary adrenal insufficiency due to central (pituitary) lesions (i.e., reduced central synthesis of ACTH) only presents with hypocortisolism, not mineralocorticoid insufficiency. Hypocortisolism may be associated with hyponatremia via increased production of corticotropin-releasing hormone, which is coexpressed with ADH. Unlike primary adrenal insufficiency, secondary adrenal insufficiency is NOT associated with hyperkalemia due to the absence of mineralocorticoid deficiency.

  - Isolated aldosterone deficiency
    - Congenital hypoaldosteronism, CYP11B2 type I: impaired hydroxylation of corticosterone at 18-carbon; CYP11B2 type II: impaired conversion of 18 hydroxyl group to an aldehyde
    - Laboratory findings for pure hypoaldosteronism: hyperkalemia, but not hyponatremia since cortisol level is normal.
  - Treatment of aldosterone deficiency:
    - Primary adrenal insufficiency:
      - Fludrocortisone (0.05 to 0.2 mg/d) *and* adequate sodium intake (i.e., $U[Na^+]$ > 20 to 40 mEq/L to indicate adequate Na^+ delivery to cortical tubules

- Glucocorticoid (hydrocortisone or prednisone) to correct cortisol deficiency
- Secondary adrenal insufficiency: Glucocorticoid replacement in divided doses daily. Fludrocortisone is generally not needed.

> **NOTE** Fludrocortisone requires tubular sodium delivery to the cortical collecting tubules to work. Salt-depleted patients cannot deliver adequate sodium to the cortical collecting tubules, rendering fludrocortisone ineffective or suboptimally effective. That is, if a patient does not adequately respond to fludrocortisone (i.e., persistent hyperkalemia +/− hypotension), make sure patient has adequate sodium intake or U[Na$^+$] > 20 mEq/L *before* increasing fludrocortisone dose.

- In patients with volume expansion and/or preexisting hypertension, consider adding low-dose loop or thiazide diuretics. This will not only reduce Na$^+$ retention, but will also enhance distal Na$^+$ delivery for optimal fludrocortisone activity.
- Aldosterone receptor mutation: pseudohypoaldosteronism type 1
  - Rare hereditary disorder, autosomal dominant, recessive, or sporadic. Autosomal dominant gives milder salt wasting than autosomal recessive form. Mutations of mineralocorticoid receptor identified in most cases. Autosomal dominant form also improves with age. Volume depletion, failure to thrive in infants
  - Laboratory findings: hyperkalemia, hyponatremia
  - Treatment: High-salt diet ± fludrocortisone 1 to 2 mg/d or carbenoxolone (antagonizes cortisol metabolism thereby allowing accumulation of cortisol to activate mineralocorticoid receptors).

> **NOTE** A much higher dose is needed in pseudohypoaldosteronism type 1 than in primary adrenal insufficiency.

Osmotic Diuresis

Cerebral Salt Wasting
- Typically associated with subarachnoid hemorrhage, thought to be associated with the following:
  - Impaired sympathetic neural input (SNS normally promotes proximal tubular Na$^+$, uric acid, and water reabsorption and renin aldosterone release), and/or
  - Increased brain natriuretic peptide → impairs renal tubular Na$^+$ reabsorption and inhibits renin release.
- Many cases diagnosed as CSW are thought to be SIADH, not CSW.
- Clinical manifestations: volume depletion, orthostatic hypotension
- Laboratory findings: hyponatremia, low serum uric acid, high urine osmolality, U[Na$^+$] > 20 to 30 mEq/L, low renin and aldosterone levels (all similar to SIADH)

> **NOTE** CSW patients present with volume depletion, in contrast to SIADH patients who present with euvolemia to slightly hypervolemica.

- Treatment of CSW:
  - Volume repletion (NS, salt tablets). Note: NS may worsen hyponatremia in SIADH when UOSM > 300 mOsm/kg, but generally improves hyponatremia in CSW. In rare severe cases of CSW, 3% saline may be required.

- Consider mineralocorticoids, for example, fludrocortisone 0.2 mg twice daily.
- Typical transient condition—long-term treatment not necessary

> **NOTE** Common features between SIADH and CSW: High ADH and natriuretic peptide levels, high U[Na$^+$], low renin and aldosterone levels, low uric acid levels.

Gastrointestinal Losses and Third-Spacing
- Clinical history
- Laboratory findings: low U[Na$^+$] < 10 to 20 mEq/L, with the exception of acute vomiting (see Metabolic Alkalosis, in Acid-Base/Potassium chapter), high U$_{OSM}$

POLYURIA

Polyuria Background
- Polyuria is typically defined as having urine volume greater than 40 mL/kg body weight/day.
- Polyuria may be due to osmotic diuresis, water diuresis, or both.
- Water diuresis is due to failure of kidneys to reabsorb water or excessive free water intake.

Basic Physiological Steps Involved in Free Water Reabsorption
- Salt and water are delivered to the thick ascending limb of loop of Henle and DCT.
- At these nephron segments where there is relative impermeability to H_2O (more so in loop of Henle than DCT), intraluminal free H_2O is "produced" when sodium chloride is reabsorbed but not H_2O.
- Free H_2O produced is delivered to the collecting tubules where it is reabsorbed via apical AQP2, and basolateral aquaporins 3 and 4. The efficiency of H_2O reabsorption depends on the presence and integrity of AQP2 and high medullary concentration gradient. The latter acts as a dry sponge which soaks up any H_2O delivered to the collecting tubules: the higher the medullary concentration gradient, the more efficient the H_2O reabsorption.
- AQP2 regulation via ADH: ADH binds to its receptor and activates adenylyl cyclase via G protein to produce cAMP. cAMP mediates the shuttling of cytoplasmic AQP2 to the apical side of principal cells along the collecting tubules where intraluminal H_2O can be reabsorbed. Prolonged ADH elevation (>24 hours) can also increase the expression of AQP2.

Based on the basic steps involved in free H_2O reabsorption above, factors that can limit effective H_2O reabsorption (Table 1.3):
- Increased distal salt and water delivery seen with poor proximal tubular function
- Reduced ADH:
  - Reduced production: cDI
  - Increased destruction: pregnancy-associated increase in vasopressinase production
- Abnormal ADH receptor: nDI (loss-of-function mutation of ADH receptor)
- Defect in cAMP production: chronic poor kidney function, hypokalemia, hypercalcemia, demeclocycline, lithium
- Problems with AQP2:
  - Mutation of AQP2 with functional defect
  - Downregulation of AQP2: Chronic poor kidney function, hypokalemia, malnutrition, lithium therapy. NOTE: Lithium has also been shown to inhibit cAMP formation by the collecting duct and downregulate the expression of AQP3 and

Table 1.3	Physiology of free water excretion and conditions associated with suboptimal water reabsorption

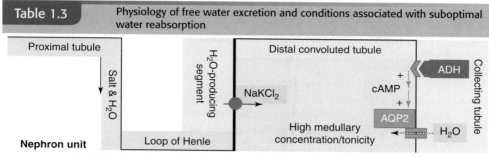

Conditions Associated with Suboptimal H_2O Reabsorption → High Free H_2O Loss	
Proximal tubular dysfunction	Poor proximal tubular function
H_2O-producing segment: Suboptimal $NaKCl_2$ cotransporter function	Chronic poor kidney function, hypokalemia, hypercalcemia
Reduced ADH level	Reduced ADH synthesis (central diabetes insipidus), pregnancy-associated increased vasopressinase production
Abnormal ADH receptor	X-linked mutation of ADH receptor
Reduced cAMP production	Chronic poor kidney function, hypokalemia, hypercalcemia, demeclocycline, lithium
Reduced AQP2 function or expression	Autosomal dominant or recessive mutation of AQP2; downregulation of AQP2: chronic poor kidney function, hypokalemia, malnutrition, lithium
Reduced medullary concentration/tonicity	Chronic poor kidney function, sickle cell disease, malnutrition, conditions leading to suboptimal $NaKCl_2$ function (see above)

the urea transporter UT-A1. The latter reduces urea accumulation in the inner medulla, hence suboptimal medullary concentration gradient for water reabsorption. More recently, the intrinsic renal purinergic system involving ATP/ADP/UTP has been shown to counteract the action of ADH on the collecting duct and reduce free water reabsorption. Blockage of the purinergic system with clopidogrel has been shown to reduce polyuria in animal models of lithium-induced NDI.

- Loss of medullary concentration gradient: chronic poor kidney function, hypokalemia, hypercalcemia, sickle cell disease, protein malnutrition

Causes of Polyuria

- Water diuresis:
  - Primary polydipsia (psychogenic polydipsia):
    - Often seen in anxious middle-aged women
    - Patients with psychiatric illness, including those taking phenothiazines which can lead to the sensation of dry mouth
    - Hypothalamic lesions affecting thirst center (sarcoidosis)
  - Central diabetes insipidus:
    - Idiopathic (autoimmune injury to ADH-producing cells). These patients can present with the lack of hyperintense T1 signal within the posterior pituitary on brain MRI.
    - Trauma, neurosurgery: typical triphasic response may be observed with severe hypothalamic or hypothalamic tract injury:
      - Initial polyuric phase beginning within 24 hours and lasting up to 4 to 5 days due to inhibition of ADH release from hypothalamic "shock"

- Antidiuretic phase due to slow release of stored ADH from degenerating posterior pituitary during days 6 to 11, (SIADH equivalent): Excessive free water intake can cause hyponatremia.
    - Permanent DI due to depletion of stored ADH in posterior pituitary
  - Pituitary surgery
  - Hypoxic/ischemic encephalopathy
  - Malignancy (metastatic disease involving hypothalamic–pituitary region, particularly lung, leukemia, lymphoma, craniopharyngioma, pinealoma)
  - Familial (rare, autosomal dominant; due to preservation of function of the normal allele, polyuria may not present until after the first year of life or even in young adulthood)
  - Infiltrative diseases:
    - Langerhans cell histiocytosis a.k.a. histiocytosis X: rare histiocytic disorderly commonly characterized by single or multiple osteolytic bone lesions with histiocytes infiltration; extraskeletal involvement: skin, lymph nodes, lungs, thymus, liver, spleen, bone marrow, CNS
    - Granulomatous diseases: sarcoidosis, tuberculosis
    - Granulomatosis polyangiitis
    - Autoimmune lymphocytic hypophysitis: lymphocytic infiltration and enlargement of pituitary followed by destruction of pituitary cells. More common in women, often associated with late pregnancy or postpartum.
  - Post-supraventricular tachycardia: due to decreased ADH secretion, presumably due to increased left atrial and systemic pressure and subsequent activation of local baroreceptors
  - Other causes of cDI: cerebral aneurysm, anorexia nervosa, infections, Guillain–Barré
- Nephrogenic diabetes insipidus:
  - Hereditary:
    - Severe polyuria and hypernatremia typically occur during first week of life
    - X-linked: mutations of *AVPR2* gene encoding the vasopressin receptor V2
    - Autosomal recessive and dominant: mutations of *aquaporin-2* gene
  - Acquired:
    - Drug-induced: chronic lithium use, demeclocycline
    - Electrolyte disturbances: hypercalcemia, hypokalemia
    - Conditions leading to reduced medullary concentration gradient: sickle cell disease/trait, protein malnutrition
- Pregnancy: DI induced by placental production of vasopressinase. In the setting of preeclampsia, twins or triplets, or subclinical cDI, a transient DI may ensue from vasopressinase-mediated degradation of N-terminal amino acids from the vasopressin molecule. Because desmopressin (DDAVP) is already deaminated at the N-terminal, it is resistant to the effect of vasopressinase and may be used to treat pregnancy associated DI. Delivery (placenta) corrects the problem.

> **NOTE**
> - In adults, the onset of cDI is usually abrupt, that is, patient can pinpoint onset, whereas onset of acquired nDI or primary polydipsia is typically gradual.
> - New onset nocturia may be a sign of defect in nocturnal urinary concentration (i.e., nocturnal need to urinate despite cessation of fluid intake), hence early sign of DI.

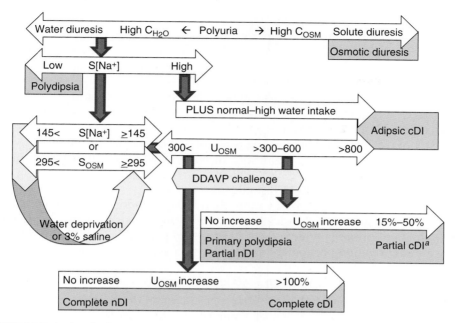

FIGURE 1.2 Evaluation of polyuria.

[a]Partial cDI may have sufficient endogenous ADH secretion with water deprivation and hyperresponsiveness to the small ADH increase due to presumed upregulation of ADH receptors. The addition of DDAVP may not further concentrate the urine. This scenario could be mistaken as polydipsia or partial nDI. Clinical history of sudden onset, however, would favor cDI.

- Solute (osmotic) diuresis:
  - Electrolytes: Excessive saline infusion, salt (Na^+, K^+) intake
  - Nonelectrolytes: glucosuria, mannitol, total parenteral nutrition, contrast dye, urea, hemoglobin, myoglobin

Diagnosis of Polyuria

- Confirm polyuria by volume: >40 mL/kg/d to rule out urinary frequency (Fig. 1.2)
- Determine water diuresis versus solute diuresis versus both
  - Solute diuresis is likely if:
    - Total urine osmolality (24-hour urine volume $\times$ U_{OSM}) >> 800 mOsm/d (800 mOsm is the daily solute load for an average American diet), or
    - C_{OSM} >> 3 L/d, or
    - U_{OSM}/S_{OSM} >> 0.7
  - Water diuresis is likely if:
    - Urine volume $\times$ $(1 - U_{OSM}/S_{OSM})$ >> 0, or
    - U_{OSM}/S_{OSM} << 0.7
  - Combined solute and water diuresis is possible if:
    - *Total* urine osmolality (= 24 hour urine volume $\times$ U_{OSM}) >> 800 mOsm/d *and*
    - Large FWC, that is urine volume $\times$ $(1 - U_{OSM}/S_{OSM})$ >> 0

Water Deprivation Testing

- Full water deprivation testing is not necessary for the following:
  - Solute diuresis without high osmolar-free water clearance
  - Low U_{OSM} and low $S[Na^+]$: Diagnosis of POLYDIPSIA is likely.
  - Adult patients with thirst sensation defect, $S[Na^+]$ > 145 mEq/L despite unlimited water access: diagnosis of adipsic DI is likely.

- There are two phases to a water deprivation test:
  - Phase 1: Aim is to induce a hyperosmolar state ($S_{OSM} > 295$ mOsm/kg or $S[Na^+]$ > 145 mEq/L) to assess the concentrating ability of the kidneys. Hypertonic saline (0.05 mL/kg/min $\times \leq 2$ hours) may be considered if water deprivation is not an option for whatever reason.
  - Phase 2: Once the patient has safely achieved the hyperosmolar goal above, DDAVP is administered and the response to DDAVP is analyzed based on the changes in U_{OSM} and urine output.
- Phase 1 of water deprivation testing is not necessary for the following:
  - $U_{OSM} < S_{OSM}$, $S[Na^+] > 145$ mEq/L in infants/children with a family history of nDI:
    - Proceed to phase 2 DDAVP challenge
    - If U_{OSM} does not increase by more than 100 mOsm/kg over baseline: diagnosis of nDI is likely. DNA testing for mutation analysis may be considered.
  - If a patient presents with $S_{OSM} > 295$ mOsm/kg or $S[Na^+] > 145$ mEq/L, omit water deprivation portion and proceed to phase 2 DDAVP challenge.

Interpretation of Water Deprivation Testing

- $U_{OSM} > 300$ to 600 mOsm/kg following phase 1 water deprivation:
  - Differential diagnoses: partial cDI, partial nDI, polydipsia
  - Response to DDAVP administration in phase 2 may set these conditions apart:
    - Partial cDI: U_{OSM} increases by 15% to 50% from phase 1. Note that partial cDI may have sufficient endogenous ADH secretion with water deprivation and hyperresponsiveness to the small ADH increase due to presumed upregulation of ADH receptors. The addition of DDAVP may not further concentrate the urine. This scenario could be mistaken as polydipsia or partial nDI. Clinical history of sudden onset, however, would favor central DI.
    - Primary polydipsia and nDI: no further increase in U_{OSM} after phase 1
- $U_{OSM} < 300$ mOsm/kg following phase 1 water deprivation:
  - Presence of either complete nDI or complete cDI
  - Response to DDAVP administration in phase 2 sets these two conditions apart.
    - Complete nDI: No further increase in U_{OSM} from phase 1
    - Complete cDI: U_{OSM} increases >100% from phase 1

Additional Diagnostic Testing: Plasma and Urine ADH

- An increase in plasma or urine ADH in response to a rising S_{OSM} excludes cDI.
- An increase U_{OSM} as ADH secretion increases excludes nDI.

Management of Polyuria

- Treat underlying cause.
- Other considerations:
  - Central diabetes insipidus: DDAVP
  - Pregnancy with placental oversecretion of vasopressinase: DDAVP, delivery
  - Nephrogenic diabetes insipidus: thiazide diuretics
  - Malnutrition: high protein intake to optimize medullary tonicity (optimize favorable concentration gradient for free H_2O reabsorption)

Access the eBook for self-assessment questions.

Acid–Base/Potassium

Phuong-Chi T. Pham and Phuong-Thu T. Pham

ACID–BASE DISORDERS

Role of Kidneys in Acid–Base Regulation

Proximal Tubules: Bicarbonate Reabsorption

- 80% to 85% of filtered HCO_3^- is reabsorbed in the proximal tubules (Fig. 2.1). Distal HCO_3^- reabsorption is small but can increase in proximal renal tubular acidosis.
- The Na^+-H^+ antiporter NHE_3 and, to a lesser extent, H^+-ATPase secrete H^+ into the lumen, where it binds filtered HCO_3^- to form bicarbonic acid (H_2CO_3). Carbonic anhydrase IV (CA IV) catalyzes the dissociation of H_2CO_3 into $H_2O + CO_2$. CO_2 diffuses into the cell, combines with H_2O to reform H_2CO_3, and then again redissociates to $H^+ + HCO_3^-$. H^+ is resecreted into the lumen, while HCO_3^- is reabsorbed via the Na^+-HCO_3^- cotransporter NBC1.
- In acute metabolic acidosis, cytoplasmic NBC1 is recruited into basolateral membranes to enhance HCO_3^- reabsorption.

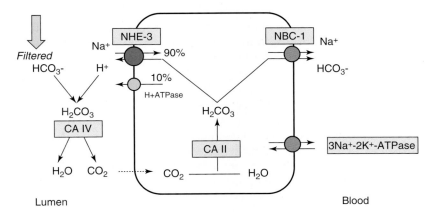

FIGURE 2.1 Bicarbonate reabsorption in the proximal tubules. Eighty to 85% of HCO_3^- is reabsorbed in the proximal tubules. NHE_3, Sodium hydrogen exchanger-3; NBC-1, Sodium bicarbonate cotransporter-1; CA IV, Carbonic anhydrase IV; CA II, Carbonic anhydrase II.

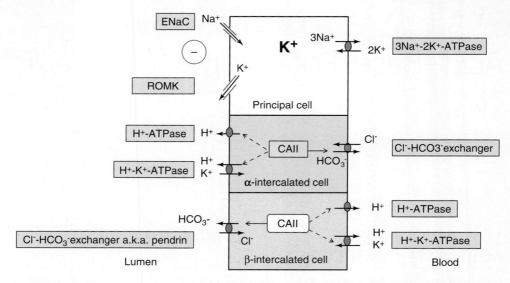

FIGURE 2.2 H^+ and K^+ secretion in the collecting tubules. ENaC, Epithelial sodium channel; ROMK, Renal outer medullary potassium channel; CA, Carbonic anhydrase.

- In metabolic alkalosis, NBC1 is redistributed into the cytoplasm to reduce HCO_3^- reabsorption.
- In respiratory acidosis, NBC1 protein synthesis is upregulated.

Distal Tubules: Hydrogen and Potassium Secretion

- H^+ secretion occurs predominantly in the late distal tubule, connecting segment, and cortical and medullary collecting tubules at approximately 1 mEq/kg/d, reflecting dietary acid load.
- Mechanisms of H^+ and K^+ secretions (Fig. 2.2):
  - Sodium enters the principal cells via the apical amiloride-sensitive epithelial sodium channel (ENaC).
    - The reabsorbed Na^+ is subsequently reabsorbed on the basolateral side in exchange for intracellular K^+ uptake via $3Na^+$-$2K^+$-ATPase. The increase in intracellular K^+ gives rise to a favorable chemical gradient for K^+ secretion.
    - The apical uptake of Na^+ also creates a relative electronegative lumen that favors the secretion of positively charged K^+ via the renal outer medullary potassium channel (ROMK in principal cells) and H^+ via H^+-ATPase and, to a lesser extent, H^+-K^+-ATPase (α-intercalated cells).
  - Optimal H^+ and K^+ secretions require sufficient Na^+ delivery to the distal nephron, intact ENaC, presence of aldosterone, and good urine flow. Aldosterone increases the number of open ENac and ROMK channels and upregulates luminal H^+-ATPase and basolateral $3Na^+$-$2K^+$-ATPase, hence upregulating both H^+ and K^+ secretion.
- Depending on the acid–base status, distal tubules can secrete either H^+ or HCO_3^- via α-intercalated cell or β-intercalated cell, respectively.
- The efficiency of H^+ urinary excretion depends on the presence of ammonia (NH_3): $H^+ + NH_3 \rightarrow NH_4^+$.

Ammoniagenesis: Proximal Tubular Production of NH_4^+, NH_3

- The substrate for ammoniagenesis is glutamine.
- Glutamine is taken up into proximal tubular cells via the sodium-dependent amino acid transporters (SNAT3), where NH_4^+ is formed in a multistep process:

$$\text{Glutamine} \xrightarrow[\text{PDG}]{NH_3} \text{glutamate} \xrightarrow[\text{PEPCK}]{NH_3} \alpha\text{-ketoglutarate} \longrightarrow \text{glucose} + CO_2 + 2HCO_3^-$$

- Rate-limiting enzymes for ammoniagenesis: phosphate-dependent glutaminase (PDG) and phosphoenolpyruvate carboxykinase (PEPCK)
- NH_3 is either transported as NH_4^+ into the lumen via NHE_3 or freely diffused into lumen as NH_3. Angiotensin II upregulates NHE_3, thereby increasing NH_4^+ secretion.
- Luminal NH_3 and NH_4^+ are reabsorbed at thick ascending limb loop of Henle into interstitium, where they are subsequently secreted into cortical collecting tubules with H^+. NH_4^+ may be reabsorbed at the loop of Henle by replacing K^+ on the Na^+-K^+-$2Cl^-$-cotransporter. Secretion of NH_3 at the connecting segments and collecting tubules is facilitated by the nonerythroid glycoproteins RhBg and RhCg.
- In metabolic acidosis, there is:
  - Mobilization of glutamine from skeletal muscle and intestinal cells
  - Increased SNAT3 expression
  - Increased expression of the rate-limiting enzymes in ammoniagenesis
- Ammoniagenesis is stimulated by intracellular metabolic acidosis and hypokalemia (Fig. 2.3).

Diagnosis of Acid–Base Disorders

Normal values: pH = 7.4, Pco_2 = 40 mm Hg, serum $[HCO_3^-]$ = 24 mEq/L, serum anion gap = 12.

Four *basic steps* in the assessment of acid–base disorders:
1. Check serum $[HCO_3^-]$.

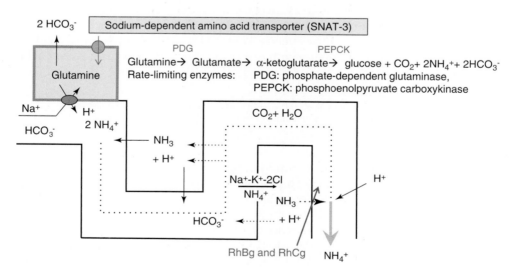

FIGURE 2.3 Ammoniagenesis.

a. If $[HCO_3^-] < 24 \rightarrow$ either metabolic acidosis or respiratory alkalosis (acute or chronic)

b. If $[HCO_3^-] > 24 \rightarrow$ either metabolic alkalosis or respiratory acidosis (acute or chronic)

2. Check pH to determine which of two possibilities (a or b) in step 1 is most likely.

Example: If a patient has $[HCO_3^-]$ 16 mEq/L, the patient can have either metabolic acidosis or respiratory alkalosis. If this patient's pH is 7.2, it would be more likely that the patient has metabolic acidosis rather than respiratory alkalosis. If, however, the patient's pH is 7.45, then it is more likely that the patient has respiratory alkalosis.

• Steps 1 and 2 give the *first* acid–base disturbance.

> **NOTE** Alternatively, one could start with, as the first step, checking pH to determine two possible acid–base disorders, and then check, as the second step, serum $[HCO_3^-]$ to determine which of the two possible acid–base disorders is more likely.

3. Calculate expected compensation for the first acid–base disturbance above. If compensation is not what is expected, there is a *second* acid–base disturbance:

	$\Delta[HCO_3^-]$	ΔP_{CO_2}
Metabolic acidosis[a]	↓1	↓1
Metabolic alkalosis	↑1	↑0.7
Respiratory acidosis (acute)	↑0.1	↑1
Respiratory acidosis (chronic)	↑0.25	↑1
Respiratory alkalosis (acute)	↓0.1	↓1
Respiratory alkalosis (chronic)	↓0.35	↓1

Note: [a]For severe metabolic acidosis (i.e., serum $HCO_3^- < 10$ mEq/L), use Winter's formula to calculate expected P_{CO_2}.
Winter's formula: Expected $P_{CO_2} = (1.5 \times$ serum $[HCO_3^-]) + 8 \pm 2$ mm Hg
Winter's formula calculates the "expected P_{CO_2}," *not* the change in P_{CO_2}.

Example 1: Patient with $[HCO_3^-]$ 37 mEq/L, pH 7.5, P_{CO_2} 34 mm Hg
Based on the high HCO_3^- and pH, the *first* acid–base disturbance is metabolic alkalosis. For every 1 increase in HCO_3^-, there is a 0.7 increase in P_{CO_2} in metabolic alkalosis. Since there is a 13 increase in $[HCO_3^-]$, there should also be a $0.7 \times 13 = 9.1$ increase in P_{CO_2}. The expected P_{CO_2} should, therefore, be 40 + 9.1 or ~49 mm Hg. The actual P_{CO_2}, however, is 34 mm Hg, a value much lower than the expected 49. This means patient also has a respiratory alkalosis as a *second* acid–base disturbance.

> **NOTE** If an "expected" $[HCO_3^-]$ is within 2 mEq/L of the actual value or expected P_{CO_2} is within 3 mm Hg of the actual value, do not consider another acid–base disorder. Clinical judgment is required.

Example 2: Patient with $[HCO_3^-]$ 18 mEq/L, pH 7.5, P_{CO_2} 18 mm Hg.
Based on the low $[HCO_3^-]$ and high pH, the *first* acid–base disturbance is respiratory alkalosis. Compensation for respiratory alkalosis: For every 1 decrease in P_{CO_2}, there is a decrease in $[HCO_3^-]$ in the range of [0.1 to 0.35], 0.1 for acute and 0.35 for chronic change. Since there is a decrease of 14 in P_{CO_2}, there should be a decrease in $[HCO_3^-]$ of $0.1 \times 14 = 1.4$ (for acute) to $0.35 \times 14 = 4.9$ (for chronic). The expected $[HCO_3^-]$ would be between 22.6 (24 − 1.4) and 19.1 (24 − 4.9). Since the actual P_{CO_2} is 18, it is likely that the patient just has a chronic respiratory alkalosis and no "second" acid–base disturbance.

4. Check serum anion gap (AG):
   - Derivation and definition of serum AG:
     - Total positive charges = total negative charges

     $$[Na^+] + \text{unmeasured cations}^+ = [Cl^-] + [HCO_3^-] + \text{unmeasured anions}^-$$

     Rearranging the equation,

     $$[Na^+] - [Cl^-] - [HCO_3^-] = [\text{unmeasured anions}^- - \text{unmeasured cations}^+] = \text{serum AG}$$

   - A normal serum AG is ~12.
   - Conditions with *high serum AG metabolic acidosis*:
     - ↑Serum AG = [↑unmeasured anions$^-$ – unmeasured cations$^+$]
     - Unmeasured anions come from methanol (converts to formic acid), uremia (accumulation of sulfates, phosphates, urates, etc.), diabetic ketoacidosis (ketone bodies), paraldehyde (causes hypotension and lactic acidosis), pyroglutamate (a.k.a. oxoproline), propylene glycol (converts to lactate), isoniazide (induces liver and mitochondrial injury leading to lactic acidosis), metformin and iron (inhibit mitochondrial function, hence lactic acid production), bacteria-producing D-lactic acidosis (if poor kidney function), L-lactic acidosis, ethylene glycol (converts to oxalate), salicylates.
   - Conditions with *normal AG metabolic acidosis*:
     - Serum AG = $[Na^+]$ – ↑$[Cl^-]$ – ↓$[HCO_3^-]$ (no change in serum AG generally due to an equivalent increase in chloride reabsorption in exchange for bicarbonate loss)
     - Bicarbonate loss from: diarrhea; poor kidney function but with eGFR > 30 mL/min/1.73 m^2; ureterosigmoid anastomosis > ileal conduit; enteric fistulas; drainage of biliary, pancreatic, or enteric secretions; renal tubular acidosis; D-lactic acidosis (if good kidney function); ingestion of NH_4Cl and/or acidic amino acids (e.g., with total parenteral nutrition); high volume normal saline infusion; toluene ingestion (if good kidney function); posthypocapnic state; and drug-induced acetazolamide, topiramate, amphotericin B, K-sparing diuretics, trimethoprim, pentamidine, $CaCl_2$, cholestyramine, etc. ($CaCl_2$ may cause metabolic acidosis because of the formation of calcium carbonate, while cholestyramine [cationic resin given as a chloride salt] may form bicarbonate salts that are eliminated in the stool). Also see Renal Tubular Acidosis.
   - Conditions with high AG but without metabolic acidosis: severe metabolic alkalosis (pH > 7.5), cellular phosphate/anion leaks in nonketotic hyperglycemia
   - Conditions with low AG that has no associated acid–base disorder:
     - Low serum AG = [↓unmeasured anions$^-$ – unmeasured cations$^+$] (e.g., hypoalbuminemia: For every drop of 1 g/dL of albumin, there is an expected drop of 2.5 for AG)
     - Low serum AG = [unmeasured anions$^-$ – ↑unmeasured cations$^+$] (e.g., excess positively charged immunoglobulins with multiple myeloma or intravenous infusion of immunoglobulins)
     - Low serum AG = [↓unmeasured anions$^-$ – ↑unmeasured cations$^+$] (e.g., primary hyperparathyroidism [elevated Ca^{2+} but low PO_4^{2-}])
     - Others due to falsely low measurements of Na^+ (e.g., hypernatremia S$[Na^+]$ > 170 mEq/L) or falsely high measurements of Cl^- (e.g., fluoride/bromide intoxication, hyperlipidemia)

- Interpretation of increased SAG:
  Imagine a patient with a SAG = 27. This may be interpreted as having 12 normal AG and 15 excess anions⁻ (A^-):
  - $27 = 12$ normal AG $+ 15 A^-$
  - One can assume that the excess 15 A^- detected enter the body with 15 acid H^+.

$$15 \, HA \leftrightarrow 15 \, H^+ + 15 \, A^-$$

  - Assume that for every H^+, one HCO_3^- will be consumed.
  - Expected $[HCO_3^-] = 24 - 15 = 9$ mEq/L. This is the *expected* $[HCO_3^-]$ based on the detected excess anions⁻.
  - Compare the calculated *expected* $[HCO_3^-]$ with the measured *actual* serum $[HCO_3^-]$:
    - If the actual serum $[HCO_3^-] =$ expected $[HCO_3^-] \pm 2$, this means there is no other acid–base process.
    - If the actual serum $[HCO_3^-] >$ expected $[HCO_3^-]$, there are more $[HCO_3^-]$ than expected. This implies patient also has metabolic alkalosis.
    - If the actual serum $[HCO_3^-] <$ expected $[HCO_3^-]$ (i.e., there are less $[HCO_3^-]$ than expected), there is "some other process" that is consuming $[HCO_3^-]$ but is not contributing any anions for detection on AG. This implies patient also has a non-AG metabolic acidosis.

Imagine another patient with a SAG = 25. This may be interpreted as having 12 normal AG and 13 excess anions⁻ (A^-):
- $25 = 12$ normal AG $+ 13 A^-$
- One can assume that the excess 13 anions⁻ detected enter the body with 13 acid H^+.

$$13 \, HA \leftrightarrow 13 \, H^+ + 13 \, A^-$$

- Assume that for every H^+, one HCO_3^- will be consumed.
- Expected $[HCO_3^-] = 24 - 13 = 11$ mEq/L. This is the *expected* $[HCO_3^-]$ based on the detected excess anions⁻.
- Compare the calculated *expected* $[HCO_3^-]$ with the measured *actual* serum $[HCO_3^-]$.
  - If the actual serum $[HCO_3^-] = 25$ mEq/L, it would mean that patient also has a metabolic alkalosis in addition to the high AG metabolic acidosis.
  - If the actual $[HCO_3^-] = 5$ mEq/L, it would imply patient also has a non-AG metabolic acidosis in addition to the high AG metabolic acidosis.

Although we typically assume a 1:1 ratio of acid consumption of HCO_3^-, this ratio is slightly higher for organic acids. For lactic acidosis, this ratio is 1.6:1.0 due to buffering of lactic acid by molecules other than $[HCO_3^-]$. That is, for every 1.6 mEq of lactate, only one HCO_3^- will be consumed, not 1.6 HCO_3^-. Example: In a patient with an increased AG of 29 due to lactate acidosis, one would expect the HCO_3^- to drop by $(29 - 12)/1.6 = 11$ instead of $(29 - 12) = 17$. The expected HCO_3^- would be $24 - 11 = 13$, not $24 - 17 = 7$.

Other Acid-Base Disorders

Lactic Acidosis

- Type A refers to tissue hypoperfusion and hypoxia-induced lactic acidosis.
- Type B refers to all other etiologies (Table 2.1).

Metabolic Alkalosis: Chloride Sensitive versus Chloride Resistant

- Chloride-sensitive metabolic alkalosis:

- This is predominantly due to reduced renal perfusion and increased proximal reabsorption of Cl^-, thus less Cl^- available for distal delivery. The limited distal Cl^- delivery reduces HCO_3^- secretion via the Cl^--HCO_3^- exchanger (a.k.a. pendrin) in the apical membranes of non-α (i.e., β- and non-α/non-β) intercalated cells within distal convoluted tubule, connecting tubule, and cortical collecting duct. It is this retention of HCO_3^- that leads to metabolic alkalosis.
- Since there is low distal Cl^- delivery, urine chloride is expected to be low (i.e., <20 mEq/L).
- Chloride infusion would increase Cl^--HCO_3^- exchange, increase HCO_3^- secretion, and correct the metabolic alkalosis, hence "chloride-sensitive" metabolic alkalosis.
- Common causes of chloride-sensitive metabolic alkalosis: vomiting, nasogastric suction, gastrocystoplasty for bladder augmentation, diuretics, villous adenoma, congenital chloride diarrhea, posthypercapnia, low dietary chloride intake.

> **NOTE** Three phases of vomiting (loss of H^+ in vomitus = HCO_3^- "loading")
>
> | Acute phase | High HCO_3^- "load" | → High urine Na^+-HCO_3^- and K^+-HCO_3^- loss |
> |---|---|---|
> | | Low volume | → Low urine Cl |
> | Later phase | Low volume | → Low urine Na^+ and Cl |
> | | | → ↑Aldosterone secretion → High urine K^+ |
> | Post phase | No more HCO_3^- loss | → Lower urine K^+ |
> | | Low volume | → Both urine Na^+ and Cl^- will be low |

- Chloride-resistant metabolic alkalosis:
  - This is due to hypersecretion of acid (H^+) due to increased mineralocorticoid activity. The high loss of acid leads to metabolic alkalosis.
  - This form of metabolic alkalosis is *not* due to the lack of chloride. Urine chloride is expected to reflect dietary chloride intake, which is typically >20 mEq/L.
  - Chloride infusion in this condition would not correct the metabolic alkalosis, hence "chloride-resistant" metabolic alkalosis.
  - Common causes of chloride-resistant metabolic alkalosis: mineralocorticoid excess, severe hypokalemia, exogenous alkali (crack cocaine with alkali load), citrate from transfusion products, transplacental transfer from mother with metabolic alkalosis, excessive calcium carbonate ingestion, Pendred syndrome [syndrome with mutation in pendrin where patients may present with goiter, sensorineural deafness, and metabolic alkalosis]. The latter is typically not clinically significant unless challenged with diuretics or alkali load.

Respiratory Alkalosis, Common Causes

Pneumonia, pulmonary embolism, head trauma, hyperthyroidism, pregnancy, cirrhosis, living at high altitude, early bacterial sepsis, meningitis, drugs (theophylline, salicylate), myocardial infarction, atrial fibrillation and flutter, tachycardia

Respiratory Acidosis, Common Causes

Chronic obstructive pulmonary disease, obstructive sleep apnea, obesity-hypoventilation syndrome, neuromuscular weakness or chest wall/diaphragm abnormality, central nervous system depression (drugs or lesions), hypothyroidism, laryngeal/tracheal stenosis

Table 2.1	Etiologies of lactic acidosis

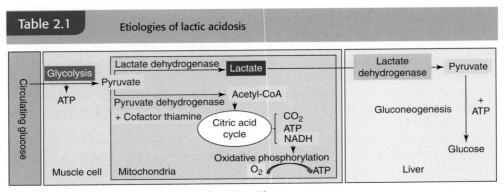

Conditions Leading to Accumulation of Lactic Acid

Excessive glycolysis, glycogenolysis, lipolysis, overwhelming mitochondrial metabolism	Thyrotoxicosis, toxic caffeine ingestion, excessive β_2-agonist stimulation (e.g., asthma treatment or pheochromocytoma), diabetic ketoacidosis, malignancies with high metabolic requirements (e.g., leukemias, lymphoproliferative malignancies, liver metastasis—may be ameliorated with thiamine)
Mitochondrial dysfunction	Inherited mitochondrial diseases; acquired/drug-induced mitochondrial injury: nucleoside reverse transcriptase inhibitors (NRTI) didanosine, stavudine, zidovudine (may be treated with uridine), possibly saquinavir, mangosteen fruit, metformin, propofol, linezolid, methanol, isoniazid, iron overload, ethylene glycol, diethylene glycol, salicylates, cyanide
Reduced pyruvate dehydrogenase activity	Metformin may interfere with pyruvate dehydrogenase activity.
Thiamine deficiency	Severe deficiency of the cofactor thiamine (e.g., may occur with high-grade malignancies above, alcoholism)
Lack of O_2 for oxidative phosphorylation	Hypoxia—type A lactic acidosis: sepsis, severe prolonged hypotension, cardiogenic shock, vigorous exercise, seizures
Liver injury	Acute fulminant liver failure
Reduced lactate dehydrogenase activity	Intralipid in propofol formulation
Others: D-lactic acidosis—*Not* L-lactic acidosis as all other etiologies above	Gut bacterial overgrowth with short-bowel syndrome (may treat with oral metronidazole or vancomycin); diabetic ketoacidosis due to accumulation of the D-lactate intermediate methylglyoxal, a metabolite of acetone and dihydroxyacetone phosphate

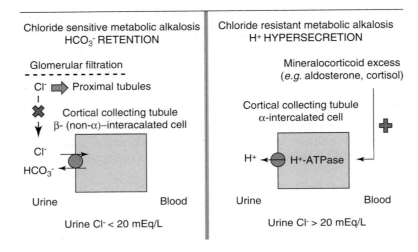

FIGURE 2.4 Chloride-sensitive versus chloride-resistant metabolic alkalosis.

Problems[1]
1. Case: 55-year-old chronically ill female with dizziness, unsteady gait:
   Blood chemistries: $[Na^+]$ 135, $[K^+]$ 4.6, $[Cl^-]$ 99, $[HCO_3^-]$ 12, blood urea nitrogen (BUN) 22 mg/dL, SCr 1.3 mg/dL. Blood gas: pH 7.34, Pco_2 22 mm Hg
   • Steps 1 and 2: Low $[HCO_3^-]$ and low pH → "first" process is metabolic acidosis
   • Step 3:

Compensation	$\Delta[HCO_3^-]$	ΔPco_2
Metabolic acidosis	↓1	↓1

   For current case, ↓$[HCO_3^-]$ by 12, Pco_2 thus ↓by 12 → expected Pco_2 = 40 − 12 = 28, which is higher than the actual Pco_2 of 22 → "second" process: respiratory alkalosis is also present
   • Step 4: Serum AG = 24 → 12 normal AG + 12 anions → 12 H^+ using up 12 $[HCO_3^-]$ → expected $[HCO_3^-]$ = 24 − 12 = 12, which is within ±2 of actual $[HCO_3^-]$ of 12 → no "third" process
   Answer: Increased serum AG metabolic acidosis and respiratory alkalosis, likely due to excess salicylate ingestion. Other possibilities: respiratory alkalosis from acute pulmonary embolism or pneumonia and high serum AG from chronic acetaminophen use (accumulation of oxoproline, a.k.a. pyroglutamic acid).
2. Case: 89-year-old thin female with nonspecific fatigue and weight loss:
   Blood chemistries: $[Na^+]$ 132, $[K^+]$ 4.6, $[Cl^-]$ 97, $[HCO_3^-]$ 13, blood urea nitrogen (BUN) 78 mg/dL, SCr 5.5 mg/dL. Blood gas: pH 7.27, Pco_2 28 mm Hg
   • Steps 1 and 2: Low $[HCO_3^-]$ and low pH → "first" process is metabolic acidosis
   • Step 3:

Compensation	$\Delta[HCO_3^-]$	ΔPco_2
Metabolic acidosis	↓1	↓1

   For current case, ↓$[HCO_3^-]$ by 11, Pco_2 thus ↓by 11 → expected Pco_2 = 40 − 11 = 29, which is within range of actual Pco_2 of 28 → no "second" process
   • Step 4: Serum AG = 22 → 12 normal AG + 10 anions → 10 H^+ using up 10 $[HCO_3^-]$ → expected $[HCO_3^-]$ = 24 − 10 = 14, which is within ±2 of actual $[HCO_3^-]$ of 13 → no "third" process.
   Answer: Increased serum AG metabolic acidosis, likely due to kidney failure and accumulation of organic anions such as sulfates, phosphates, urates, etc.
3. Case: 52-year-old male with nausea, vomiting, and lethargy in the park[2]:
   Blood chemistries: $[Na^+]$ 130, $[K^+]$ 3.1, $[Cl^-]$ 85, $[HCO_3^-]$ 24, blood urea nitrogen (BUN) 32 mg/dL, SCr 1.2 mg/dL. Blood gas: pH 7.40, Pco_2 40 mm Hg
   • Steps 1 and 2: Normal $[HCO_3^-]$ and normal pH → "first" process: not detectable
   • Step 3:

Compensation	$\Delta[HCO_3^-]$	ΔPco_2
Unknown process	?	?

   For current case, there is no obvious "first" process; thus, no compensation can be calculated → no detectable "second" process.
   • Step 4: Serum AG = 21 → 12 normal AG + 9 anions → 9 H^+ using up 9 $[HCO_3^-]$ → expected $[HCO_3^-]$ = 24 − 9 = 15, which is much lower than the actual $[HCO_3^-]$ of 24 → "third" process: metabolic alkalosis

---

[1]Units for electrolytes are mEq/L.
[2]This is a favorite BOARDS case.

Answer: The increased serum AG likely arises from a high AG metabolic acidosis and the higher actual $[HCO_3^-]$ compared with expected $[HCO_3^-]$ indicates a concurrent metabolic alkalosis.

4. Case: 57-year-old male with chronic obstructive pulmonary disease and congestive heart failure presents with fluid overload:

   Blood chemistries: $[Na^+]$ 145, $[K^+]$ 3.1, $[Cl^-]$ 100, $[HCO_3^-]$ 32 mEq/L, blood urea nitrogen (BUN) 15 mg/dL, SCr 1.2 mg/dL. Blood gas: pH 7.44, P_{CO_2} 45 mm Hg. Urine Cl^- 57

   • Steps 1 and 2: High $[HCO_3^-]$ and high pH → "first" process is metabolic alkalosis
   • Step 3:

Compensation	$\Delta[HCO_3^-]$	ΔP_{CO_2}
Metabolic alkalosis	↑1	↑0.7

   For current case, $[HCO_3^-]$ ↑ by 8, P_{CO_2} thus ↑ by $8 \times 0.7 = 5.6$ → expected $P_{CO_2} = 40 + 5.6 = 45.6$ ~46, which is within range of actual P_{CO_2} of 45 → no "SECOND" process.
   • Step 4: Serum AG = 13, which is within ±2 of normal AG of 12. → no "third" process
   Answer: Metabolic alkalosis, with urine $Cl^- >> 20$, suggesting chloride-resistant metabolic alkalosis. Evaluation for mineralocorticoid excess is necessary in this case given the triad hypertension, hypokalemia, and metabolic alkalosis.

5. Case: 89-year-old thin female with nonspecific fatigue and weight loss:

   Admitting arterial blood gas: pH 7.29, P_{CO_2} 60 mm Hg, P_{O_2} 70 mm Hg on 2 L of O_2. After net negative fluid balance of 7 L over 2 days on a bumetanide drip, patient eats less and sleeps more. Repeat blood gas: pH 7.34, P_{CO_2} 85 mm Hg. Patient is still volume overloaded, and kidney function is still adequate with good response to diuretics.

   Which one of the following would be the best treatment for her worsening hypercapnia?
   a. Replace fluid loss with normal saline
   b. Correct diuretic-induced metabolic alkalosis with intravenous 100 mM HCl
   c. Initiate hemodialysis with ultrafiltration
   d. Initiate noninvasive positive pressure support, add acetazolamide, and reduce bumetanide dose.
   Answer: D. The rise in P_{CO_2} is likely a compensatory response to loop-induced volume loss and metabolic alkalosis. Since patient is still volume overloaded, more fluid needs to be removed. Since patient still responds to diuretics, hemodialysis/ultrafiltration is not yet necessary. Acetazolamide is a diuretic, which induces bicarbonaturia. This may be added transiently to reduce the severity of bumetanide-induced metabolic alkalosis while continuing medical diuresis.

6. True or false: A person walking in the street with $[HCO_3^-]$ 38 can have either a metabolic alkalosis or acute respiratory acidosis as the *only* acid–base disorder.
   Answer: False. Although a pure metabolic alkalosis is possible, it is unlikely that a pure acute respiratory acidosis can raise the serum bicarbonate to 38. For acute respiratory acidosis, the change in HCO_3^- is an increase in 0.1 for every 1 increase in P_{CO_2}. An increase in HCO_3^- of 14 (38 − 24) would imply an increase in P_{CO_2} of 14/0.1 or 140 mm Hg from 40 mm Hg. The expected P_{CO_2} would be 40 + 140 = 180 mm Hg. This is unlikely in an ambulating patient.

Rare Acid–Base Disorders, Pearls, and Calculations for Boards

- High acetaminophen use in malnourished chronically ill patients is associated with high AG metabolic acidosis due to excess production of oxoproline, a.k.a. pyroglutamic acid (OXO/PA), due to the lack of negative feedback from gluta-thione. Other notable associated labs include increased serum osmolality gap due to accumulation of OXO/PA and absence or low levels of lactate and ketones that could normally explain increased AG. Consider acetylcysteine therapy to replete glutathione.

- Infusion of high dose lorazepam (Ativan) can lead to accumulation of propylene glycol (constituent in intravenous lorazepam formulation), which can metabolize to L-lactate, hence high AG metabolic acidosis. Suspect this condition in admitted alcoholics with new-onset high AG metabolic acidosis mimicking sepsis/tissue hypoperfusion, but with negative evaluation. Other notable associated signs/symptoms: high serum osmolality, hemolysis, arrhythmias, seizures, and coma.

- Drugs associated with mitochondrial dysfunction and L-lactic acidosis (Table 2.1)

- D-Lactic acid produced by gut bacterial overgrowth in short bowel syndrome. This is *not* the same as what humans produce, which is L-lactate. D-Lactate is filtered quickly and not reabsorbed well because human kidneys only recognize and reabsorb only the L-form of lactate. This can lead to a low or normal AG in those with D-lactate and good kidney function. Patients with D-lactate can present with altered mental status and cerebellar dysfunction, mimicking a "drunk."

- Toluene intoxication presents as non-AG metabolic acidosis in patients with good kidney function because its metabolite, the anion hippuric acid, is freely filtered and excreted. There will thus be excess anions in the urine. The excess anions lead to an increase in the excretion of the cations Na^+ and K^+, giving rise to a positive
  - $U_{AG} = \uparrow U_{Na} + \uparrow U_K - U_{Cl} > 0$

- The presence of hippurate in the urine also increases urine osmolality. Thus, when the urine osmolality is measured, it will be much higher than what is normally expected in the urine. That is, {Measured $U_{OSM} - [U_{[Na+K]} \times 2 + U_{urea}/2.8 + U_{glucose}/18]$}, defined as urine osmolality gap, will be increased. The increased osmolal gap accounts for hippurate $+$ associated $NH4^+$. Normal urine osmolality gap is <150 mEq/L. With toluene intoxication, urine osmolality gap will be >150 mEq/L.

$$\{\text{Measured } U_{OSM} - [U_{[Na+K]} \times 2 + U_{urea}/2.8 + U_{glucose}/18]\} > 150$$

- Serum ketones may be seen with starvation ketosis and diabetic ketoacidosis, but it may also be seen with isopropyl alcohol (a.k.a. isopropanol, rubbing alcohol) intoxication. With isopropyl alcohol, however, there is *no metabolic acidosis*. (NOTE: Serum ketones can give fruity breath odor.)

- Serum osmolality gap (SOG) interpretation:

$$[\text{Measured } S_{OSM} - \{(S[Na^+] + S[K^+]) \times 2 + \text{blood urea nitrogen}/2.8 + \text{glucose}/18\}] > 12 \text{ mOsm/kg}$$

Presence of SOG implies presence of extra osmoles not normally present in serum. Increased SOG should raise concerns for presence of other osmoles, i.e., intoxications (ethanol, methanol, ethylene glycol, isopropanol, or toluene), oxoproline, ketones, and/or lactate. Example: If ethanol is suspected, total mosmoles of ethanol should match SOG. If not the case, look for other concurrent ingestions (e.g., methanol, isopropanol etc.) or oxoproline if chronic acetaminophen use.

- Acidification: Calculating mEq of NH_4Cl or HCl needed to correct severe metabolic alkalosis (i.e., pH > 7.55):
  - = HCO_3 excess (mEq) = 0.5 × lean body weight (kg) × [serum HCO_3^- − 24], for female
  - = HCO_3 excess (mEq) = 0.6 × lean body weight (kg) × [serum HCO_3^- − 24], for male
- Alkalinization: Calculating mEq of $NaHCO_3$ needed to correct metabolic acidosis:
  - HCO_3 deficit (mEq) = [0.4 + 2.6/actual serum HCO_3^-] × lean body weight (kg) × [24 − serum HCO_3^-]
  - In less severe cases of metabolic acidosis, the term [0.4 + 2.6/actual serum HCO_3^-] is ~0.5.

RENAL TUBULAR ACIDOSIS

Renal tubular acidosis (RTA) may be suspected when there is a non-AG gap metabolic acidosis, positive urine AG, and urine osmolality gap < 150 mEq/kg. In chronic metabolic acidosis where there is no concern for toluene ingestion or D-lactic acidosis (from gut bacterial overgrowth seen in short bowel syndrome), calculation of urine osmolal gap is not necessary (Fig. 2.5).

Proximal Renal Tubular Acidosis (pRTA): Impairment of HCO_3^- Reabsorption
Clinical Presentation of pRTA
- Serum [HCO_3^-] (S_{HCO3}) is typically greater than 15 mEq/L.
- Urine pH varies with serum [HCO_3^-] (i.e., urine pH > 5.5) if receiving alkalinization therapy, but appropriately low (i.e., pH < 5.5) in the presence of metabolic acidosis.
- Hypokalemia

Etiologies of pRTA
- Isolated defects (Review Proximal Tubules: Bicarbonate Reabsorption. See Fig. 2.1):
  - Autosomal dominant pRTA (*SCL9A3* gene), encoding NHE₃ transporter; autosomal recessive pRTA (*SLCA4A4* gene), encoding NBC1—associated with mental retardation, ocular abnormalities (glaucoma, cataracts, band keratopathy); sporadic pRTA—nonfamilial, transient type described in infancy, no defect isolated; possibly immaturity of NHE₃ function
  - Isolated defects are rare; typically associated with other proximal tubular transport defects (Fanconi syndrome).
- Fanconi syndrome: multiple proximal tubular transport defects (See Tubular, Interstitial, and Cystic Disorders chapter, Fanconi syndrome)

Diagnosis of pRTA
- Fractional excretion of HCO_3^- ($FeHCO_3$) > 15% and urine pH typically >7.5 following HCO_3^- load (0.5 to 1.0 mEq/kg body weight/hour to increase serum [HCO_3^-] concentration > 20 mEq/L)
- $FeHCO_3 = [(U_{HCO_3} \times S_{Cr}) / (S_{HCO_3} \times U_{Cr})] \times 100\%$

Management of pRTA
- Bicarbonate replacement 5 to 15 mEq/kg/d (NOTE: this can worsen hypokalemia)
- Potassium replacement

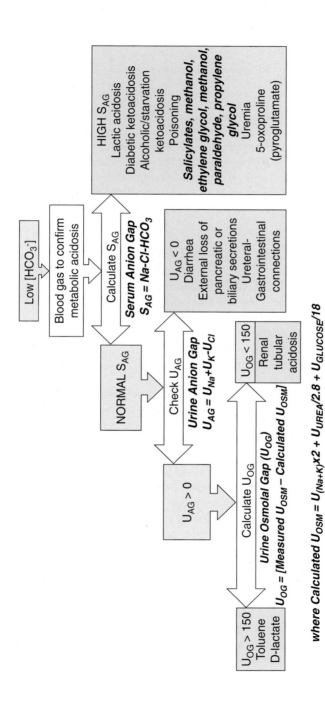

FIGURE 2.5 Evaluation of metabolic acidosis and renal tubular acidosis.

- Thiazide diuretics → induces volume contraction → enhances proximal reabsorption of bicarbonate (NOTE: this can also worsen hypokalemia)
- Vitamin D and phosphate for patients with rickets and hypophosphatemia

Distal Renal Tubular Acidosis (dRTA): Impairment of H^+ Secretion
Clinical Presentation of dRTA

- Metabolic acidosis may be severe (i.e., serum $[HCO_3^-]$ may be <15 mEq/L).
- Growth impairment
- Polyuria
- Hypercalciuria, nephrocalcinosis, nephrolithiasis—due to increased bone resorption and reduced urinary citrate secretion from chronic metabolic acidosis, high urine pH facilitating calcium phosphate precipitation
- High urine pH (e.g., >5.5), but pH could be lower if ammoniagenesis is suboptimal (e.g., seen in dRTA with concurrent hyperkalemia as hyperkalemia inhibits ammoniagenesis). NH_3 is needed to buffer/facilitate H^+ secretion: $NH_3 + H^+ \rightarrow NH_4^+$. The lack of NH_3 leaves more free H^+, which lowers urine pH.

Etiologies of dRTA

- Normo-, hypokalemic dRTA (Review Distal Tubules: Hydrogen and Potassium Secretion. See Fig. 2.2):
  - Isolated defect of H^+-ATPase: Autosomal recessive, mutation of *ATP6B1* gene coding for β_1-subunit of H^+-ATPase; different gene defect in H^+-ATPase, renal specific, with normal hearing
  - Defective anion exchange (AE-1): Autosomal dominant, mutation of *SLC4A1* gene coding for Cl^-/HCO_3^- exchanger AEI
  - Incomplete dRTA (mutation involving CA II)
    - Rare, autosomal recessive
    - Coexistence of pRTA and dRTA (a.k.a. type 3 RTA)
    - Failure to maximally acidify urine, decreased NH_4^+ excretion, high urinary citrate level (thought to be due to concurrent proximal tubular dysfunction)
    - Osteopetrosis (increased bone calcification, thick dense bones on plain X-ray films) due to failure of osteoclasts to secrete acid to dissolve bone mineral
    - Cerebral calcification, mental retardation, sensorineural deafness
  - Autoimmune: Sjögren's, rheumatoid arthritis, hypergammaglobulinemia
  - Medications: lithium, ifosfamide (more commonly pRTA than dRTA)
  - H^+ back-leak: amphotericin can insert itself into tubular cell membrane and act as an ionophore, allowing urinary H^+ to leak back into cell and get reabsorbed. Liposomal formulation of amphotericin reduces the drug ability to insert itself into cell membrane, thus reducing this H^+ back-leak effect.
- Hyperkalemic dRTA:
  - Aldosterone deficiency or resistance (type 4 RTA associated with diabetes), tubulointerstitial nephropathy, nephrocalcinosis, obstruction, lupus nephritis
  - Medications: spironolactone, eplerenone, amiloride, triamterene, trimethoprim, calcineurin inhibitors, NSAIDS, ACEI, ARB, heparin
  - Factors affecting transmembrane voltage (e.g., obstructive uropathy, K-sparing diuretics)
  - Pseudohypoaldosteronism types 1 and 2 (see Hyperkalemia)

Diagnosis of dRTA

- Measurement of [urine P_{CO_2}-blood P_{CO_2}] following bicarbonate load
  - If [urine P_{CO_2}-blood P_{CO_2}] > 30 mm Hg → normal

- If [urine P_{CO_2}-blood P_{CO_2}] < 10 mm Hg → dRTA
- NH_4Cl (100 mg/kg lean body weight) oral load over 1 hour, or furosemide (40 mg) and fludrocortisone (1 mg) orally with ad lib fluid:
  - If there is increased urine NH_4^+ secretion and titratable acid within 2 to 3 hours → normal
  - Otherwise → dRTA
- Management of dRTA:
  - Treatment of underlying disease
  - Bicarbonate supplement 1 to 2 mEq/kg lean body weight/day
  - If hyperkalemic, hypoaldosterone: consider fludrocortisone ± furosemide, dietary K^+ restriction

POTASSIUM

Potassium Physiology and Homeostasis

Potassium Background

- Total body K^+ stores in adults: ~3,000 to 4,000 mEq (50 to 55 mEq/kg body weight)
- Unlike Na^+, 98% of K^+ is intracellular. Intracellular K^+ concentration is ~140 mEq/L whereas plasma K^+ is ~4 to 4.5 mEq/L.
- The differential location of Na^+ and K^+ is maintained by (3)Na^+- (2)K^+-ATPase in cell membrane, which pumps 3 Na^+ out in exchange for 2 K^+ into cell (3:2 ratio).
- Functions of K^+:
  - Cell metabolism (i.e., regulation of protein and glycogen synthesis)
  - Major determinant of resting membrane potential across cell membrane → necessary for generation of action potential required for normal neural and muscular function
- Plasma K^+ concentration ($P[K^+]$), typically measured as serum K+ ($S[K+]$) and total body content depend on:
  - Input: blood transfusions (particularly old blood products due to extracellular K^+ leakage), dietary supplements (salt substitutes [KCl], high K^+-containing foods)

> **NOTE** K^+ loss associated with GI fluid loss occurs via:
> - Direct K^+ loss from vomitus/gastric fluids is relatively low—~5 to 20 mEq/L of fluid loss.
> - More significantly, there is renal K^+ loss via associated volume depletion, compensatory hyperrenin, and hyperaldosteronism.

- Output (i.e., bodily loss): skin (sweats, extensive burns), respiratory (airway secretions), gastrointestines (large volume vomiting, nasogastric suctions, fistulas/drainages, diarrhea, renal excretion)
- Cellular K^+ shift: major determinants (Fig. 2.6):
  - Extracellular pH:
    - Low extracellular pH shifts K^+ out of cells in exchange for H^+ and vice versa (K^+/H^+ exchange).
    - This effect is most pronounced with kidney failure–associated metabolic acidosis and less pronounced with organic acidoses (lactic acid, ketoacids), metabolic alkalosis, and respiratory acidosis/alkalosis.

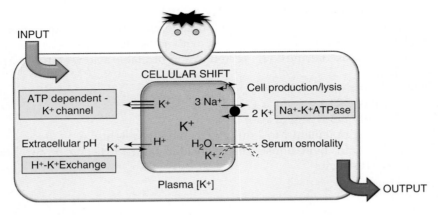

FIGURE 2.6 Mechanisms of cellular potassium shift: intra- versus extracellular distribution.

- Extracellular osmolality: Hyperosmolality shifts water out of cells, which leads to:
  - Higher intracellular K^+ concentration, hence more favorable gradient for K^+ exit into plasma
  - Extracellular K^+ shift due to solvent drag effect
- Na^+-K^+-ATPase:
  - Stimulated by insulin, aldosterone, β_2-agonists (e.g., drug-induced cellular K^+ uptake, thus hypokalemia: albuterol, terbutaline, dobutamine, isoproterenol)
  - Inhibited by α-agonists, presumably via inhibition of renin release, thus downstream hypoaldosteronism and hyperkalemia. (NOTE: α-agonists are vasoconstrictive agents such as phenylephrine and the commonly used agent norepinephrine in the critical care setting. These agents may cause hyperkalemia via their α-agonistic activity). Dopamine has weak to moderate α-1 activity and could contribute to minimal increase in $S[K^+]$ if used in high doses.
- ATP-dependent K^+ channels: ATP depletion with exercise opens up more K^+ channels $\rightarrow K^+$ leaves cells $\rightarrow$ local increase in plasma K^+ enhances vasodilatation, hence blood flow and energy delivery to exercising muscles. This effect is impaired with K^+ depletion.
- Plasma K^+ concentration: Passive movement in or out of cells depends on acute plasma K^+ concentration changes.
- Cell lysis: Cellular K^+ release into plasma: tumor lysis, rhabdomyolysis, hemolysis, bowel infarction
- Cell production/anabolism: K^+ uptake for cell production (i.e., red blood cells, platelets) with folic acid or vitamin B_{12} therapy for megaloblastic anemia; refeeding syndrome

Renal potassium handling (Fig. 2.7): K^+ balance depends on K^+ reabsorption and secretion:
- K^+-reabsorption:
  - Proximal tubules: passive reabsorption; follows Na^+ reabsorption

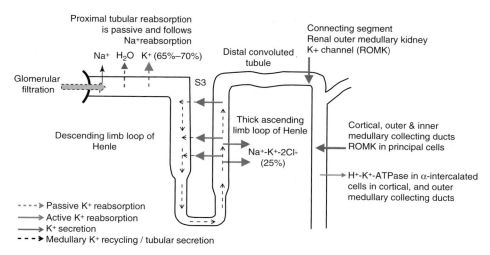

FIGURE 2.7 Renal handling of potassium.

- Thick ascending limb loop of Henle: active reabsorption via Na^+-K^+-$2Cl$
- Cortical and outer medullary collecting ducts α-intercalated cells H^+-K^+-ATPase reabsorbs K^+ in exchange for H^+; Activity of this pump is increased with K^+ depletion and reduced with K^+ loading and facilitated by aldosterone
- K^+ secretion:
  - Medullary K^+ recycling:
    - Reabsorbed medullary K^+ is secreted back into the lumen at the S3 segment of late proximal tubules and descending limb loop of Henle for subsequent reabsorption at thick ascending limb loop of Henle.
    - Maintenance of high medullary K^+ concentration is thought to minimize passive K^+ back-leak
  - Regulated K^+ secretion via the renal outer medullary potassium channel (ROMK) at the connecting and collecting tubules:
    - Efficiency depends on plasma K^+ concentration *and* (1) distal Na^+ delivery, (2) generation of transepithelial potential difference (negative lumen) via Na^+ entry into ENaC in principal cells at aldosterone-sensitive distal nephron segment, (3) distal urine flow (to maintain the favorable electrochemical gradient for K^+ secretion), (4) presence of aldosterone (regulates expression of ENaC, Na^+-K^+-ATPase), (5) sensitivity to aldosterone, and (6) kidney mass.
    - ADH is also thought to increase the number of luminal ROMK channels.

Diagnosis of Potassium Disorders (Dyskalemias)

Common indices used to determine renal versus extrarenal causes of potassium disorders (Table 2.2)

> **NOTE** The first response to a K^+ load is intracellular uptake, a process facilitated by basal levels of catecholamines and insulin. Subsequently, the kidneys will excrete any excess K^+.

Table 2.2	Commonly used urinary indices in the evaluation of potassium disorders					
Hyperkalemia	**Renal Cause**	**Extrarenal Cause**	**Hypokalemia**	**Renal Cause**	**Extrarenal Cause**
Spot [K$^+$] (mEq/L)	<20	>30	Spot [K$^+$] (mEq/L)	>30	<20
Spot [K$^+$]/[Cr] (mEq/g Cr)	<20	>30	Spot [K$^+$]/[Cr] (mEq/g Cr)	>30	<20
24-h urine K$^+$ (mEq/d)	<30	>40	24-h urine K$^+$ (mEq/d)	>40	<30
Transtubular K$^+$ gradient (TTKG)	<3	>7	Transtubular K$^+$ gradient (TTKG)	>7	<3

Note: Transtubular K$^+$ gradient is no longer thought to be valid but may still be useful with clinical judgment. Use of several indices concurrently may improve diagnostic sensitivity and specificity.

HYPERKALEMIA

Clinical Manifestations

- Muscle weakness, cardiac arrhythmias
- ECG changes:
  - Peaked T waves: tall peak (sharp tented) T waves; T wave taller than R wave in ≥2 leads
  - Flattened P waves; Prolonged PR interval
  - Changes associated with high risk of cardiac arrest: widened QRS complex; merging of S and T waves; bradycardia, idioventricular rhythm; sine wave formation; ventricular fibrillation

Causes and Mechanisms of Hyperkalemia

Pseudohyperkalemia

- In vitro (test tube) hyperkalemia, *not* in vivo hyperkalemia
- Correction (treatment) of hyperkalemia is not necessary.
- Common conditions associated with pseudohyperkalemia (Fig. 2.8):
  - Excessive fist clinching with blood draw: exercising (of hand) reduces local ATP and opens up ATP-dependent K$^+$ channels, and allows extracellular K$^+$ shift.
  - Mechanical trauma, hemolysis with blood draw: release of intracellular K$^+$
  - Thrombocytosis, e.g., for every 100,000 platelets/µL, serum K$^+$ can increase by ~0.15 mEq/L because K$^+$ moves out of platelets after clotting has occurred in test tube. Diagnosis: obtain plasma [K$^+$] (i.e., [K$^+$] measured from blood sample collected in heparin-containing tube to avoid clotting process). If serum [K$^+$] (i.e., [K$^+$] measured in usual manner in nonanticoagulated blood) is greater than P[K$^+$] (i.e., S[K$^+$] − P[K$^+$] > 0.3 mEq/L), pseudohyperkalemia is likely present.
  - Pseudohyperkalemia may also be seen with erythrocytosis and leukocytosis, with the following exception:
  - "Reverse" pseudohyperkalemia:
    - Condition where P[K$^+$] > S[K$^+$] (not the usual S[K$^+$] > P[K$^+$] with "regular" pseudohyperkalemia)

Rule out PSEUDOHYPERKALEMIA: Check for good blood draw technique, presence of thrombocytosis, leukocytosis, history of familial pseudohyperkalemia

INCREASED INPUT:
Diet, transfusions, K⁺-containing drugs

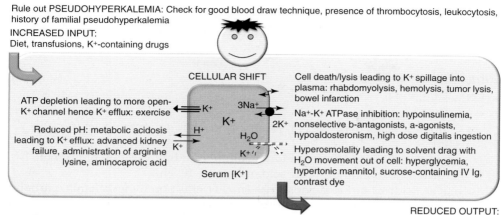

CELLULAR SHIFT

ATP depletion leading to more open-K⁺ channel hence K⁺ efflux: exercise

Reduced pH: metabolic acidosis leading to K⁺ efflux: advanced kidney failure, administration of arginine lysine, aminocaproic acid

Serum [K⁺]

Cell death/lysis leading to K⁺ spillage into plasma: rhabdomyolysis, hemolysis, tumor lysis, bowel infarction

Na⁺-K⁺ ATPase inhibition: hypoinsulinemia, nonselective b-antagonists, a-agonists, hypoaldosteronism, high dose digitalis ingestion

Hyperosmolality leading to solvent drag with H_2O movement out of cell: hyperglycemia, hypertonic mannitol, sucrose-containing IV Ig, contrast dye

REDUCED OUTPUT:
Reduced collecting tubules K⁺ secretion: 1) Low Na⁺ delivery: low effective circulating volume; 2) ENaC inhibition: amiloride, triamterene, trimethoprim, pentamidine; 3a) Hypoaldosteronism: adrenal insufficiency, heparin, ketoconazole, calcineurin inhibitors; 3b) Aldosterone resistance: pseudohypoaldosteronism: type I (aldosterone receptor mutation) and type II (Gordon syndrome); 4) Low urine flow: obstructive uropathy
Advanced kidney disease ± constipation
Isolated reduced K⁺ secretion (due to tubulointerstitial nephritis, lupus nephritis), sickle cell disease

OTHERS:
Succinyl choline administration in patients with conditions associated with increased acetylcholine receptor expression (burn patients, chronic infections/immobilization, neuromuscular disease)
Ureterojejunostomy (increased jejunal K⁺ reabsorption)
Hyperkalemic periodic paralysis

FIGURE 2.8 Summary of causes of hyperkalemia.

- Due to cell fragility and lysis with centrifugation, traumatic blood handling (shuttling pneumatic tube system) – heparin-induced K⁺ leakage from white blood cells
- Reported with chronic lymphocytic leukemia
- To minimize cell lysis, hand-carry specimen to lab immediately following blood draw and avoid heparin-containing tubes
- Benign familial (autosomal dominant) pseudohyperkalemia ± associated stomatocytosis: Passive K⁺ leaks from red blood cells into serum when the blood sample is left at room temperature. This K⁺ leakage does not occur in vivo. Diagnosis: serial S[K⁺] measurements while blood is allowed to cool down to normal temperature leads to increasing S[K⁺] levels.

Increased K⁺ Input

- Dietary: High K⁺-containing foods, salt substitutes (typical salt-substitute contains 10 to 13 mEq KCl/g or 283 mEq of KCl/tablespoon), mixed fruit juice
- K⁺-containing medications: KCl, high-dose penicillin K, K-citrate, polycitrate
- Supplements: fruit/herbal extracts
- Red blood cell transfusion due to K⁺ leakage, particularly problematic with massive transfusions or transfusions of prolonged stored blood

> NOTE   Hyperkalemia from intake is not common except in cases of accidental large quantity ingestion, or moderate ingestion in those with poor kidney function and/or reduced mineralocorticoid activity.

Reduced Bodily K⁺ Loss/Output

- Gastrointestinal: severe, chronic constipation with concurrent poor kidney function
- Kidneys: See Reduced Renal K^+ Loss below.

Extracellular K⁺ Shift

- Extracellular pH:
  - Metabolic acidosis:
    - Inorganic acids (e.g., HCl or sulfuric acid), but not organic acids, cause K^+ shift.
    - Organic acidosis seen with kidney failure or administration of arginine hydrochloride or aminocaproic acid may cause K^+ shift.
    - Lactic acidosis or ketoacidosis has smaller effect on hyperkalemia, partially due to concurrent entry of both anion and hydrogen ion into cells via a sodium-organic anion cotransporter, thus eliminating the need for K^+ shifting out of cells to maintain electroneutrality.
  - Respiratory acidosis:
    - No significant effect on extracellular K^+ shift unless severe and prolonged
    - Mechanisms for difference on K^+ shift compared with metabolic acidosis are not well understood.
  - Extracellular osmolality:
    - Increased osmolality (e.g., hyperglycemia, sucrose containing intravenous immune globulin, radiocontrast media, hypertonic mannitol) leads to extracellular K^+ shift due to:
      - Extracellular H_2O shift with hyperosmolality increases intracellular K^+ concentration, hence greater concentration gradient favoring extracellular shift.
      - Extracellular H_2O shift drags K^+ along: "solvent drag" effect.

> **NOTE** Hyperkalemia is often observed in fasting (e.g., immediate preoperative) blood draws in type 2 diabetic patients. This is thought to be due to the lack of endogenous insulin secretion with fasting, hence reduced insulin-stimulated cellular K^+ uptake as well as hyperglycemia/hyperosmolality-induced hyperkalemia, as described above. To correct this hyperkalemia, administer 5% dextrose (D5) saline solutions $\pm$ insulin depending on degree of hyperglycemia. The administration of D5 alone can induce sufficient endogenous insulin secretion and ameliorate hyperkalemia.

- Therapy with somatostatin or somatostatin agonist (octreotide) can lead to a fall in insulin and hyperkalemia in susceptible individuals.
- Cell death/increased tissue catabolism: e.g., tumor lysis (cytotoxic or radiation therapy), hemolysis, rhabdomyolysis, bowel infarction, soft tissue trauma, severe accidental hypothermia, etc.
- Altered Na^+-K^+-ATPase activity:
  - Reduced insulin
  - Reduced β_2-adrenergic activity reduces cellular K^+ uptake:
    - Digitalis overdose (digoxin, ingestion of common oleander or yellow oleander): inhibition of Na^+-K^+-ATPase
    - β-Antagonists and hyperkalemia: (1) inhibits catecholamine-stimulated renin release, hence aldosterone; (2) most important: inhibits Na^+-K^+-ATPase activity via β_2-inhibition. Nonselective agents, therefore, cause more hyperkalemia compared with β_1-selective antagonists.

- Nonselective β-antagonists: alprenolol, bucindolol, carteolol, carvedilol (+ α-antagonism), labetalol (+ α-antagonism), nadolol, penbutolol, pindolol, propranolol, timolol
  - Selective β_1-antagonists: acebutolol, atenolol, betaxolol, bisoprolol, celiprolol, esmolol, metoprolol, nebivolol
- Exercise-induced hyperkalemia:
  - Delay between K^+ exit from cells during depolarization and subsequent cellular reuptake via Na^+-K^+-ATPase
  - Exercise-induced reduction in ATP reduces ATP-dependent inhibition of K^+-channels, hence more open K^+ channels, and increases K^+ leak extracellularly.
  - Extracellular K^+ shift is thought to be adaptive since higher K^+ concentration has a vasodilatory effect, hence improved blood flow and energy supply to exercising muscles.
  - Exercise-induced hyperkalemia is reversed within a few minutes of rest.
- ATP-dependent K^+ channels: Opening of K^+ channels leads to K^+ efflux.
  - Lack of ATP as seen with exercise
  - Medications: calcineurin inhibitors (cyclosporine, tacrolimus), diazoxide, minoxidil, isoflurane

Others

- Hyperkalemic periodic paralysis:
  - Autosomal dominant, varying penetrance
  - Rare channelopathy involving α_1-subunit of skeletal muscle Na^+ (SCN4A) channels
  - Age of onset: infancy to second decade of life
  - May be associated with prolonged QT interval (Anderson syndrome), malignant hyperthermia, or paramyotonia congenital von Eulenburg (paradoxical myotonia may be prominent feature, which is worsened with activity or aggressive lowering of $S[K^+]$).
  - Episodic weakness or paralysis may be precipitated by rest after activity, changes in daily level of activity especially in cool temperature, K^+ administration
  - Attacks last 10 to 60 minutes, rarely 1 to 2 days; abrupt paralysis onset may result in falls
  - Stiffness may be aborted with walking, high carbohydrates (candy) intake
  - $S[K^+]$ most often normal, may be high (minimally high), or even low during recovery
  - Diagnosis:
    - Compound muscle amplitude test
    - Genetic testing for a *small number* of mutations available
  - Treatment: Diet—high carbohydrates, candy; avoid high K^+-containing foods; consider diuretics (thiazides, loop diuretics), β-agonists such as albuterol.
- Administration of succinylcholine to susceptible patients with conditions where there is upregulation of acetylcholine receptors (e.g., neuromuscular disease, severe trauma, burns, chronic immobilization, or infections). Succinylcholine activation of acetylcholine receptors causes cell depolarization and large K^+ efflux.
- Heparin may cause hyperkalemia by several mechanisms:
  - Inhibition of aldosterone production via reduction in the number and affinity of angiotensin II receptors in zona glomerulosa
  - Inhibition of the final enzymatic steps of aldosterone formation (18-hydroxylation)
  - Adrenal hemorrhage

Reduced Renal K^+ Loss

- Recall renal K+ secretion depends on: (1) distal Na^+ delivery, (2) generation of transepithelial potential difference (negative lumen) via Na^+ entry into ENaC in principal cells at aldosterone-sensitive distal nephron segment, (3) distal urine flow, (4) presence of aldosterone, (5) sensitivity to aldosterone, and (6) kidney mass. See Distal Tubules: Hydrogen and Potassium Secretion and Fig. 2.2.
- Reduced renal K^+ secretion occurs when:
  - Distal Na^+ delivery to cortical and corticomedullary collecting tubules is reduced:
    - Reduced effective circulating volume (heart failure, cirrhosis, volume depletion, etc.), dietary sodium restriction
    - Diagnosis: clinical history, $U[Na^+] < 20$ mEq/L, improved urinary K^+ ($U[K^+]$) excretion with saline infusion
    - Increased proximal Na^+ uptake at distal convoluted tubules, hence reduced Na^+ delivery to the more distal collecting tubules (pseudohypoaldosteronism type 2/Gordon syndrome).
  - Reduced generation of transepithelial potential difference (negative lumen) generated by Na^+ entry into ENaC in principal cells at aldosterone-sensitive distal nephron segment: inhibitors of ENaC—triamterene, amiloride, trimethoprim, pentamidine
  - Compromised urine flow: obstructive uropathy.
  - Lack of aldosterone:
    - Hypoaldosteronism: diabetes mellitus → type 4 RTA, primary adrenal insufficiency
    - Medications: renin angiotensin aldosterone system inhibitors, nonsteroidal anti-inflammatory drugs, COX-2 inhibitors, calcineurin inhibitors, heparin (low molecular weight as well), ketoconazole, drospirenone-containing oral contraceptives (e.g., Yaz, Yasmin): drospirenone has mineralocorticoid antagonist activity
  - Resistance to aldosterone:
    - Medications: aldosterone antagonists (spironolactone, eplerenone)
    - Pseudohypoaldosteronism type 1 (PHA 1)
      - Hyperkalemia associated with metabolic acidosis and salt-wasting
      - Autosomal dominant form (AD PHA1):
        - Aldosterone receptor mutation
        - Treatment: high-dose fludrocortisone, salt support
      - Autosomal recessive form (AR PHA1):
        - Inactivating mutations in α, β, or γ subunits of ENaC; associated with pulmonary infections
        - More severe than AD PHA1
        - Salt-wasting in organs requiring ENaC for salt transport (lungs, kidneys, colon, sweat, salivary glands)
        - High sodium chloride content in sweat and salivary testing
      - Treatment: high salt support; NSAIDS have been reported to be beneficial in AR PHA1
    - Pseudohypoaldosteronism type 2 (Gordon syndrome, a.k.a. familial hyperkalemic hypertension [FHH])
      - Enhanced paracellular Cl^- reabsorption

- Enhanced Na^+ reabsorption via NaCl cotransporter (NCC) in distal convoluted tubules (DCT), leading to reduced Na^+ availability for delivery to cortical collecting tubules (CCT). Reduced Na^+ availability at CCT reduces CCT ability to secrete K^+ and H^+ → hyperkalemia and metabolic acidosis.
  - The increased Na^+ and Cl^- reabsorption leads to volume-expanded state, which suppresses renin angiotensin aldosterone system. Reduced aldosterone also contributes to hyperkalemia and metabolic acidosis.
  - Clinical manifestations: hypertension in early adulthood, non-AG metabolic acidosis and hyperkalemia, hypercalciuria, osteoporosis, nephrolithiasis
  - Reported NCC regulatory molecules with mutations leading to FHH: with-no-lysine (WNK) 1-4 (inactivating mutations of WNK4 or activating mutations of WNK1), Kelch-Like 3 (KLHL3), and Cullin 3 (CUL3). Mutations in WNK4 also downregulate the transient receptor potential V5 channel (TRPV5, calcium channel) and decrease Ca^{2+} reabsorption in DCT, thus hypercalciuria and osteoporosis. (See Hypertension)
  - Treatment: thiazide diuretics
  - Kidney mass/function is reduced:
    - Reduced overall capacity for renal K^+ secretion
    - Reduced Na^+-K^+-ATPase activity with uremia, thus reduced cellular uptake

Others

- Ureterojejunostomy: increased absorption of urinary K^+ by jejunum
- Selective impairment of K^+ secretion of unclear mechanisms: interstitial disease—lupus nephritis, sickle cell disease

> **NOTE**   Common clinical scenarios with multiple reasons for hyperkalemia:
> - Diabetic patient: (1) neurogenic bladder leading to urinary stasis; (2) low aldosterone state due to reduced sympathetic stimulation for renin release, adrenal atrophy, and use of renin angiotensin aldosterone inhibitors; and (3) insulin deficiency leading to reduced cellular K^+ uptake via Na^+-K^+-ATPase, hyperosmolality from hyperglycemia leading to cellular K^+ efflux, metabolic acidosis with diabetic ketoacidosis leading to K^+ efflux, and hypovolemia leading to reduced Na^+ delivery to collecting tubules
> - Patient with cirrhosis or heart failure: (1) use of spironolactone, (2) low effective circulating volume leading to poor Na^+ delivery to collecting tubules, and (3) recurrent kidney injuries

Management of Hyperkalemia: Temporizing Measures

- For patients with relatively good kidney function and nonthreatening ECG changes, consider volume resuscitation with normal saline and administration of loop diuretics.
- For severe hyperkalemia with high-risk ECG changes and kidney failure, emergent hemodialysis is indicated.
- Consider nutritional consult for low-K^+ diet if applicable.
- Good bowel regimen and other emergent measures (Table 2.3)

Table 2.3   Treatment of hyperkalemia

Therapeutic Options		Dose	Onset	Duration	Caution
Stabilize cardiac membrane potential.	Calcium chloride (or three times of suggested dose if calcium gluconate is used)	10 mL of 10% of $CaCl_2$ given intravenously over 10 min NOTE: 1 ampule of calcium chloride = 3 ampules of calcium gluconate in terms of elemental calcium.	1–3 min	0.5–1 h	Irritating; do not give calcium in HCO_3 line; avoid in digoxin toxicity (risk and benefit unclear)
Increase intracellular shift.	Insulin *plus* glucose	10 units *plus* glucose supplement if serum level < 250 mg/dL (25 g glucose [50 mL of dextrose 50%] +/– 10% dextrose continuous infusions)	15–30 min	4–6 h	Hypoglycemia in advanced CKD
	Albuterol	10–20 mg nebulizer	15–30 min	4–6 h	Risk of tachycardia, precipitation of myocardial infarction
	$NaHCO_3$	1 mEq/kg (if pH < 7.2 or advanced CKD—$NaHCO_3$ is not effective if patient is not acidotic)	15–30 min	Prolonged	Do not give in calcium line; avoid if high $CaxPO_4$ product or volume overload
Increase excretion.	Gastrointestines: Sodium polystyrene sulfonate	Sodium polystyrene sulfonate: 30 g oral or per rectum × up to q.i.d. ± laxative (20% sorbitol) if oral	Variable; hours	4–6 h	Risk of colonic ischemia; contraindicated in bowel obstruction or ileus, postanesthesia
	Patiromer	8.4 g/d with food, titrate weekly as needed up to 24.2 g/d	Variable	Variable	Avoid taking any other medication within 6 h of taking patiromer; may bind magnesium and cause hypomagnesemia
	Kidneys: Volume re-expansion as needed; diuretics (loop and or thiazides); fludrocortisone in hypoaldosteronism	Titration per clinician discretion	Variable	Variable	Per selected therapy and response

HYPOKALEMIA

Clinical Manifestations

- Muscle weakness, rhabdomyolysis, fatigue, ileus, constipation, leg cramps, respiratory difficulty
- ECG changes: U waves, T-wave flattening, ST-segment depression, arrhythmias, asystole
- Nephrogenic diabetes insipidus, hypokalemic nephropathy
- 40% of patients with hypokalemia also have hypomagnesemia: possible mechanisms:
  - Underlying abnormality/pathology can cause both (e.g., cisplatin, amphotericin, diuretics use, poor dietary intake, diarrhea)
  - Mg^{2+} is a gate-keeper for ROMK. Low Mg^{2+} level leaves ROMK open, thus K^+ wasting
  - Mg^{2+} is a cofactor in Na^+-K^+-ATPase, H^+-K^+-ATPase
  - Enhanced aldosterone state leading to renal wasting of both cations.

Causes and Mechanisms of Hypokalemia

Pseudohypokalemia

- In vitro (test tube) hypokalemia, *not* in vivo hypokalemia
- Pseudohypokalemia may be seen in patients with acute (or chronic) myeloid leukemia due to continuing cellular K^+ uptake into rapidly proliferating cells even after the blood is drawn. There may be associated pseudohypoglycemia and hypophosphatemia.
- Seasonal pseudohypokalemia: due to increased intracellular K^+ uptake via increased Na^+-K^+-ATPase activity with transport of blood tubes in warm ambient temperatures (Fig. 2.9)

Decreased K^+ Input

- Inadequate dietary intake, severe malnutrition (rare due to kidneys' ability to minimize K^+ loss to 5 to 20 mEq/L)
- Clay ingestion "geophagia." Clay binds K^+.

Increased Bodily K^+ Loss/Output

- Gastrointestinal loss: severe diarrhea, vomiting[3]/nasogastric suction, bowel cleansing (phenolphthalein laxatives, sodium polystyrene sulfonate), acute colonic obstruction, Ogilvie syndrome (acute colonic pseudo-obstruction associated with a secretory diarrhea with very high K^+ content due to activation of colonic K^+ secretion. This condition is associated with various acute illnesses/stressors. Associated electrolyte abnormalities include hypokalemia, hypomagnesemia, and hypocalcemia).
- Excessive sweats, extensive burns
- Dialysis, plasmapheresis
- Urinary loss: See "Increased Renal K^+ Loss" below.

---

[3]Hypokalemia associated with vomiting predominantly occurs via renal K^+ loss due to volume depletion-induced hyperrenin, hyperaldosteronism, and bicarbonaturia. Gastric fluid [K^+] is only 5 to 20 mEq/L. Diarrhea [K^+] is higher at 10 to 40 mEq/L, and up to >100 mEq/L in colonic fluid in Ogilvie syndrome.

Rule out PSEUDOHYPOKALEMIA: Check for leukocytosis from acute myeloid leukemia

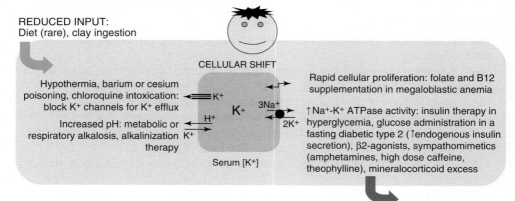

REDUCED INPUT:
Diet (rare), clay ingestion

CELLULAR SHIFT

Hypothermia, barium or cesium poisoning, chloroquine intoxication: block K⁺ channels for K⁺ efflux

Increased pH: metabolic or respiratory alkalosis, alkalinization therapy

Serum [K⁺]

Rapid cellular proliferation: folate and B12 supplementation in megaloblastic anemia

↑Na⁺-K⁺ ATPase activity: insulin therapy in hyperglycemia, glucose administration in a fasting diabetic type 2 (↑endogenous insulin secretion), β2-agonists, sympathomimetics (amphetamines, high dose caffeine, theophylline), mineralocorticoid excess

INCREASED OUTPUT:
Increased K⁺ secretion at collecting tubules: 1) High Na⁺ delivery: high fluid intake/infusion, diuretics, Bartter, Gitelman, nonreabsorbable anions (penicillins, bicarbonate, β-hydroxybutyrate, hippurate); 2) Increased ENaC activity: Liddle syndrome; 3) Mineralocorticoid excess; 4) High urine flow: high fluid intake, diuretics, hypercalcemia

OTHERS:
Hypomagnesemia: multifactorial. See text
Amphotericin B: self-insertion into tubular membranes and acting as ionophores allowing intracellular electrolyte leakage into tubular lumen and H⁺ back-leak from urine into tubular cells and circulation. Salt-wasting nephropathies, tubulointerstitial diseases, tubular injuries: cisplatin, aminoglycosides, acute monocytic or myelomonocytic leukemia with lysozyme induced tubular injury leading to K⁺ wasting. Hypercalcemia (blocks ROMK in thick ascending limb of loop of Henle and induces diabetes insipidus)

FIGURE 2.9 Summary of causes of hypokalemia.

Intracellular K⁺ Shift Due to Increased Extracellular pH

- Increased extracellular pH (e.g., metabolic or respiratory alkalosis) leads to K⁺ shifting into cells in exchange for H⁺ efflux to reduce the extracellular pH.

> **NOTE**   In patients with severe hypokalemia and metabolic acidosis (e.g., patient with proximal RTA), replace K⁺ to safe level *prior* to alkalinization!!!

- Increased Na⁺-K⁺-ATPase activity:
  - Insulin administration or endogenous insulin release with glucose administration (e.g., dextrose 5% saline solution)

> **NOTE**   In diabetic patients with poorly controlled glucose and preexisting life-threatening hypokalemia, provide K⁺ replacement prior to insulin administration to avoid further fall in preexisting low S[K⁺]!!!

- Increased β₂-adrenergic activity increases cellular K⁺ uptake: stress, coronary ischemia, delirium tremens, thyroid hormone, β₂-agonists (albuterol, terbutaline, dopamine, dobutamine, pseudoephedrine), sympathomimetic stimulants (e.g., amphetamines, high-dose caffeine), theophylline toxicity.
- Inhibition of ATP-dependent K⁺ channels blocks K⁺ efflux during repolarization: hypothermia, barium/cesium poisoning, chloroquine intoxication.

Others

- Hypokalemic periodic paralysis:
  - Rare channelopathy (autosomal dominant, varying penetrance):
  - 90% with mutation of the α_1-subunit of dihydropyridine-sensitive Ca^{2+} channel; 10% with mutation of the skeletal muscle Na^+ (SCN4A) channel
  - Muscle weakness or paralysis in association with a fall in $S[K^+]$
    - Upper > lower extremity; proximal > distal weakness
    - May be associated with hypophosphatemia and hypomagnesemia
  - Attacks often begin in adolescence
  - Triggered by strenuous exercise followed by rest; high-carbohydrate and high-sodium meals or administration of glucose, insulin, or glucocorticoids; sudden changes in temperature, excitement, loud noise, or flashlights
  - Associated conditions:
    - Andersen syndrome: periodic paralysis occurring with either hypo- or hyperkalemia; associated with prolonged QT and sudden death
    - Thyrotoxicosis due to Graves disease: more common in Asian or Latin/Native American males (propranolol may reverse attacks pending definitive therapy). Of note, patients with thyrotoxicosis hypokalemia periodic paralysis may also have elevated bone alkaline phosphatase for unclear reason.
  - Diagnosis: Electromyograms during attacks or with exercise
  - Treatment:
    - Potassium supplement (slow and low dose due to rebound)
      - If can swallow and breathe adequately: oral KCl, K-citrate, or K-bicarbonate 15 to 30 mEq in 30- to 60-minute intervals as needed.
      - If cannot swallow and life-threatening: KCl 15 mEq over 15 minutes, then 10 mEq/h in 500 mL dilutant; 5% mannitol dilutant is preferred over normal saline (sodium may worsen condition). Never use glucose (due to endogenous insulin secretion and exacerbation of hypokalemia).
    - Cardiac monitoring is required with intravenous KCl administration.
    - Prevention: β_2-blockers, K^+ supplement, low carbohydrate diet, K^+-sparing diuretics, CA inhibitor (acetazolamide)

Increased Renal K+ Loss

- Recall renal K^+ secretion depends on: (1) distal Na^+ delivery, (2) generation of transepithelial potential difference (negative lumen) via Na^+ entry into ENaC in principal cells at aldosterone-sensitive distal nephron segment, (3) distal urine flow, (4) presence of aldosterone, (5) sensitivity to aldosterone, and (6) kidney mass
- Enhanced renal K^+ secretion occurs with:
  - Increased distal Na^+ delivery to cortical and corticomedullary collecting tubules:
    - Diuretics, high fluid intake/intravenous fluid infusion
    - Bartter and Gitelman syndromes
  - Generation of transepithelial potential difference (negative lumen) via Na^+ entry into ENaC in principal cells at aldosterone-sensitive distal nephron segment is increased:
    - Liddle syndrome
      - Autosomal dominant, gain-of-function mutation in the β- and γ-subunits of ENaC (PY motif) that reduces the "housekeeping" recognition of ENaC by Nedd4-2 for internalization and degradation, resulting in an increased number of functioning apical ENaC.

- Affected patients present with HTN due to excess Na^+ retention; hyporenin, hypoaldosteronism due to volume expansion; but hypokalemia and metabolic alkalosis due to facilitated renal K^+ and H^+ secretion following increased Na^+ entry into the undegraded apical ENaC.
    - Treatment: ENaC inhibition with amiloride. Since this is an end-organ defect, kidney transplantation is curative.
  - Nonreabsorbable anions delivery to collecting tubules can enhance K^+ secretion due to the favorable electrical gradient. Additionally, the increased Na^+ delivery associated with the anions will also enhance the generation of the favorable electrochemical gradient for K^+ secretion. Examples of nonreabsorbable anions: bicarbonate (vomiting and proximal RTA), β-hydroxybutyrate in diabetic ketoacidosis, high-dose penicillin/penicillin derivative administration, hippurate from toluene with glue sniffing.
- High distal urine flow: high volume intake/infusion, diuretics
- Increased mineralocorticoid activity (Fig. 2.10)
  - Clinical manifestations: classically seen with triad of hypertension, hypokalemia, and metabolic alkalosis
  - Mineralocorticoid excess may be categorized as aldosterone dependent, cortisol dependent, or non-aldosterone, non-cortisol dependent
  - Aldosterone dependent:
    - Secondary aldosteronism:
      - High renin level leads to aldosterone synthesis.
      - Source of renin: hypoxia-induced (renovascular hypertension) or unregulated synthesis (renin-secreting tumors)
    - Primary aldosteronism:
      - Aldosterone synthesis is independent of renin levels.

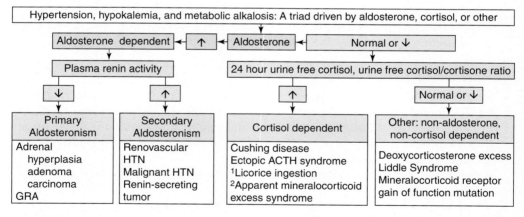

FIGURE 2.10 Evaluation of mineralocorticoid excess in patients with the triad of hypertension, hypokalemia, and metabolic alkalosis.

HTN, Hypertension; GRA, Glucocorticoid-remediable aldosteronism; ACTH, Adrenocorticotropin hormone.

[1]Glycyrrhizic acid and its hydrolytic product glycyrrhetinic acid from licorice are potent competitive inhibitors of 11 β-hydroxysteroid dehydrogenase, the enzyme required to metabolize cortisol to its inactive form, cortisone.

[2]Apparent mineralocorticoid excess: mutation of 11 β-hydroxysteroid dehydrogenase enzyme

- Sources of aldosterone: adrenal hyperplasia, adenoma, or carcinoma, glucocorticoid-remediable aldosteronism
- Glucocorticoid-remediable aldosteronism:
  - Autosomal dominant with formation of a chimeric gene due to unequal crossover of sequences at meiosis, where the hybrid gene contains both the promoter of 11-β-hydroxylase enzyme (enzyme for cortisol synthesis) and aldosterone synthase gene (enzyme for aldosterone synthesis)
  - Stimulation of the promoter with ACTH upregulates both cortisol and aldosterone synthesis. Recall that aldosterone is normally upregulated by angiotensin II.
  - Clinical manifestations: early moderate to severe HTN, hemorrhagic stroke and ruptured aneurysms (brain MRA every 5 years after puberty has been recommended), normo- to hypokalemia (the former due to the diurnal variation of ACTH).
  - Diagnosis: genetic testing for crossover between aldosterone-synthetase and 11-β-hydroxylase; biochemical evaluation: suppressed plasma renin activity and high serum aldosterone, increased levels of 18-hydroxy-cortisol, ACTH and 18-oxo-cortisol.
  - Treatment: glucocorticoid (to suppress ACTH) or mineralocorticoid receptor antagonism (spironolactone, eplerenone) ± ENaC antagonism (amiloride) to counteract the effect of excess aldosterone.
- Cortisol dependent: (cortisol has mineralocorticoid activity)
  - Sources of cortisol: excess production (Cushing's); reduced inactivation of cortisol to cortisone by the enzyme 11-β-hydroxysteroid dehydrogenase type 2 11-βHSD2).
  - Reduced 11-β-hydroxysteroid dehydrogenase activity:
    - Licorice: glycyrrhizic acid and its hydrolytic product, glycyrrhetinic acid, from licorice are potent competitive inhibitors of 11-βHSD2.
    - Mutation of 11-βHSD2: Syndrome of apparent mineralocorticoid excess (AME)
- Non-aldosterone, non-cortisol dependent:
  - Liddle syndrome (see above)
  - Deoxycorticosteroid excess (associated with congenital adrenal hyperplasia)
  - Activating mutation of mineralocorticoid receptor (MR):
    - Autosomal dominant disorder where the MR is constitutively activated
    - Hypertension may worsen with pregnancy due to progesterone
    - Spironolactone (normally an MR antagonist) now acts as an agonist!

Others

- Amphotericin B: This is a multiplanar molecule that is lipophilic on the outside and hydrophilic on the inside. The molecule inserts itself into tubular cell membrane and acts as an ionophore, allowing electrolytes to flow in the direction of favorable chemical gradient. The formulation of liposomal amphotericin covers up the lipophilic surface of amphotericin and reduces its insertion into tubular membranes, thus minimizing intracellular electrolyte losses into the urinary space and back-leak of H^+ into circulation (Fig. 2.11).

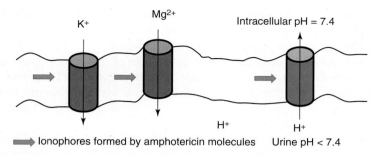

K+

Mg²⁺

Intracellular pH = 7.4

H⁺   H⁺

➡ Ionophores formed by amphotericin molecules   Urine pH < 7.4

FIGURE 2.11 Amphotericin: metabolic acidosis and electrolyte wasting. Intracellular concentrations of K^+ and Mg^{2+} are much higher than those in the urine, thus favoring K^+ and Mg^{2+} leakage/wasting into the urine. Urine concentration of H^+, however, is much greater than that intracellularly, thus favoring H^+ "back-leak" and development of metabolic acidosis. The aim of "liposomal" amphotericin is to minimize insertion of the molecule into tubular membranes.

- Magnesium deficiency can lead to K^+ wasting at the thick ascending limb of loop of Henle. Mg^{2+} is a "gate-keeper" against K^+ exit via ROMK into the lumen.
- Salt-wasting nephropathies, tubular injuries (tubulointerstitial diseases, cisplatin, aminoglycosides), acute monocytic or myelomonocytic leukemia with lysozyme-induced tubular injury leading to K^+ wasting)
- Hypercalcemia (inhibits ROMK in thick ascending limb of loop of Henle and induces a form of nephrogenic diabetes insipidus)

Management of Hypokalemia: Routine Considerations
- If S[K+] < 3 mEq/L, STAT ECG, cardiac monitor
- If safe, avoid glucose-containing solutions until *life-threatening* hypokalemia has been corrected.
- If safe, avoid correction of hyperglycemia with insulin administration until *life-threatening* hypokalemia has been corrected.
- If safe, avoid alkalinization until *life-threatening* hypokalemia has been corrected.
- Use central lines if >10 mEq/h replacement is needed.
- Consider femoral line over internal jugular or subclavian line if >20 mEq/h replacement is needed to avoid cardiac irritation.
- Check magnesium levels and replace as necessary.

BARTTER VERSUS GITELMAN SYNDROMES

Think furosemide (Bartter) versus thiazides (Gitelman). As these syndromes are equivalent to taking diuretics, they can induce salt loss and relative volume depletion, hence "compensatory" hyperrenin hyperaldosteronism without associated hypertension. As mutations of Bartter syndromes can lead to greater salt-wasting compared with Gitelman, hyperrenin and hyperaldosteronism are more marked in the former. Increased vasodilating prostaglandin E2 production is also thought to play a role in maintaining normotension in Bartter syndromes. Similar to taking diuretics, both Bartter and Gitelman syndromes are associated with hypokalemia and metabolic alkalosis.

Mutations in Bartter Syndromes
- Neonatal Bartter syndromes: types I (NKCC2) and II (ROMK—renal outer medullary K^+ channel)

- Classic Bartter syndrome: type III (ClC-Kb)
- Bartter syndrome and sensorineural deafness (BSND): type IV Bartter (β-subunit of ClC-Ka and ClC-Kb); ClC-Ka is present in inner ear.
- Calcium-sensing receptor (CaSR) gain-of-function mutation (inhibits ROMK): type V Bartter, associated with autosomal dominant hypocalcemia. Activation of CaSR inhibits ROMK activity (Fig. 2.12).

> **NOTE** K^+ recycling back into the lumen via ROMK creates a positively charged lumen which facilitates divalent cation (Ca^{2+}, Mg^{2+}) reabsorption paracellularly. This process is facilitated by tight junction proteins claudin 16 and 19. Any transporter defect leading to suboptimal K^+ recycling (e.g. loss of function mutation of ROMK or gain of function mutation of CaSR) or mutation of claudin 16/19 induces Ca^{2+} and Mg^{2+} wasting (Fig. 2.12).

Mutation in Gitelman Syndrome Mutation of NCC a.k.a. TSC Fig. 2.13.

Clinical Manifestations of Bartter and Gitelman Syndromes

See Table 2.4.

> **NOTE**   CLC-Kb is present in both loop of henle and distal convoluted tubule. This may explain minimal or absence of nephrocalcinosis in classic Bartter and BSND, respectively.

> **NOTE**   Hypomagnesemia is a prominent feature with Gitelman, but not typical with bartter syndromes. Reasons are not clear but suggested below:
> - There are apoptotic and/or histologic changes in DCT in patients with Gitelman that could affect DCT Mg^{2+} reabsorption, but not in patients with Bartter syndrome. These changes are thought to occur later than other electrolyte changes, hence the absence of hypomagnesemia observed in early disease.
> - Compensatory DCT Mg^{2+} reabsorption with loop Mg^{2+} wasting

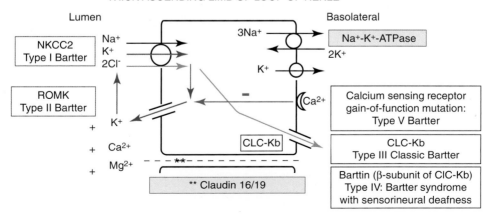

FIGURE 2.12 Transport mutation in Bartter syndrome.

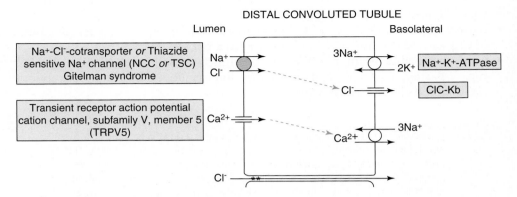

FIGURE 2.13 Transport mutations in Gitelman syndrome.

Table 2.4	Clinical manifestations of Bartter and Gitelman syndromes			
	Neonatal Bartter (I, II)	**Classic Bartter (III)**	**BSND Bartter (IV)**	**Gitelman**
Age at presentation	Prenatal	Childhood	Prenatal	Early adult
Polyhydramnios				
Growth retardation	+	±	+	−
Delayed cognitive development, dysmorphia				
Polyuria, volume depletion	+	+	+	±
Concentrating ability	+	+	+	−
Muscle weakness, cramps, tetany	−	−	−	±
Chondrocalcinosis	−	−	−	±
Nephrocalcinosis	+	±	−	−
Sensorineural deafness	−	−	+	−
Laboratory Findings				
Serum Mg^{2+}	Low to normal	↓ in 20%	Normal	↓ in 100% Normal in early disease
Urinary Ca^{2+}	↑↑↑	=/↑	Normal	↓ majority
Urinary prostaglandin E_2	↓↓↓	↑	↑↑↑	Normal

Gain of function mutation of CaSR is associated with hypocalcemia, hypercalciuria, hypoparathyroidism, and varying degree of Bartter-like syndrome (Bartter type V).

Management of Bartter and Gitelman Syndromes

- Potassium and magnesium supplement as needed
- Consider renin angiotensin aldosterone inibitors

Access the eBook for self-assessment questions.

Calcium, Phosphorus, Magnesium, and Kidney Stones

Phuong-Chi T. Pham, Monica S. Deshmukh, and Phuong-Truc T. Pham

DISORDERS OF CALCIUM METABOLISM

Calcium Background

- Calcium is mostly bound and associated with bones (~99% of total body calcium, ~1 kg)
- Extracellular calcium concentration range: 9.0 to 10.6 mg/dL
  - 40% to 50% is protein bound (mostly albumin). Corrected total serum calcium concentration (SCa) for patients with hypoalbuminemia may be estimated as:

Measured SCa (mg/dL) + 0.8 × (4.0 − serum albumin concentration (g/dL))

  - 55% is diffusible (ultrafilterable)
    - 40% to 50% exists as free ionized calcium
    - 10% is complexed (e.g., to bicarbonate, citrate, phosphate anions)
- Intracellular calcium concentration is minute at approximately 100 nmol/L, but may increase up to 10- to 100-fold during various cellular functions.
- Physiologic roles of calcium: skeletal composition, neuromuscular excitation, cardiac and muscle contractility/function

Calcium Metabolism

- Gastrointestinal (GI) (Fig. 3.1):
  - Dietary calcium intake is approximately 1 g/d. Twenty percent is absorbed by the GI tract.
    - *Paracellular* absorption does not depend on vitamin D, but the favorable intraluminal gradient at the jejunum and ileum when calcium intake is high.
    - *Transcellular* absorption occurs primarily in the duodenum when calcium intake is low:
      - Apical uptake by enterocytes is via the transient receptor potential TRPV6 calcium channel.

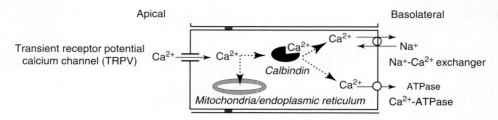

FIGURE 3.1 Epithelial calcium transport is similar in both enterocytes and renal distal tubules. In enterocytes, the responsible calcium channel is TRPV6. In renal distal tubules, the channel is TRPV5.

- Cytoplasmic Ca^{2+} is taken up into mitochondria or endoplasmic reticulum, or transported into the basolateral side via Ca^{2+}-ATPase, or in the presence of high intracytoplasmic Ca^{2+} concentration, via the Na^+-Ca^{2+} exchanger.
  - Calbindin D_{9k} mediates Ca^{2+} transport across enterocytes into circulation.
- Hormonal regulations of GI absorption:
  - Calcitriol (1,25 vitamin D): 1,25 vitamin D binds to its receptor (VDR) to increase TRPV6 expression, calbindin D9k, and Ca^{2+}-ATPase, all acting in concert to increase Ca^{2+} absorption.
  - Other hormones that may contribute to increased GI absorption of calcium: estrogens, prolactin, growth hormone, parathyroid hormone (PTH)
- Intestinal Ca^{2+} absorption may be
  - Increased in acromegaly and excess vitamin D ingestion
  - Decreased in patients whose diet has low Ca^{2+}/PO_4^{2-} ratio, high vegetable fiber, or high fat content, older patients, patients with estrogen deficiency, corticosteroid use, or various medical conditions including diabetes, kidney failure, gastrectomy/bowel malabsorption.
- Renal handling (Fig. 3.2):
  - Glomerular filtration: 8 to 10 g/d
    - Ultrafilterable Ca^{2+} load is determined by glomerular filtration rate (GFR), glomerular surface, ultrafiltration coefficient K_f, and ultrafilterable calcium load. PTH reduces K_f.

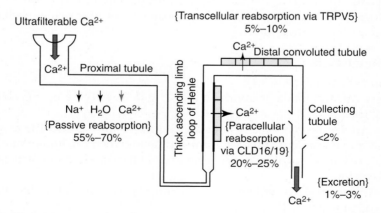

FIGURE 3.2 Renal handling of calcium. Ultrafilterable Ca^{2+} load is determined by glomerular filtration rate, glomerular surface, PTH-regulated ultrafiltration coefficient, acid–base status.

- Respiratory and metabolic acidosis increase plasma ionized Ca^{2+}, hence increased ultrafilterable Ca^{2+} load and wasting.
  - Metabolic acidosis enhances bone release of Ca^{2+}, hence increased ultrafilterable Ca^{2+} load and wasting.
- Proximal tubules: Ca^{2+} is absorbed via convection (parallels Na^+ and water absorption). Any osmotic diuretic agent, for example, mannitol, reduces Ca^{2+} reabsorption.
- Thick ascending limb of Henle loop: paracellular reabsorption, facilitated by claudin 16/19 and positive tubular lumen (created by K^+ recycling via ROMK)
  - PTH enhances paracellular reabsorption.
  - Activation of calcium-sensing receptors (CaSR) by high extracellular Ca^{2+} or calcimimetics inhibits ROMK, hence reduced intraluminal K^+ recycling and the associated positively charged lumen that drives paracellular Ca^{2+} reabsorption.
  - Loop diuretics reduce paracellular Ca^{2+} reabsorption due to reduced NKCC activity and subsequent ROMK activity. Downstream effect is similar to above.
- Distal tubules: luminal uptake is via the apical TRPV5 calcium channel, followed by reabsorption into the basolateral side via Ca^{2+}-ATPase and Na^+-Ca^{2+} exchanger.
  - Both PTH and calcitriol increase distal calcium reabsorption.
  - Thiazides and amiloride increase Ca^{2+} reabsorption in distal tubules.
- Despite the high amount of glomerular filtration of calcium, daily urinary excretion is minimal, <0.3 g/d, due to its effective reabsorption along the entire nephron.

Calcium Regulation

Vitamin D Metabolism

- UV light (skin exposure) converts 7-dehydrocholesterol to *cholecaliferol* (Fig. 3.3).
- Liver hydroxylates cholecalciferol at the 25 carbon position to *25-OH vitamin D.*
- Kidney hydroxylates 25-OH vitamin D (via 1α-hydroxylase) to *1,25 (OH)$_2$ vitamin D.* This is the most biologically active form of vitamin D.
- 24-hydroxylation of 1,25 or 25 vitamin D (by 24-hydroxylase) to 1,24,25 or 24,25 vitamin D respectively renders the vitamin D inactive.
  - Overactivity of 24-hydroxylase leads to 1,25 vitamin D deficiency.
  - Underactivity of 24-hydroxylase (e.g., loss of function mutation of the enzyme) leads to 1,25 vitamin D excess.
  - Regulation of vitamin D-24-hydroxylase
    - PTH decreases 24-hydroxylase activity.
    - Vitamin D receptor (VDR) agonist (VDRA) (e.g., 1,25 vitamin D) increases 24-hydroxylase activity.
    - The fibroblast growth factor-23 (FGF-23) increases 24-hydroxylase activity while decreasing1α-hydroxylase activity. The former results in increased inactivation of 1,25-vitamin D while the latter leads to lower 1,25-vitamin D formation.

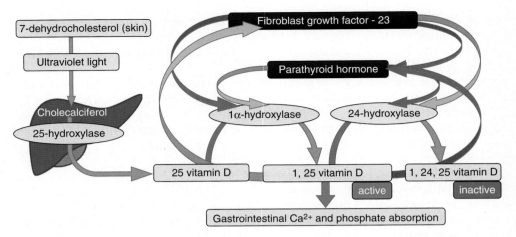

FIGURE 3.3 Regulation of vitamin D metabolism. Green arrows indicate stimulatory and red arrows indicate inhibitory effects. Blue arrows indicate the ultraviolet light conversion of 7-dehydrocholesterol to cholecalciferol and other major enzymatic steps involved in vitamin D metabolism.

- Of note, 1,25 vitamin D synthesis increases during puberty, pregnancy, and lactation.
- Physiologic effects of 1,25 vitamin D:
  - Increases GI absorption of calcium and phosphate
  - Stimulates FGF-23 and 24-hydroxylase
  - Provides negative feedback on PTH via
    - Reducing *PTH* gene transcription
    - Increasing VDR and CaSR expressions on parathyroid cells
    - Reducing parathyroid cell proliferation
  - Maintains healthy bone formation and mineral homeostasis

Parathyroid Hormone

- Primary function is to increase ionized calcium level in response to hypocalcemia (Fig. 3.4).
  - Increases 1,25 vitamin D:
    - Stimulates 1-α hydroxylase
    - Inhibits 24-hydroxylase
  - Increases calcium reabsorption at distal tubules
- Phosphaturic effect: PTH induces phosphaturia.

Fibroblast Growth Factor-23 (FGF-23)

- FGF-23 is a peptide produced by osteocytes and osteoblasts.
- Induces phosphaturia by suppressing *NPT2a* and *NPT2b* (genes encoding two different sodium phosphate transporters in renal proximal tubules)
- Reduces 1,25 vitamin D activity via inhibition of 1α-hydroxylase and stimulation of 24-hydroxylase activity
- Inhibits PTH
- FGF-23 expression is upregulated by increased phosphate "burden" (not necessarily actual hyperphosphatemia) and 1,25 vitamin D.

> **NOTE** In chronic kidney disease (CKD), FGF-23 level increases before PTH.

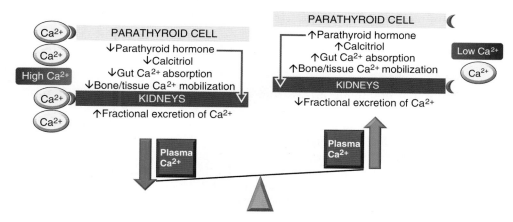

FIGURE 3.4 Calcium regulation: Plasma ionized Ca^{2+} levels are sensed by calcium-sensing receptors present in both kidneys and parathyroid glands, both of which act to maintain Ca^{2+} balance.

Calcium Intake and Outcomes: "Too Much of a Good Thing May Be Bad. . ."

- Recent prospective longitudinal cohort study revealed that women with *dietary calcium intake > 1400 mg/d* had increased rate of all-cause-mortality, hazard ratio (HR) 1.4, and increased rate of cardiovascular disease, HR 1.49. All-cause-mortality HR increases to 2.57 if these women also took calcium supplements.
- Recent short-term studies revealed that patients with CKD stage 3 or 4 can develop positive calcium balance when consuming dietary calcium ≥ 2,000 mg/d or receiving calcium carbonate supplement ≥ 1,500 mg daily.

HYPERCALCEMIA

Causes of Hypercalcemia

- Ingestions:
  - Calcium-containing products (calcium carbonate "TUMS," → "milk-alkali syndrome," Nicorette gum, calcium-supplemented bottled carbonated water, etc.)
  - Excessive vitamin D (recent report of over-the-counter vitamin supplement "Soladek" containing high dose of both vitamins D and A)
- Malignancy:
  - Direct invasion (bone metastatic disease)
  - Osteoclastic activating factors: PTH-related peptides, calcitriol, transforming growth factors, prostaglandin E (PGE), tumor necrosis factor α, PTH (parathyroid malignancy)
  - Immobilization due to pain, deconditioning (increased bone resorption)
- Primary hyperparathyroidism (hPTH):
  - Parathyroid adenoma (80%), diffuse hyperplasia (10% to 15%) or carcinoma (5%)
  - Multiple endocrine neoplasia type 1 (MEN-1):

- Autosomal dominant, arises from inactivating germ line mutations of a tumor-suppressor gene (*MEN-1* gene)
  - May involve parathyroid, anterior pituitary, enteropancreatic, and other endocrine tumors
- MEN-2A:
  - Autosomal dominant, arises from activating mutations of the *RET* proto-oncogene.
  - May involve thyroid medulla, adrenal medulla, parathyroid with associated increase in calcitonin, catecholamines, and PTH, respectively.
- Latent primary hPTH (diagnosis of exclusion):
  - May present as either normocalcemic hPTH (normal SCa, high PTH level) or normoparathyroid hypercalcemia (normal PTH level, high SCa)
  - High likelihood for eventual development of overt hPTH. Close monitoring recommended.
- Granulomatous diseases (e.g., tuberculosis, sarcoid, berylliosis):
  - Due to increased 1α-hydroxylase activity in macrophages within granulomas
  - Sarcoid may increase plasma Ca^{2+} further with high sun exposure
  - Laboratory findings: low PTH, high 1,25 vitamin D
- Medications: lithium (may lead to hPTH), thiazide diuretics, antacids (calcium carbonate—patients present with both hypercalcemia and metabolic alkalosis), vitamin A overload (due to increased bone resorption)
- Familial Hypocalciuric Hypercalcemia (FHH):
  - Rare autosomal-dominant hereditary condition due to inactivating mutations of the gene encoding CaSR. Recall that normally CaSR senses hypercalcemia and inhibits ROMK in the thick ascending limb of Henle loop, which leads to the loss of the favorable positive luminal charge necessary for paracellular calcium reabsorption. Thus, normal activation of CaSR induces calciuria. In contrast, inactivating mutations of CaSR cannot sense the presence of ionized calcium/hypercalcemia to induce facilitated calciuria.
  - Laboratory findings:
    - Moderate chronic hypercalcemia, normo- to hypophosphatemia, hypermagnesemia
    - Plasma PTH is normal to moderately high - thus association with hypophosphatemia (this is why FHH may be mistaken for primary hPTH). (Normal CaSR activity inhibits PTH secretion. Inactivating mutation of CaSR leads to uninhibited PTH secretion.)
    - 1,25 vitamin D level may be high in response to elevated PTH levels.
    - NOTE: Fractional calcium excretion is *low* (e.g., <0.01) in FHH but HIGH in primary hPTH. This is the differentiating point for FHH versus primary hPTH. Do *not* perform parathyroidectomy if hypercalcemia is due to FHH.
    - Fractional excretion of calcium may be calculated based on 24-hour clearance and referred to as "calcium-to-creatinine-clearance ratio" (CCCR):
      - CCCR = [(24-hour urine calcium) × (SCr)]/[(24-hour urine creatinine) × (SCa)]
      - CCCR < 0.010 indicates FHH, whereas a CCCR > 0.020 is likely consistent with primary hPTH.
- Activating mutation of the PTH/PTHrP receptor gene (Jansen disease):
  - Laboratory findings are similar to those with primary hPTH.

- Clinical manifestations: short-limbed dwarfism, severe hypercalcemia, hypophosphatemia, and metaphyseal chondrodysplasia
- Loss of function mutation of vitamin D-24-hydroxylase:
  - Loss of function mutation of vitamin D-24-hydroxylase leads to high levels of 1,25 vitamin D and hypercalcemia (both of which suppress PTH).
  - Resultant phenotype: hypercalcemia with associated nephrocalcinosis and/or nephrolithiasis
  - Treatment: ketoconazole (inhibitor of vitamin D-1α-hydroxylase) corrects hypercalcemia.

> **NOTE** Corticosteroids ameliorate hypercalcemia in patients with high 1,25 vitamin D level due to ingestion and granulomatous disease, but not in those with inactivating mutation of vitamin D-24-hydroxylase.

- Sunitinib and imatinib may induce secondary hPTH, presumably by inducing bone resistance to PTH.
  - Sunitinib (Sutent) and imatinib (Gleevac) are tyrosine kinase inhibitors that inhibit the actions of vascular endothelial growth factors. These agents are used in the treatment of various malignancies including pancreatic neuroendocrine tumors, gastrointestinal stromal tumors, and advanced renal cell carcinoma, and Philadelphia chromosome-positive chronic myelogenous leukemia.
  - Affected patients typically have marked hypocalciuria and normal to high SCa, hypophosphatemia, elevated 1,25 vitamin D.
  - Reversal of this form of secondary hPTH is possible with drug discontinuation.
- Other cause of hypercalcemia: Paget disease

Clinical Manifestations, Complications of Hypercalcemia

- Fatigue, poor concentration, headaches, depression, anxiety
- Ocular: conjunctivitis, band keratopathy
- Cardiac: shortened QT, arrhythmias
- Gastrointestinal: constipation, nausea, vomiting, peptic ulcer disease, pancreatitis
- Kidney-related complications: polyuria, nephrogenic diabetes insipidus, kidney stones, medullary and cortical calcium depositions (nephrocalcinosis).

Management of Hypercalcemia

- Volume repletion with normal saline as tolerated
- Loop diuretics may be added once euvolemic or hypervolemic to enhance paracellular Ca^{2+} excretion from thick ascending loop of Henle.
- Bisphosphonates:
  - Inhibit bone resorption
  - Preferred agents for hypercalcemia associated with cancer
  - Commonly used agents:
    - Intravenous pamidronate, oral alendronate
    - Calcitonin: rapid onset of action (within hours), but only short-term benefit due to tachyphylaxis

- Mithramycin: cytostatic drug
  - Potent inhibitor of bone resorption
  - Rapid onset of action, effect lasts days, but high adverse effects (transaminitis, thrombocytopenia)
  - Reserved for malignant hypercalcemia. Prostaglandin antagonists (e.g., aspirin, indomethacin) may also be considered in malignant hypercalcemia.
- Corticosteroids: (0.5 to 1.0 mg/kg prednisone daily)
  - Reduces GI absorption of calcium
  - May be used in hypervitaminosis D (either endogenous source such as sarcoid/granulomatous diseases or exogenous vitamin D ingestion)
  - Corticosteroid is ineffective in patients with vitamin D-24-hydroxylase mutations. Ketoconazole is used instead (see Ketoconazole).
  - May be considered in lymphoproliferative malignancies such as lymphoma, multiple myeloma, or even solid organ malignancy such as breast CA.
- Ketoconazole:
  - Inhibits calcitriol synthesis via inhibition of 1-α hydroxylase
  - May be used for patients with vitamin D-24-hydroxylase loss of function mutation
- Others:
  - Propranolol for thyrotoxicosis-induced hypercalcemia
  - Estrogens in women with primary hPTH to reduce bone resorption.
  - Calcimimetics (CaSR agonists such as cinacalcet) for hPTH (primary, secondary, or even parathyroid carcinoma), particularly for nonsurgical patients
- Treatment consideration for malignancy-associated hypercalcemia:
  - Denosumab (Prolia, Xgeva) is a human mAb that binds to and inhibits the bone-resorption mediator *Receptor Activator of NF-kB Ligand* (RANKL). RANKL is normally secreted by osteoblasts to stimulate osteoclastic proliferation and activity (increase bone resorption). Inhibition of RANKL by denosumab inhibits osteoclastic activity.
  - Current data suggest that denosumab may ameliorate malignancy-associated hypercalcemia due to bone involvement.
  - May cause severe hypocalcemia in patients with end-stage renal disease (ESRD) and should be avoided
- Parathyroidectomy for primary hPTH (National Institute of Health Consensus Guidelines):
  - Indications:
    - SCa level > 1.0 mg/dL above upper limit of normal
    - Hypercalciuria > 400 mg/d or kidney stones
    - Creatinine clearance < 30% of normal
    - Marked bone density reduction with T-score < −2.5 at any site
    - Age < 50 due to eventual significant complications if left untreated
    - Patient surgical preference due to difficult/impossible follow-up
  - Presurgical considerations for hPTH:
    - Localization with imaging studies to allow minimal invasive surgery is now preferred over four-gland exploration without presurgical imaging.
    - Localization studies: combination ^{99m}Tc-sestamibi scintigraphy ± single-photon emission computed tomography (SPECT) and ultrasound
      - If positive for adenoma → focused surgery
      - Otherwise, consider 4D-computed tomography, exploratory surgery

- Hungry bone syndrome:
  - Definition: profound (SCa < 6 mg/dL) and prolonged (>4 days postoperative) hypocalcemia following parathyroidectomy for severe hPTH.
  - Risks: severe hPTH with associated skeletal manifestations, preoperative indices of high bone turnover, osteitis fibrosa cystica, and/or "brown tumors"
  - Pathogenesis:
    - Continuing high skeletal calcium uptake from plasma without the opposing calcium leaking back into plasma from bone resorption due to acute fall in PTH with parathyroidectomy
  - Management:
    - Intravenous calcium supplement (6 to 12 g/d), followed by oral therapy when safe, plus
    - Calcitriol (2 to 4 mcg/d), plus
    - Correction of hypomagnesemia if present

HYPOCALCEMIA

Causes of Hypocalcemia

- Pseudohypocalcemia:
  - Acute respiratory alkalosis or severe metabolic alkalosis: clinically significant reduction in ionized Ca^{2+} may occur due to increased Ca^{2+} complexing to the increased levels of organic anions associated with alkalemia. Total SCa levels remain the same.
  - Hypoalbuminemia: low total SCa with normal ionized Ca^{2+} levels due to reduced albumin-bound calcium fraction.
- Differential diagnoses of true hypocalcemia may be categorized based on serum phosphate:
  - Hypocalcemia in association with normal to low phosphate:
    - Hungry bone syndrome: due to reduced bone resorption with acute surgical removal of PTH.
    - Magnesium deficiency reduces PTH synthesis/release and induces bone resistance to PTH (no release of bone calcium or phosphorus into circulation).
    - Malnutrition
    - Acute pancreatitis (likely due to compensatory hPTH and resultant phosphaturia)
    - Vitamin D deficiency (vitamin D 25 or calcitriol (1,25) deficiency or liver disease or anticonvulsants with associated reduced 25-hydroxylation)
    - Vitamin D resistance
  - Hypocalcemia in association with hyperphosphatemia:
    - Kidney failure
    - Rhabdomyolysis (calcium is sequestered into injured tissue, thus hypocalcemia; intracellular phosphate is released from injured muscle cells, thus hyperphosphatemia)
    - Pseudohypoparathyroidism: resistance to PTH. PTH level is high.
    - Hypoparathyroidism (neck irradiation, amyloid infiltration of parathyroids, idiopathic, sporadic, or postoperative hypoparathyroidism)

> **NOTE** Treatment of rhabdomyolysis-induced hypocalcemia is *not* recommended unless neurologic symptoms or ECG changes (i.e., prolonged QT, tetany) because
> - Hypocalcemia associated with rhabdomyolysis is transient as Ca^{2+} sequestered in injured tissue will be released back into circulation with recovery.
> - PTH is stimulated during the initial hypocalcemic phase and can contribute to recovery phase "overshoot" hypercalcemia.
> - Calcium infusion in the presence of hyperphosphatemia may facilitate intravascular and soft-tissue calcifications.

- Autosomal dominant hypoparathyroidism:
  - Arises from activating mutation of CaSR
  - Renal effects: hypercalciuria, thus hypocalcemia
  - Parathyroid effects: PTH suppression, thus hyperphosphatemia and reduced 1,25 vitamin D. The latter leads to hypocalcemia.

Diagnosis of Hypocalcemia, Notable Laboratory Findings

- Urinary calcium excretion during treatment with calcium and vitamin D derivatives:
  - Increased in the treatment of hypoparathyroidism and may lead to nephrocalcinosis
  - Decreased in all other causes of hypocalcemia
- Calcium-to-creatinine-clearance ratio:
  - High, that is ratio > 0.020 in hPTH, post-AKI diuresis, diuretics (except thiazides and amiloride), and severe CKD
  - Low in all other etiologies of hypocalcemia
- Urinary phosphate excretion:
  - High in vitamin D deficiency (due to increased PTH), steatorrhea, CKD, active phosphate infusion
  - Low in hypoparathyroidism (recall the opposite is true in primary hPTH, where phosphaturia and hypophosphatemia are observed), pseudohypoparathyroidism, magnesium deficiency
- Intracranial calcifications, particularly within basal ganglia, are observed more frequently in idiopathic hypoparathyroidism compared with other forms of hypoparathyroidism.

Management of Hypocalcemia

- NOTE:
  - In the case of concurrent acidemia and clinically significant hypocalcemia, correct hypocalcemia FIRST. Do *not* correct acidemia prior to the correction of hypocalcemia. Alkalinization may acutely reduce circulating levels of ionized Ca^{2+} and induce life-threatening neurologic complications and/or arrhythmias.
  - Calcium CANNOT be given in the same IV line as sodium bicarbonate due to calcium precipitation as calcium carbonate.
- Correct underlying etiology
- Calcium supplement:
  - Calcium gluconate is generally preferred over calcium chloride ($CaCl_2$) because it is less irritating to tissue.
  - Calcium chloride may be used if there is central venous access.
  - NOTE: 1 g of $CaCl_2$ contains 272 mg (13.2 mEq) of elemental calcium, whereas 1 g of calcium gluconate contains 94 mg (4.7 mEq). THUS, 1 ampule

of calcium chloride = 3 ampules of calcium gluconate in terms of elemental calcium content.
- In severe cases of hypocalcemia where there are neurologic complications (i.e., tetany, seizures, arhythmias), administer calcium gluconate as follows:
  - Intravenous bolus: 10 mL of 10% diluted in 50 mL of either 5% dextrose water or isotonic saline given over 5 to 10 minutes, followed by
  - Continuous infusion of a solution mixture containing 8 to 10 amps of calcium gluconate in 1 L of normal saline or 5% dextrose to run over the next 24 hours
- Thiazide diuretics may be used concurrently with calcium supplementation in patients with hypoparathyroidism to reduce urinary calcium excretion and nephrocalcinosis. As with calcium stone management, high fluid intake and low sodium intake should be advised.
- Vitamin D supplement: Active forms of vitamin D such as calcitriol or 1α-hydroxycholecalciferol are the treatment of choice for idiopathic or acquired hypoparathyroidism because they can minimize large calcium supplement.

DISORDERS OF PHOSPHATE METABOLISM

Phosphate Background
- 99% of total body phosphates (700 g) exist intracellularly and in bones.
- 1% of total body phosphates exist extracellularly as HPO_4^{2-} and $H_2PO_4^-$ in a 4:1 ratio, with normal serum phosphate concentrations of 2.8 to 4.5 mg/dL.
- Daily phosphate intake is ~1 to 1.5 g/d, where 60% to 80% is absorbed by the GI tract and 10% is secreted back into the GI tract.
- Kidney excretes 60% to 70% of dietary intake.
- Less than 1% of total body phosphate is involved in constant bone turnover.
- Physiologic roles of phosphate: bone mineralization, phospholipid bilayers, ATP, DNA/RNA synthesis, glycolysis, cell function, unloading of O_2 via 2,3-bisphoglycerate

Phosphate Metabolism
- Gastrointestines:
  - GI phosphate absorption is linear and nonsaturable function of phosphate intake.
  - Absorption ccurs via both paracellular and transcellular pathways.
  - Transcellular absorption occurs via sodium–phosphate (Na-Pi) cotransporters, type 2b in the small intestines.
    - *NPT2b*, the gene encoding Na-Pi 2b, is upregulated by calcitriol.
    - Niacin inhibits Na-Pi 2b and has been used to reduce GI phosphate absorption. Niacin may reduce phosphate by 0.4 mg/dL.
    - Deletion of NPT2b has no phosphate phenotype in humans. It is possible that paracellular absorption alone may be sufficient to maintain phosphate levels.
- Kidney:
  - Phosphate is minimally protein bound and freely filtered in the glomeruli.
  - Total renal reabsorption is approximately 80% to 95%, leaving fractional excretion of phosphate (FE_{PO4}) to be 5% to 20%.

- Proximal tubules:
  - Absorption of phosphate occurs via Na-Pi, types 2a and 2c, at the brush borders of proximal tubules.
  - FGF-23 and PTH downregulates *NPT2a* (gene encoding Na-Pi 2a), thus enhances phosphaturia.
  - NOTE: For optimal FGF-23 binding and function in the kidneys, FGF-23 requires the cofactor klotho. Mutations of either FGF-23 or klotho can reduce phosphaturia.
  - Typically, kidneys excrete 5% to 20% of filtered phosphate load to maintain phosphate balance, that is FE_{PO4} is 5% to 20%.
  - In CKD, when GFR is reduced, each of the remnant nephrons will have to reabsorb more phosphate per filtered load to maintain balance. FE_{PO4} can exceed 50%.
  - $FE_{PO4} = (U_{PO4} \times S_{Cr})/(S_{PO4} \times U_{Cr})$,
    - where U_{PO4} = urine phosphate concentration
    - S_{Cr} = serum creatinine
    - S_{PO4} = serum phosphate concentration
    - U_{Cr} = urine creatinine concentration
    - NOTE: This is similar to the calculation of FeNa.

HYPERPHOSPHATEMIA

Causes of Hyperphosphatemia

- Pseudohyperphosphatemia:
  - Heparin-containing blood samples due to phosphate-containing preservatives
  - Paraproteinemia (multiple myeloma) if phosphate is measured with the phosphomolybdate ultraviolet assay
- Exogenous sources (usually in association with poor kidney function and excretion):
  - Excessive ingestion of phosphate salts, for example, accidental ingestion of phosphate-containing enemas
  - Treatment with vitamin D (increase GI absorption of phosphates)
- Extracellular shift:
  - Cell death, extracellular release of phosphate: rhabdomyolysis, hemolysis, malignant hyperthermia, heavy tumor burden with necrotic cell death, tumor lysis syndrome, bowel infarction
  - Acid–base status:
    - Lactic acidosis
    - Diabetic ketoacidosis
    - Chronic respiratory alkalosis (associated with prolonged hyperventilation) may lead to renal resistance to PTH, hyperphosphatemia, hypocalcemia, and possibly reduced PTH secretion.
  - Reduced kidney excretion:
    - Reduced kidney function (typically with GFR < 25 to 30 mL/min/1.73 m^2)
    - Hypoparathyroidism (idiopathic, postsurgical, pseudohypoparathyroidism, PTH resistance, abnormal forms of plasma PTH)
    - Drug-induced: bisphosphonates
    - Acromegaly: Increased growth hormone and insulin-like growth factor-1 in acromegaly can increase tubular reabsorption of phosphate.
    - Familial tumoral calcinosis:
      - Rare autosomal recessive disorder affecting Middle Eastern or African ancestries

- Thought to involve inactivating mutations of *GALnt3*, *FGF-23*, or *klotho* genes, all of which are necessary for optimal FGF-23 activity. (*GALnt3* codes for glycosyltransferase, an enzyme necessary for post-translational processing and stabilization of FGF-23.)
- The lack of active FGF-23 (low FGF-23) leads to the following:
  - Hyperphosphatemia
  - Loss of FGF-23 inhibitory effect on 1,25 vitamin D synthesis → elevated 1,25 vitamin D (increased GI calcium absorption) → low PTH → hypercalciuria
  - Normal SCa due to opposing effects of 1,25 vitamin D and PTH
  - Ectopic calcifications due to combination of positive calcium balance and hyperphosphatemia

Clinical Manifestations of Hyperphosphatemia

- Soft tissue, vascular calcium phosphate depositions
- Hyperphosphatemia inhibits the conversion of 25-vitamin D to 1,25-vitamin D (calcitriol).

Management of Hyperphosphatemia

- Dietary restriction
- Fluid resuscitation to ensure good renal excretion
- Phosphate binders with meals to reduce GI absorption (See Secondary Hyperparathyroidism)
- Intravenous dextrose and insulin to increase intracellular phosphate shift

HYPOPHOSPHATEMIA

Causes of Hypophosphatemia

- Reduced intake: alcoholics, eating disorders (anorexia, bulimia), old/debilitated/poor patients with poor access to high-phosphate-containing food
- Reduced GI absorption:
  - Vitamin D deficiency
  - Vitamin D-dependent rickets:
    - Defect in renal 1α-hydroxylase (vitamin D-dependent rickets type 1)
      - Laboratory findings: low 1,25 vitamin D, hypocalcemia, secondary hPTH, hypophosphatemia
      - 50% of patients may have alopecia.
      - Treatment: low-dose calcitriol
    - VDR deficiency (vitamin D-dependent rickets type 2):
      - Laboratory findings: high 1,25 vitamin D level
      - Treatment: high-dose calcitriol
  - Malabsorptive GI disorders, extensive bowel resection
- Cellular shift:
  - *Acute* respiratory alkalosis: acute respiratory alkalosis leads to extracellular CO_2 diffusion which in turn leads to a rise in intracellular pH. The increased intracellular pH increases glycolysis, a process where phosphates are needed to produce adenosine triphosphates (ATP). The requirement for cellular phosphate uptake leads to hypophosphatemia. Acute metabolic alkalosis does *not* cause hypophosphatemia because bicarbonate cannot freely cross cell membranes to cause a rapid rise in intracellular pH.
  - NOTE: *Chronic* respiratory alkalosis is associated with HYPERphosphatemia due to renal resistance to PTH +/− reduced PTH secretion.

- Refeeding syndrome
- Total parenteral nutrition with insulin-mediated intracellular phosphate shift or low phosphate content
- Diabetic ketoacidosis following insulin administration
- Increased renal excretion:
  - Volume expansion
  - Mutations leading to increased levels of FGF-23 and resultant downregulation of Na-Pi 2a expression in the proximal tubules. Affected individuals present with various skeletal deformities.
    - Autosomal-dominant hypophosphatemic rickets:
      - Mutation in FGF-23 that renders FGF-23 resistant to proteolysis
      - Associated skeletal abnormalities: bowing of long bones and widening of costochondral joints
    - Autosomal-recessive hypophosphatemic rickets: Mutations in DMP1 can lead to increased FGF-23 levels. *DMP1* is gene encoding the dentin matrix protein 1, a molecule thought to normally suppress bone secretion of FGF-23.
    - X-linked hypophosphatemic rickets:
      - Mutations of the *PHEX* gene encoding the phosphate-regulating endopeptidase (on X chromosome). PHEX is thought to play a role in the proteolysis of FGF-23.
      - Associated skeletal deformities: short stature, osteomalacia
  - Intrinsic renal defect leading to reduced renal phosphate reabsorption: Fanconi syndrome:
    - Mutation of NPT2a: autosomal-recessive Fanconi syndrome with associated hypophosphatemic rickets and renal failure
    - Mutation of NPT2c: hereditary hypophosphatemia with rickets and hypercalciuria (HHRH)
      - Phenotype: hypophosphatemia, normal SCa, normal PTH, low FGF-23, high 1,25 vitamin D, and hypercalciuria
      - NOTE: Hypophosphatemia is independent of FGF-23 or PTH.
      - Secondary hypercalciuria is due to FGF-23 suppression, followed by 1,25 vitamin D activation, and hypercalciuria.
  - Oncogenic hypophosphatemic osteomalacia:
    - Mostly associated with benign mesenchymal tumors (e.g., hemagiopericytoma, fibroma, angiosarcoma, and more recently, metastatic prostate carcinoma)
    - Malignant tissue secretion of phosphatonins (i.e., FGF-23 and other phosphaturic factors)
    - Laboratory findings:
      - Affected individuals present with impaired bone mineralization and hypophosphatemia caused by reduced renal phosphate reabsorption, paradoxically low levels of calcitriol, the production of which is typically enhanced by hypophosphatemia. Calcitriol is inappropriately low to normal in this condition due to reduced 1α-hydroxylase activity with increased FGF-23 levels.
      - Intact PTH may be elevated due to low 1,25-vitamin D levels or excessive phosphate replacement.
      - Alkaline phosphatase levels are often elevated.
      - SCa levels are normal to low.
    - Diagnosis: clinical presentation above, elevated FGF-23 (commercially available)

- Post-renal transplant hypophosphatemia:
  - Persistent secondary hPTH in new functioning allograft
  - Persistently high circulating levels of FGF-23—although this is more commonly seen in patients with markedly elevated pretransplant FGF-23 levels
  - Note, however, that persistent hypophosphatemia beyond 1 year post-transplant has been attributed to persistent hPTH rather than increased FGF-23 levels.
- Others:
  - Drugs: corticosteroids, diuretics, bicarbonate, sunitinib/imatinib (tyrosine kinase inhibitors associated with hPTH, normal to high SCa levels, hypophosphatemia)
  - Ferric carboxymaltose injection: It is thought that carboxymaltose can inhibit the cleavage and inactivation of FGF-23 within osteocytes, resulting in increased levels of active FGF-23, phosphaturia, hypophosphatemia, and decreased 1,25-vitamin D.
  - Alcoholism: malnutrition, hypomagnesemia-associated renal phosphate wasting, intracellular shift due to hyperventilation or glucose infusion
  - Hungry bone syndrome
  - Hypophosphatemia following hepatectomy: This is thought to be due to increased proximal tubular expression of nicotinamide phosphoribosyl-transferase (Nampt), a protein associated with reduced renal expression of the sodium phosphate transporter.

Clinical Manifestations of Hypophosphatemia

- Symptoms typically not evident unless serum phosphate level is <2.0 mg/dL.
- Respiratory distress/arrest due to poor-functioning/weak diaphragm presumably because of inability to produce adequate ATPs, rhabdomyolysis (alcoholics with underlying alcoholic myopathy are particularly at risk), cardiomyopathy, metabolic encephalopathy, hemolysis, red and white blood cell dysfunction.

Management of Hypophosphatemia

- Phosphate supplementation: Estimating phosphate deficit (i.e., repletion dose): Phosphate dose (mmol) = 0.5 body weight (kg) $\times$ (1.25 − [serum phosphate mmol/L]). The factor 0.5 indicates that the volume of distribution of phosphate is approximately 50% of total body weight.
- Treatment of underlying etiology whenever possible

SECONDARY HYPERPARATHYROIDISM

Clinical Implications of Secondary hPTH

- Renal osteodystrophy with increased risk of fractures:
  - Osteomalacia
  - Osteopenia
  - Adynamic bone disease
  - Mixed bone disease
- Calcific uremic arteriolopathy, a.k.a. calciphylaxis: See End-stage renal disease
- Accelerated atherosclerosis
- Refractory anemia
- Tertiary hPTH
- Increased morbidity and mortality: 1% increase in relative risk of all-cause mortality per 100 pg/mL increase in PTH and a 2% increase in cardiovascular mortality (0.007).

Diagnosis of Secondary hPTH

- Secondary hPTH may be diagnosed in patients with CKD and is characterized by elevated serum PTH levels with associated normal to high serum phosphate and normal to low SCa (prior to the administration of calcium-containing agents and/or vitamin D supplementation).
- Measurements of PTH:
  - Clinical significance (e.g., regarding bone health) and treatment of secondary hPTH should depend on "trending" of PTH levels, *not* on a single value.
  - Clinical assays for measuring PTH levels are not standardized and may give a wide range of values. This variation is thought to be due to the ability of some assays to measure more (or less) circulating PTH fragments than others.
  - Current commercially available PTH measurements cannot differentiate biologically inactive oxidized forms of PTH from active nonoxidized forms.

Pathogenesis of Secondary Hyperparathyroidism

- Reduced kidney mass results in:
  - Reduced 1α-hydroxylase level thus reduced 1,25-vitamin D levels.
  - Reduced glomerular filtration leading to phosphate retention
- Phosphate retention leads to: (Fig. 3.5)
  - Increased FGF-23 synthesis. FGF-23 in turn reduces 1,25 vitamin D production by inhibiting 1α-hydroxylase and increasing 24-hydroxylase.
  - Hyperphosphatemia has direct effects on the parathyroid gland to increase PTH secretion and parathyroid cell growth.
  - Hyperphosphatemia is also associated with the following:
    - Skeletal resistance to PTH which contributes to hypocalcemia
    - Parathyroid cell resistance to calcitriol
    - Reduced calcitriol synthesis (feedback phenomenon: calcitriol increases phosphate level while hyperphosphatemia reduces calcitriol synthesis)
- Reduced 1,25-vitamin D leads to:
  - Reduced GI absorption of calcium, thus hypocalcemia and subsequent hPTH
  - Reduced repression of *PTH* gene transcription and parathyroid cell proliferation

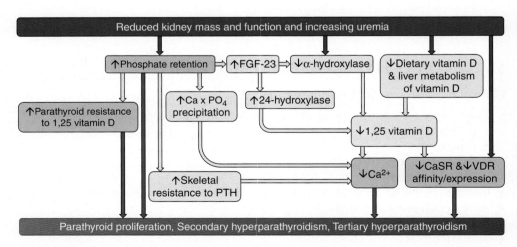

FIGURE 3.5 Pathogenesis of secondary hyperparathyroidism. Severe reduction of CaSR and VDR can lead to eventual tertiary hyperparathyroidism. CaSR, Calcium-sensing receptor; VDR, Vitamin D receptor; FGF-23, Fibroblast growth factor-23; PTH, Parathyroid hormone.

- Reduced expression of parathyroid VDR and CaSR
- Increased set point for calcium-regulated PTH secretion
- Patients with kidney disease may also have low 25-vitamin D due to reduced skin conversion of 7-dehydrocholesterol to cholecaliferol and liver hydroxylation of cholecalciferol 25-OH vitamin.
- Hypocalcemia due to reduced vitamin D, poor dietary intake, and $CaPO_4$ precipitation leads to uninhibited parathyroid proliferation and PTH secretion.
- Intrinsic parathyroid cell abnormalities in CKD below can also contribute to hPTH:
  - Decreased expression of VDR and CaSR
  - Increased set point for calcium-regulated PTH secretion

Other notes regarding FGF-23 in CKD

- Binding of FGF-23 and its cofactor klotho to the receptor complex klotho-FGFR1 **in the kidney** leads to phosphaturia via suppression of Na-Pi 2a and 2c expressions in the brush border of proximal tubules. NOTE: Recall FGF-23 has low affinity for its receptor (FGFR) and requires the cofactor klotho to effectively bind and activate the receptor. Of interest, klotho expression is reduced early in the course of CKD. This is thought to be the reason for reduced phosphaturia in patients with CKD. Reduction of klotho has also been implicated in inducing a more rapid progression of CKD.
- **FGF-23 also acts on parathyroid** cells via the FGF-23-klotho complex to reduce PTH synthesis and secretion and PTH proliferation.
  - Increase expression of CaSR and VDR.
- FGF-23 in CKD:
  - FGF-23 level is increased early in CKD, even before the rise in PTH levels.
  - FGF-23 level is increased in association with an increased phosphate "burden" alone and not necessarily high serum phosphate levels.
  - FGF-23 is an independent predictor of mortality, progression of kidney disease, left ventricular hypertrophy, vascular dysfunction, and kidney transplant outcomes.
  - FGF-23 levels may remain increased post-kidney transplant with resultant hypophosphatemia and relative 1,25-vitamin D deficiency.

Management of Secondary hPTH

- Consistent control of mineral biochemical profile (PTH, calcium, phosphorus) is associated with improved survival.
- Recommended goals:
  - KDIGO guidelines:
    - Maintain PTH levels, SCa, and phosphate levels within normal range for all CKD stages up to stage 5. However,
    - For dialysis dependent patients, PTH levels should be kept at two to five times upper-normal limit.
  - KDOQI guidelines:
    - Maintain PTH level at 35 to 70 pg/mL for stage 3, 70 to 110 pg/mL for stage 4 CKD, and 300 to 500 pg/mL for stage 5 CKD.
    - Maintain SCa and phosphate levels within normal range for CKD stages 3 to 4.
    - Maintain calcium between 8.5 and 9.5 mg/dL and serum phosphate between 3.5 and 5.5 mg/dL for stage 5 CKD.
  - 25-vitamin D levels > 30 ng/mL (not evidence based)

- Phosphate control:
  - Dietary phosphorus restriction (typically 1,000 mg/d):
    - Of the 1,000 mg phosphorus ingested daily, ~60% is absorbed (600 mg/d or 4,200 mg/wk). A typical thrice weekly hemodialysis regimen removes 2,400 mg/week. Removal of the remaining weekly net gain of 1,800 mg requires the use of phosphate binders.
    - The most efficient phosphate binder is lanthanum which has twice the binding capacity for phosphate compared to most other agents (90 mg of phosphate removed per 1 g of lanthanum versus 45 mg of phosphate per 1 g of other commonly used agents).
    - Dietary phosphate:
      - Organic phosphorus:
        - Found in protein-rich foods from both animal and vegetarian sources of protein.
        - Organic phosphorus are highly protein bound, which limits absorption. Phosphorus derived from plants (phytate) has lower bioavailability compared to that from animal source.
      - Inorganic phosphorus commonly found in food preservatives or flavor enhancers have 90% to 100% bioavailability because they are not protein bound.
      - NOTE: Active vitamin D increases GI absorption of phosphorus.
    - Examples of high-phosphate-containing foods:
      - Dairy products: cheese, cream, custard, ice cream, milk, pudding, yogurt
      - Vegetables: beans, dried peas, lentils, mixed vegetables, soybeans and soy products
      - Protein foods: liverwurst, eggs, liver, salmon, sardines, tuna
      - Breads, cereals
      - Beverages: beer, colas (typically dark colas), some fruit punch
      - Others: chocolate, nuts, processed foods
  - Phosphate binders:
    - Commonly available agents: calcium carbonate, calcium acetate, magnesium carbonate (low efficacy), sevelamer HCl or carbonate (reduces low-density lipoproteins, reduces FGF-23, may attenuate progression of vascular calcifications), lanthanum carbonate, nicotinic acid/niacin (binds to gut Na-Pi 2b and reduces phosphate absorption)
    - Newer agents:
      - Iron-containing agents:
        - Ferric citrate (Auryxia)
        - Stabilized polynuclear iron(III)-oxyhydroxide (PA21)
      - Colestilan (non–calcium-based phosphate binder that also binds bile acids and reduces LDL cholesterol)
    - Special NOTES regarding various phosphate binders:
      - The use of phosphate binders in hemodialysis patients has been shown to reduce both cardiovascular and all-cause mortality by 20% to 30% in several large studies. Nonetheless, the use of phosphate binders in stages 3B to 4 CKD may be associated with an increase in annualized coronary artery and abdominal aortic calcium scores. This is thought to be due to the use of calcium-containing agents. Further studies are needed.
      - Lanthanum, a non–calcium, non–resin-based binder:
        - May increase bone turnover

- High phosphate-binding capacity, thus lower pill burden compared to others
  - Sevelamer, a non–calcium binder, may bind vitamin D. Higher vitamin D supplements may be necessary.
  - Sevelamer-treated hemodialysis patients have been shown to experience lower cardiovascular and all-cause mortality (but not if analyzed for non-cardiovascular mortality alone) compared to calcium-containing phosphate binders (Dialysis Outcomes and Practice Patterns Study (DOPPS)).
  - The use of >1.5 g/d of calcium-based phosphate binders can lead to positive calcium balance and is not recommended.
- Dialysis removal
  - Hemodialysis removes approximately 800 mg of phosphorus per treatment
  - Peritoneal dialysis removes approximately 300 mg of phosphorus per treatment
  - Since phosphorus is predominantly intracellular, there is a rebound phenomenon after dialysis due to extracellular shift.
  - Prolonged and frequent dialysis (i.e., nocturnal or daily hemodialysis) are superior in phosphorus removal than conventional hemodialysis.
  - NOTE: Increasing blood flow rate in hemodialysis is not effective in increasing phosphorus removal.
- Vitamin D supplementation:
  - Ergocalciferol (25-Vitamin D2 - plant source) or cholecalciferol (25-Vitamin D3 animal source)
    - Rationale:
      - Potential benefits other than for CKD-MBD: inflammation, immunity, cardiac function (reduced ventricular mass), response to erythropoietin stimulating agents, malignancy.
      - Serves as substrate for 1,25 vitamin D synthesis
      - Does help with CKD-MBD, but insufficient to reduce PTH levels, particularly in later CKD stages 4 and 5. Therefore, concurrent use of active vitamin D analogs may also be required in later CKD stages.
    - NOTE: Prior to any vitamin D supplementation, serum phosphate levels should be reduced to below 5.5 mg/dL, because vitamin D does increase GI absorption of phosphate and may worsen existing hyperphosphatemia.
  - Active vitamin D a.k.a. vitamin D receptor activator (VDRA) supplementation:
    - Calcitriol (Rocaltrol): $1,25(OH)_2D_3$
    - Doxercalciferol (Hectoral): $1(OH)D_2$ (needs to be converted to $1,25(OH)_2D_3$ in liver)
    - Pericalcitol (Zemplar): $19\text{-nor}1,25(OH)_2D_2$
  - Comparative effects of commercially available VDRA:
    - Doxercalciferol and paricalcitol may have less calcemic and phosphatemic effects compared to calcitriol. However, all three agents have similar PTH-lowering effect.
    - Intravenous paricalcitol:
      - May reduce PTH faster with fewer sustained episodes of hypercalcemia and/or $CaPO_4$ precipitation compared with calcitriol.
      - May confer less-vascular calcification and better-vascular wall remodeling compared with calcitriol and doxercalciferol
    - Despite the potential advantage of VDRA on left ventricular mass noted in animal studies, the Paricalcitol Capsules Benefits in Renal Failure Induced Cardiac Morbidity in Subjects with CKD Stage 3/4 (PRIMO) study did *not*

show a significant reduction in LV mass index at 48 weeks in paricalcitol treated versus placebo group.

- NOTE: doxercalciferol 1(OH)-vitamin D needs to be hydroxylated at the 25 position to 1,25-vitamin D in the liver before it becomes an active vitamin D. Thus, doxercalciferol may not be optimally effective in advanced liver patients.
- Calcimimetics:
  - Cinacalcet (30 to 180 mg/d):
    - May be indicated for secondary hPTH in patients with CKD and on dialysis
    - May lower SCa and should only be used in patients with SCa > 8.4 mg/dL
    - May increase serum phosphorus levels in CKD stages 3 and 4
  - Mechanism of action: acts directly on CaSR as a positive allosteric modulator to increase cellular sensitivity to extracellular calcium.
  - Effective in controlling difficult-to-treat secondary hPTH in both hemo- and peritoneal dialysis patients (i.e., cases resistant to optimal doses of VDRA and phosphate binders)
  - Cinacalcet has been shown to reduce FGF-23 levels whereas VDRA increase FGF-23 levels.
  - Cinacalcet effects on morbidity and mortality:
    - Reduction in risk of parathyroidectomy, fractures, and hospitalization based on post-hoc analysis of four randomized controlled trials, $n = 1,184$, follow-up 6 to 12 months.
    - There are data to suggest that cinacalcet-centered therapy (i.e., cinacalcet + low-dose vitamin D-based regimen) may be advantageous in controlling secondary hPTH.
    - Cinacalcet has been suggested to reduce the incidence of calcific uremic arteriolopathy.
    - Recent Cochrane analysis revealed no survival benefit.
- New agent being reviewed by FDA: velcalcetide, an intravenously administered agent that directly activates CaSR (unlike cinacalcet whose action requires calcium for CaSR activation). Velcalcetide has also been shown to reduce both PTH and FGF-23 levels.
- Indications for parathyroidectomy in patients with CKD and secondary hPTH (Table 3.1):
- Management of hypocalcemia:
  - As per KDIGO and KDOQI guidelines, maintain SCa levels in normal range. Calcium supplement should not exceed 1,000 mg/d.
  - Avoid excess calcium supplement due to concerns for increased vascular calcifications and increased cardiovascular and all-cause mortality.
  - For hemodialysis patients, dialysate calcium concentration of 1.25 mmol/L (2.5 mEq/L) provides neutral calcium balance, whereas calcium concentration of 1.5 mmol/L (3 mEq/L) may lead to significantly positive balance and potential increased associated complications.

DISORDERS OF MAGNESIUM METABOLISM

Magnesium Background

- Second most abundant intracellular and fourth most abundant cation in body
- 70% to 80% exists as free ionized Mg^{2+} and 20% to 30% as protein-bound or complexed

Table 3.1	Indications for parathyroidectomy in patients with CKD and secondary hyperparathyroidism

Non–renal transplant patients:

1. Elevated intact PTH levels > 800 pg/mL associated with hypercalcemia and/or hyperphosphatemia that are refractory to medical therapy (K/DOQI)[a]
2. Clinical signs and symptoms associated with refractory hyperparathyroidism:

    Hypercalcemia

    Uncontrollable hyperphosphatemia

    Evidence of osteitis fibrosa by bone biopsy, classic radiologic findings, or bone metabolic markers

    Enlarged ± nodular parathyroid glands (>500 mg)

    Calciphylaxis

    Intractable pruritis

    Progressive calcification of blood vessels

    Severe skeletal deformity

    Severe bone pain

    Anemia resistance to erythropoietin

    Peripheral neuropathy

Indications for parathyroidectomy are opinion based.
[a]K/DOQI, Kidney Disease Outcome Quality Initiative.

Physiological Functions of Magnesium

- Serves as cofactor for all enzymatic reactions requiring ATP (ATP-ase) "kinases"
- Enzyme activator for neuromuscular excitability and cell permeability
- Regulator of ion channels and mitochondrial function
- Critical element in cellular proliferation and apoptosis
- Important factor in both cellular and humoral immune reactions

Magnesium Metabolism

- Input: GI absorption:
  - Passive paracellular absorption when there is a high concentration gradient between intestinal lumen and epithelial cells
  - Active transport via transient receptor potential melastatin channel TRPM6 in large intestines where there is a low intraluminal magnesium content. TRPM6 is also present in the distal convoluted tubules in the kidneys where it determines the final urinary magnesium loss.
    - Autosomal recessive mutation of TRPM6 is associated with hypomagnesemia with secondary hypocalcemia. Hypomagnesemia results from both poor GI absorption and urinary loss.
    - Affected individuals may present with seizures/tetany perinatally.
    - Treatment is high-dose oral administration of magnesium sulfate for absorption via passive paracellular pathway.
- Cellular shift, redistribution:
  - Bones are the principal reservoirs of Mg^{2+} and do not readily exchange with extracellular Mg^{2+}. In negative Mg^{2+} balance, bone Mg^{2+} shift into plasma does not occur for weeks. Acute maintenance of plasma Mg^{2+} relies on renal reabsorption.

- Cellular influx increases with catecholamines, refeeding syndrome, treatment of metabolic acidosis, hungry bone syndrome seen after parathyroidectomy or in patients with diffuse osteoblastic metastases.
- Redistribution: Mg^{2+} deposition in necrotic tissues, for example, acute pancreatitis
- Output:
  - There is a physiologic GI magnesium loss of ~40 mg/d from pancreatic and salivary secretions.
  - GI loss: chronic diarrhea, steatorrhea
  - Renal loss

Renal Metabolism of Magnesium

- Glomerular filtration:
  - 70% to 80% of plasma Mg^{2+} is ultrafilterable in the ionic form.
  - Ultrafilterability of Mg^{2+} is dependent on glomerular filtration, volume and acid–base status, serum content of anions, and glomerular basement membrane integrity (Fig. 3.6).
- Proximal tubules: 15% to 25% is reabsorbed, mainly passive, and proportional to Na^+ and H_2O reabsorption
- Thick ascending limb loop of Henle (TALH):
  - 65% to 75% is reabsorbed paracellularly. Recall this is facilitated by the positively charged lumen created via K^+ recycling through ROMK and the tight junction protein claudin 16 (CLD) + CLD19 (See Bartter and Gitelman Syndromes)
  - Mutation of CLD16 or CLD19 is associated with severe hypomagnesemia, hypercalciuria, and nephrolithiasis.
- Distal convoluted tubules: 5% to 10% of total filtered Mg^{2+} (or 70% to 80% of Mg^{2+} delivered from TALH) is reabsorbed via TRPM6. Mg^{2+} reabsorption may be facilitated by the positive intraluminal voltage created by K^+ secretion via Kv1.1 and the negative intracellular voltage created by Na^+/K^+ exchange via $3Na^+$-$2K^+$-ATPase. Binding of epidermal growth factor (EGF) to its receptor in DCT induces shuttling of cytoplasmic TRPM6 to the apical cell surface for efficient Mg^{2+} reabsorption (Fig. 3.7).

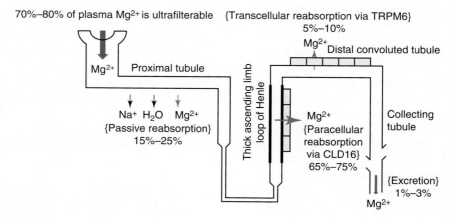

FIGURE 3.6 Renal magnesium handling. Reprinted with permission from Pham et al. Hypomagnesemia: a clinical perspective. *Int J Nephrol Renovasc Dis*. 2014;7:219.

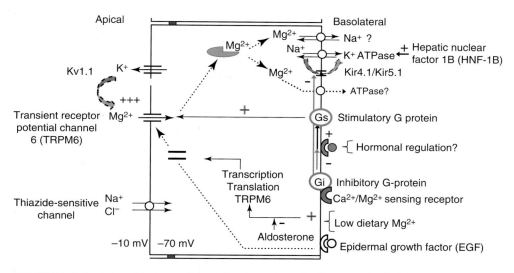

FIGURE 3.7 Active and regulated transcellular Mg^{2+} reabsorption at the distal convoluted tubule. Reprinted with permission from Pham et al. Hypomagnesemia: a clinical perspective. *Int J Nephrol Renovasc Dis.* 2014;7:219.

HYPOMAGNESEMIA

Clinical Manifestations of Hypomagnesemia

- Signs/symptoms (typically <1.2 mg/dL): Muscular tremors, fasciculations, nystagmus, tetany, altered mentation, depression, psychosis, migraine, ataxia, vertigo, seizures, dysphagia, asthma, chronic fatigue syndrome
- Electrolyte disturbances associated with hypomagnesemia:
  - Hypokalemia: thought to be due to hypomagnesemia induced hyperaldosteronism and impaired Na^+-K^+-ATPase at the DCT and ROMK at TAL (Mg^{2+} is a cofactor for the former and negative regulator for the latter—i.e., Mg^{2+} keeps ROMK closed. The lack of Mg^{2+} leads to K^+ leakage via ROMK).
  - Hypocalcemia: impaired PTH secretion and tissue sensitivity to PTH
- ECG changes:
  - Prolonged QT and PR intervals
  - Flattening or inversion of precordial P waves
  - ST-depression
  - T-wave inversion
  - Widening of QRS
  - Torsades de pointes
  - Treatment-resistant ventricular fibrillation (and other arrhythmias)
  - Worsening of digitalis toxicity
- Other associated adverse effects: altered glucose homeostasis, increased insulin resistance, atherosclerotic vascular disease, hypertension, myocardial infarction, osteoporosis, worse GFR decline in patients with diabetes type 2 and CKD, worse recovery potential in AKI in ICU setting, asthma, osteoporosis
- The protective effects of magnesium is thought to be via its anticalcification property, antioxidant activity on endothelial function, and mesangial smooth muscle relaxation effect among others.

Causes of Hypomagnesemia

- Decreased intake: malnutrition, prolonged intravenous therapy without Mg^{2+} supplementation
- Decreased intestinal absorption: surgical resection of small intestine, familial Mg^{2+} malabsorption (TRPM6)
- Excessive fluid loss: prolonged nasogastric suction, ulcerative colitis, laxative abuse, intestinal and biliary fistulas
- Excessive urinary losses:
  - Diuretics, postobstructive, post-transplant diuresis.
  - NOTE: The use of proton pump inhibitors has been reported to be associated with hypomagnesemia in patients receiving concurrent diuretics.
  - Hypercalcemia
  - RTA
  - Hypophosphatemia
  - Drugs aminoglycosides, amphotericin, cisplatin $>>$ carboplatin, cyclosporine, EGF receptor inhibitors (e.g., cetuximab, panitumumab, matuzumab), antituberculous drugs (e.g., viomycin, capreomycin), ritodrine, β-adrenergic agonists (e.g., theophylline, salbutamol, riniterol), other drugs (amphotericin B, pentamidine, foscarnet, pamidronate, anascrine)
  - Inherited disorders:
    - Hypomagnesemia with secondary hypocalcemia: autosomal recessive mutation of TRPM6
    - Mutation affecting pro-EGF processing: normal EGF-binding to its receptor is necessary for normal trafficking of TRPM6 to the apical surface in distal convoluted tubules. Absence of EGF or presence of antibodies directed against the EGF receptor (e.g., cetuximab) can lead to urinary magnesium wasting.
    - Gitelman syndrome
    - Familial hypomagnesemia with hypercalciuria and nephrocalcinosis: Mutation of claudin 16 or 19 (tight junction proteins), autosomal recessive, age of onset: children, renal Mg^{2+} and Ca^{2+} wasting, hypomagnesemia but normal serum Ca^{2+} and K^+, nephrolithiasis and nephrocalcinosis
    - Isolated dominant hypomagnesemia (IDH): Mutation of γ-subunit of Na^+-K^+-ATPase, autosomal dominant, urine Mg^{2+} wasting but hypocalciuria. Clinically, affected individuals have hypomagnesemia but normal serum Ca^{2+} and K^+.
    - Hepatic nuclear factor 1-β mutation: HNF1B regulates transcription of FXYD2, a gene encoding γ-subunit of Na^+-K^+-ATPase; clinically same as IDH.
    - Kv1.1 mutation: reduces K^+ exit into lumen, hence reduced positive voltage that would normally favor Mg^{2+} entry via TRPM6.
    - Kir4.1/5.1: loss of function reduces basolateral K^+ recycling, hence reduced $3Na^+$-$2K^+$-ATPase activity, and favorable negative voltage for Mg^{2+} apical entry. CaSR activation reduces Kir4.1 expression.
- Others: acute pancreatitis, transfusion of citrated blood, severe burns, continuous ambulatory peritoneal dialysis, chronic alcoholism (multifactorial)
- Congenital Causes of Hypomagnesemia (Table 3.2)
- Acquired Causes of Hypomagnesemia (Table 3.3)

Table 3.2	Congenital causes of hypomagnesemia		
	Sites of Defect in Magnesium Metabolism	**Congenital**	
Gastrointestinal absorption	Passive reabsorption	—	
	Active reabsorption	TRPM6	Hypomagnesemia with secondary hypocalcemia
Cellular shift; tissue sequestration	—		—
Kidney handling	Glomerular filtration		—
	Proximal tubular reabsorption		Proximal renal tubular acidosis with or without associated Fanconi syndrome
	Thick ascending limb of loop of Henle	Claudin-16	Familial hypomagnesemia with hypercalciuria, and nephrocalcinosis
		Claudin-19	Familial hypomagnesemia, with hypercalciuria, nephrocalcinosis, and ocular manifestation
		NKCC2	Antenatal Bartter syndrome type I with low–normal serum magnesium
		ROMK	Antenatal Bartter syndrome type II with low–normal serum magnesium
		ClC-Kb	Classic Bartter syndrome type III, hypomagnesemia in 20%
		CaSR	Bartter syndrome type V
	Distal convoluted tubule:	TRPM6	Hypomagnesemia, secondary hypocalcemia
		Apical regulators/effectors of TRPM6	
		Kv1.1	Isolated autosomal-dominant hypomagnesemia
		Kir4.1/Kir5.1	Kir4.1 mutation: SeSAME/EAST syndrome; Kir5.1 mutation: hypomagnesemia, hypokalemia, hyperchloremic metabolic acidosis and hypercalciuria
		NCCT	Gitelman syndrome
		Basolateral regulators/effectors of TRPM6	
		Na$^+$-K$^+$-ATPase	FXYD2: autosomal-dominant hypomagnesemia with hypocalciuria; HNF1B: renal cysts and diabetes mellitus with renal magnesium wasting and hypocalciuria
		EGF	Isolated recessive hypomagnesemia with normocalciuria
		CaSR	Activating mutations
		CNNM2	Autosomal-dominant hypomagnesemia
		Hormonal regulators of TRPM6	
		Insulin	TRPM6 polymorphisms Ile1393Val and Lys1584Glu: reduced insulin activation of TRPM6, particularly if low dietary magnesium intake; tendency for diabetes mellitus
Other sources of loss	Nonspecific tubular injury/cellular leak		—
	Other		—

Reprinted with permission from Pham et al. Hypomagnesemia: a clinical perspective. *Int J Nephrol Renovasc Dis.* 2014;7:219.

Table 3.3	Acquired causes of hypomagnesemia		
	Sites of Defect in Magnesium Metabolism		**Acquired**
Gastrointestinal absorption	Passive reabsorption		Low dietary Mg^{2+} intake; prolonged nasogastric suction; diarrhea; enteric fistulas; steatorrhea; short-gut syndrome; alcoholism; proton pump inhibitors?
	Active reabsorption	TRPM6	Proton pump inhibitors?
Cellular shift; tissue sequestration	–		Acute pancreatitis (magnesium and calcium saponification in necrotic fat); hungry bone syndrome; refeeding syndrome; Foscarnet (magnesium incorporation into bone matrix following complex formation with foscarnet); massive blood transfusions; third trimester pregnancy; lactation; excessive parenteral alimentation; cardiopulmonary bypass
Kidney handling	Glomerular filtration		Hyperfiltration (diabetes mellitus, postobstructive or acute tubular necrosis diuresis, osmotic diuresis, post-kidney transplantation); Extracellular volume expansion; Increased filterable Mg (metabolic acidosis, low organic anions)
	Proximal tubular reabsorption		Acquired Fanconi syndrome, drug toxicity (cisplatin, gentamicin, pentamidine); high dietary salt intake
	Thick ascending limb of loop of Henle	Claudin-16	–
		Claudin-19	–
		NKCC2	Loop diuretics; hypokalemia
		ROMK	Hypokalemia
		ClC-Kb	–
		CaSR	Increase in serum calcium and magnesium; aminoglycosides
	Distal convoluted tubule:	TRPM6	Calcineurin inhibitors (cyclosporine and tacrolimus shown to reduce renal TRPM6 expression); Rapamycin (reduced TRPM6 mRNA stability); metabolic acidosis
		Apical regulators/effectors of TRPM6	
		Kv1.1	Hypokalemia
		Kir4.1/ Kir5.1	–
		NCCT	Thiazide diuretics; cyclosporine
		Basolateral regulators/effectors of TRPM6	
		Na$^+$-K$^+$-ATPase	Hypophosphatemia; calcineurin inhibitors (cyclosporin shown to inhibit Na+-K+-ATPase); ethanol (inhibits Na+-K+-ATPase activity)
		EGF	Anti-EGF receptor antibodies (cetuximab, panitumumab); cisplatin (reduced EGF and TRPM6 mRNA); cyclosporine (reduce TRPM6, NCC, EGF mRNA)
		CaSR	Increase in serum calcium and magnesium; aminoglycoside (gentamicin, amikacin); cinacalcet
		CNNM2	–
		Hormonal regulators of TRPM6	
		Insulin	Diabetes mellitus?
Other sources of loss	Nonspecific tubular injury/ cellular leak		Amphotericin; pentamidine
	Other		Severe burns (skin loss)

Reprinted with permission from Pham et al. Hypomagnesemia: a clinical perspective. *Int J Nephrol Renovasc Dis.* 2014;7:219.

Diagnosis of Hypomagnesemia: Evaluation Indices

- Total magnesium urinary loss in hypomagnesium:
  - Urinary magnesium > 20 mg/d indicates urinary Mg^{2+} wasting.
  - Urinary magnesium < 10 mg/d indicates total body Mg^{2+} depletion.
- Urinary Mg excretion may be measured as fractional excretion of Mg (FeMg) = [(urine Mg $\times$ SCr)/(0.7 $\times$ serum Mg $\times$ urine Cr)] $\times$ 100
  - Factor of 0.7 indicates only ~70% of plasma Mg is filterable.
  - Equation should only be used with relatively good kidney function.
  - FeMg $> 2\%$ to 4% indicates excessive renal Mg loss.
  - FeMg $< 2\%$ to 2.5% indicates nonrenal Mg loss.
- For GI causes of magnesium, 24-hour urine magnesium < 20 mg
- For renal magnesium loss , 24 hour urine magnesium > 20 mg
  - Conditions involving defective magnesium reabsorption at the loop of Henle will have concurrent calcium wasting, that is, urinary calcium > 250 mg/d. Examples: loop diuretics, CaSR agonists (e.g., gentamicin, cinacalcet), familial hypomagnesemia with hypercalcemia and nephrocalcinosis (claudin 16/19 mutations)
  - Conditions involving defective magnesium reabsorption at the distal tubules will have hypocalciuria, that is, urinary calcium < 200 mg/d. Examples: thiazides, Gitelman syndrome, IDH

Management of Hypomagnesemia

- Severe deficiency: Intravenous repletion for severe but non–life-threatening hypomagnesemia: 1 to 2 g/h for 3 to 6 hours then 0.5 to 1 g/h as needed to correct deficiency
- Symptomatic deficiency: Intravenous: 1 to 2 g over 15 to 60 minutes; maintenance intravenous therapy may be required to correct deficiency (0.5 to 1 g/h).
- Severe or symptomatic
  - 1 to 2 g $MgSO_4$ (in 100 mL 5% dextrose water) intravenously over 15 minutes
  - Torsades: 1 to 2 g $MgSO_4$ intravenously over 1 to 2 minutes
  - Seizures: 2 g $MgSO_4$ intravenously over 10 minutes; administration of calcium may be necessary (separate line).

> **NOTE** Intravenous magnesium supplementation causes an abrupt rise in serum Mg^{2+} level which leads to reduced reabsorption of Mg^{2+} across the thick ascending limb of the loop of Henle. This limits efficient magnesium repletion with intravenous supplementation.

- Aldosterone has been suggested to induce renal Mg^{2+} wasting, an effect that may be ameliorated by aldosterone antagonists (spironolactone, eplerenone).

Caution with Excessive Mg^{2+} Supplementation

- Drug interactions: central nervous system (CNS) depressants (barbiturates, hypnotics, narcotics, antihistamines, antidepressants); cardiac glycosides; neuromuscular blocking agents (pancuronium)
- Side effects (dose related): flushing, sweating, hypotension, depressed reflexes, flaccid paralysis, hypothermia, circulatory collapse, cardiac and CNS depression proceeding to respiratory paralysis. Hypocalcemia with signs of tetany secondary to $MgSO_4$ therapy for eclampsia has been reported.

HYPERMAGNESEMIA

Clinical Manifestations of Hypermagnesemia

- Signs/symptoms: Muscular weakness, paralysis, ataxia, drowsiness, confusion, paralytic ileus, bladder paralysis, nausea/vomiting, hypotension, bradycardia, absent tendon reflexes, hypoventilation (everything slows down)
- Associated electrolyte changes: hypocalcemia (due to suppressed PTH secretion and possible Mg^{2+} binding and activation of CaSR)
- ECG changes:
  - Increased PR and QT
  - Increased QRS duration
  - Variable decrease in P-wave voltage
  - Variable degree of T-wave peaking
  - Complete AV block
  - Asystole
- Other effects: hypoparathyroidism, vascular relaxation, interference with platelet adhesiveness, thrombin-generation time and clotting time.
- NOTE: Hyperkalemia may occur due to suppression of K^+ secretion. This is possibly due to Mg^{2+}-gate keeping function in ROMK: Mg^{2+} normally keeps ROMK closed and limits K^+ wasting.

Causes of Hypermagnesemia

- Kidney failure, rhabdomyolysis, tumor lysis
- Excessive intake: oral, infusion, magnesium-containing enemas, Dead Sea water drowning (very high content of both calcium and magnesium), parenteral, urethral irrigation; common Mg^{2+}-containing medications: laxatives (milk of magnesia), antacids (extra-strength Rolaids)
- Redistribution: acute acidosis
- Others: familial hypocalciuric hypercalemia, diabetic ketoacidosis, lithium, milk-alkali syndrome, theophylline toxicity, adrenal insufficiency, hypothyroidism

Treatment of Hypermagnesemia

- Antagonizing magnesium:
  - Calcium: ~100 to 200 mg *elemental* Ca^{2+} infused over 5 to 10 minutes
  - One 10 mL ampule of Ca^{2+} gluconate contains 90 mg of elemental calcium
  - One 10 mL ampule of Ca^{2+} chloride contains 272 mg of elemental calcium
- Removal of magnesium:
  - Dialysis
  - Use of loop diuretics (NOTE: loop diuretics can lower Ca^{2+} and facilitate development of arrhythmias in patients with hypermagnesemia!!! Calcium is a natural antagonist of Mg^{2+}.)
- Cardiopulmonary support

NOTE
- Magnesium can potentiate the hypotensive effect of calcium channel blockers (CCB) and can cause severe hypotension in preeclamptic/eclamptic patients treated with both. Treatment: calcium gluconate
- Both hypo- and hypermagnesemia can reduce PTH secretion.

KIDNEY STONES

Definitions

- Nephrolithiasis refers to *intratubular* stone deposits.
- Nephrocalcinosis refers *to interstitial* stone deposits in cortex and medulla.
- Both may occur in the same patient.

Epidemiology

- Lifetime risks: 5% to 10% of US women, 10% to 20% of US men
- Male-to-female ratio = 2:1
- Prevalence: 2% to 7%; prevalence increases until age 70 in males and 60 in females.
- Annual incidence: 0.6% to 1.5%
- Age: peak incidence at third to fourth decade
- Race: More common in Caucasians, followed by African Americans, Hispanics, Asians
- More prevalent in Southeast United States: thought to be due to hot climate, inadequate fluid intake
- Recurrence: probability of second stone at 1 year: 15%; 5 years: 35% to 40%; 10 years: 50% to 65%, 20 years: 70% to 85%
- Medical conditions associated with increased stone risk: hypertension, diabetes, obesity, metabolic syndrome, gout
- Risks for eventual ESRD are thought to be associated with urologic complications (e.g., history of hydronephrosis, recurrent urinary tract infections, acquired single kidney, neurogenic bladder, ileal conduit).
- There are data to suggest increased fracture incidence and risk of cardiovascular disease associated with kidney stones.

Stone Types and Prevalence in the United States

- Calcium (60% to 80%): of all calcium stones, most common type is mixed calcium oxalate and phosphate (37%), followed by calcium oxalate (26%), and calcium phosphate (7%) (Fig. 3.8)

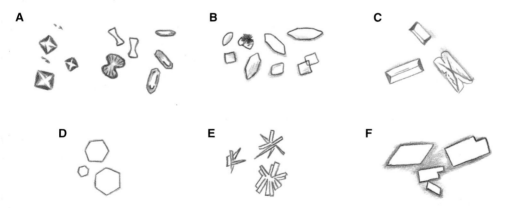

FIGURE 3.8 Stone crystals. **A.** Calcium oxalate (octahedral, dumbbell, or picket fence-shaped): may be seen with ethylene glycol toxicity or hypercalciuria. **B.** Uric acid (platelike, rhomboid, or square-shaped): seen in pH < 7.0; may be seen in tumor lysis syndrome; **C.** Struvite ("coffin lid" or fern-leaf like if freshly formed): consist of ammonium, magnesium, and phosphate; **D.** Cystine (hexagonal): seen in cystinosis, not seen in normal urine. **E.** Calcium phosphate (blunt-ended needles, prisms, or rosette): may also appear amorphous as urate, but unlike urate, they precipitate at urine pH > 7.0. Additionally, unlike the pinkish color with urate, calcium phosphate crystals are colorless or white. **F.** Cholesterol plates.

- Uric acid (10% to 15%); NOTE: The incidence of uric acid stone is on the rise in the United States and thought to be associated with the increased incidence of metabolic syndrome.
- Struvite (10% to 15%)
- Cystine (<1%)
- Other (<1%)

Stone Inhibitors and Promoters

- Inhibitors:
  - Inorganic:
    - Mg^{2+}
      - Mg^{2+} complexes with oxalate thereby decreases calcium oxalate supersaturation.
      - Mg^{2+} may also reduce gut oxalate absorption.
      - Higher dietary Mg^{2+} has been shown to be associated with a 30% lower risk of stone formation in men, but not in women.
    - Pyrophosphate: forms highly soluble complexes with Ca^{2+}
    - Citrate: citrate binds to calcium to form a soluble complex in urine, thus reduces Ca^{2+} availability for calcium phosphate/oxalate formation.
  - Organic: nephrocalcin, urinary prothrombin fragment 1, protease inhibitor: inter-α-inhibitor, glycosaminoglycans
  - High urine flow: MOST effective inhibitor (i.e., intervention) in stone prevention.
- Promoters:
  - Randall plaque: subepithelial calcification in the renal papilla that acts as an anchor for calcium oxalate crystals and is considered to be the initiating event in renal stone formation
  - Urinary factors that can promote supersaturation and crystallization:
    - Sodium: Ca^{2+} is reabsorbed passively in parallel with Na^+ in the proximal tubules. Low dietary sodium leads to enhanced proximal tubular Na^+ reabsorption, hence Ca^{2+} reabsorption, thus leaving less intratubular Ca^{2+} for stone formation.
    - High levels of stone substrates: calcium, oxalate, urate, phosphate, cystine
    - Low urine pH: facilitates uric acid, cystine precipitation
    - High urine pH: facilitates calcium phosphate precipitation. NOTE: although triple phosphate stones (also known as magnesium ammonium phosphate or struvite) are seen in high urine pH, it is the ammonia concentration that is the primary factor for the triple phosphate crystals formation. Alkalinization of a urine specimen with ammonia generates triple phosphates while alkalinization with sodium hydroxide does not.
    - Low urine flow
    - Bacterial products

Clinical Manifestations

- Pain depends on stone location:
  - Intrarenal stone: asymptomatic unless pyelonephritis or obstruction with distention of renal capsule
  - Proximal ureter: colicky flank or anterior abdominal pain
  - Distal third ureter: flank pain radiating to groin/genitals
  - Ureterovesicular junction: suprapubic pain, urgency, dysuria
  - Bladder neck: suprapubic pain, anuria, gross hematuria

- Hematuria: ranges from none to microscopic to gross hematuria
- Pyuria: may be sterile due to inflammation or occur with concurrent urinary tract infection/pyelonephritis

General Dietary Advice for Unknown Stone Types

- Increase fluid intake to assure urine output > 2.0 to 2.5 L/d or a volume of approximately 3% of body weight (kg) daily. Example: 70 kg person should drink enough to ensure a urine volume of at least $0.03 \times 70 = 2.1$ L/d.
- Good dietary dairy calcium, potassium, and phytate. Avoid grapefruit juice (particularly if calcium oxalate stone, mechanism unknown) and high volume of cranberry juice (increased urinary saturation of calcium oxalate) daily. Coffee, tea, milk, and alcohol increase urine flow, which effectively inhibit stone formation.
- Decrease intake of animal protein, sucrose, fructose, (sodas), sodium, excessive supplemental calcium, vitamin D, and vitamin C (metabolize to oxalate).

> **NOTE**   *Dietary* calcium (e.g., dairy) is protective, whereas *supplemental* calcium (medication) may increase stone risk. Dietary calcium may bind oxalate and prevent gut oxalate absorption. Supplemental calcium, particularly when taken in between meals, predominantly leads to increased gut Ca^{2+} absorption and subsequent hypercalciuria, hence potential for increased stone risk. Dietary calcium restriction is *not recommended*. For patients who require calcium supplement, monitor urine calcium and titrate calcium supplement to keep urine calcium excretion < 70% of upper limit of normal.

Specific Stones

Calcium Stones

- Mixed calcium oxalate and phosphate are most common, followed by calcium oxalate, then calcium phosphate in the US.
- When calcium phosphate is main constituent, that is >50% composition:
  - Urine pH is higher than that observed with calcium oxalate
  - Types of calcium phosphate stones: calcium apatite (main constituents of bones/teeth), calcium brushite (Calcium monohydrate phosphate: physically resistant to extracorporeal shock-wave lithotripsy (ESWL); may need repeated treatments)
- Nephrocalcinosis is common in patients with distal RTA (type 1) (Fig. 3.9)

Metabolic factors for calcium stones:
- Hypercalciuria (40% to 60%):
  - Idiopathic
  - Absorptive hypercalciuria: autosomal dominant, jejunal mucosa is hyperresponsive to vitamin D
  - Renal hypercalciuria:
    - Impaired renal tubular Ca^{2+} reabsorption, for example, Dent disease (hypercalciuria with nephrocalcinosis), neonatal Bartter syndromes, familial hypomagnesemia with hypercalciuria and nephrocalcinosis (mutation of claudin 16/19—See Hypomagnesemia section), distal RTA, medullary sponge kidney, horseshoe kidney
    - Loss of function mutation of vitamin D-24-hydroxylase, the enzyme that inactivates 1,25-vitamin D. Recall treatment is ketoconazole. See Hypercalcemia Section.

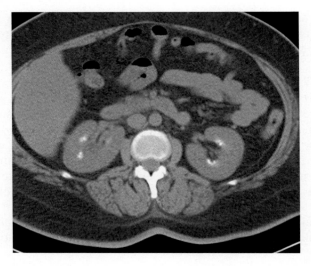

FIGURE 3.9 Medullary nephrocalcinosis. Axial and coronal noncontract CT images showing amorphous and course pyramidal calcifications in both kidneys consistent with medullary nephrocalcinosis.

- To be proven: Altered CaSR function that could lead to: (1) reduced Ca^{2+} reabsorption at the thick ascending limb of Henle loop, (2) reduced proximal tubular reabsorption of phosphate, and (3) reduced both urinary acidification and inhibitory activity against ADH at the collecting duct, all of which act in concert to increase calcium phosphate precipitation in distal nephrons.
- Resorptive hypercalciuria: increased bone resorption in primary hPTH
- Hyperuricosuria: Dissolved uric acid salts appear to increase calcium oxalate precipitation via unclear mechanism(s).
- "Renal phosphate leak" due to the following:
  - Mutations in the renal phosphate cotransporters
  - Either increased FGF-23 or presence of an allelic variant (FGF23716T)
- Hyperoxaluria
  - Dietary causes of hyperoxaluria:
    - Low calcium in diet allows free oxalate to be absorbed readily in gut which is then eliminated into urine. In contrast, concurrent high dietary calcium intake, for example, dairy products, leads to calcium oxalate formation in gut and is eliminated.
    - High intake of protein, oxalate, or its precursor (ethylene glycol, methoxyflurane anesthesia, or large doses of ascorbic acid in susceptible individuals)
  - Enteric causes of hyperoxaluria:
    - Slc26a6 anion transporter: knockout mice model has increased gastrointestinal oxalate absorption.
    - Fat malabsorption (e.g., inflammatory bowel disease/resection/bypass, exocrine pancreatic insufficiency). Undigested fatty acids bind calcium, hence less calcium availability to bind oxalate in gut for gut elimination. This leads to increased intestinal oxalate absorption, hence urinary oxalate excretion.

> **NOTE** Although inflammatory bowel disease (e.g., Crohns disease) is associated with increased risk of calcium oxalate stones, chronic diarrhea or colitis (e.g., ulcerative colitis) with resultant chronic metabolic acidosis may also lead to increased risk for uric acid stones.

> **NOTE** Presence of gut *Oxalobacter formigenes is thought to be protective against the risk of kidney stones: O. formigenes* is a gram-negative bacteria that degrade gut oxalate. Colonized patients have been shown to have reduced oxaluria under controlled, standardized diet. An association between *O. formigenes* colonization and reduced number of stone episodes (recurrence) has also been shown.

- Primary hyperoxaluria:
  - Autosomal recessive disorders due to mutations of enzymes involved in hepatic glyoxylate metabolism, resulting in excessive production and urinary excretion of oxalate (PH types 1 and 2, PH1 and PH2)
  - PH1: Mutation or mistargeting of alanine glyoxylate aminotransferase (AGT) results in buildup of glyoxylate and increased oxalate. Since pyridoxine (vitamin B6) is a cofactor for the causative enzyme (AGT) in PH1, pyridoxine administration can reduce urine oxalate levels in a subset of PH1 patients (i.e., patients with the AGT C.508 G > A allele).
  - PH2: Mutation of a protein with dual enzymatic activities, glyoxylate reductase and hydroxypyruvate reductase, results in the accumulation of hydroxypyruvate and glyoxylate, precursors of L-glycerate and oxalate, respectively
  - PH3: Another yet-to-be-identified genetic cause of hyperoxaluria.
  - Wide outcome variability for PH patients, but typically result in death from kidney failure and oxalosis without aggressive therapy
- Hypocitriuria:
  - Chronic metabolic acidosis, RTA (reduces luminal citrate):
    - Citrate exists as a divalent ($citrate^{2-}$) or trivalent ($citrate^{3-}$) anion.
    - $Citrate^{2-} + HCO_3^- \rightarrow Citrate^{3-} + CO_2 + H_2O$. In metabolic acidosis (i.e., lack of HCO_3^-), there are more $citrate^{2-}$ than $citrate^{3-}$.
    - Proximal tubular reabsorption of $citrate^{2-}$ occurs more readily than that of $citrate^{3-}$, leaving less citrate in tubular lumen.
    - Intracellular acidosis associated with metabolic acidosis also promotes citrate mitochondrial uptake and metabolism, hence lower cytoplasmic concentration. This results in a more favorable chemical gradient for tubular citrate reabsorption, leaving less citrate in tubular lumen.
  - Inflammatory bowel disease
  - Idiopathic
- Others: Vitamin A deficiency (associated with reduced urinary concentration of stone inhibitors glycosaminoglycans and citrate and increased urinary calcium and oxalate excretion), hot climates, immobilization, urinary tract anomalies

Management of Calcium Stones

- Dietary advice:
  - Fluid intake to ensure urine volume ≥ 2.0 to 2.5 L/d or volume of approximately 3% of body weight (kg) daily.

- Protective fluids: coffee, tea, beer, wine which can increase urine output and flow
  - Fluids that can increase stone risks: sugar-sweetened sodas, fruit punch, grapefruit juice, cranberry juice.
  - Sugar-sweetened drinks (sucrose, fructose) can increase stone risk; likely via increased urinary calcium, uric acid, and/or oxalate excretion
- Sodium restriction (2 to 2.3 g or 88 to 100 mmol daily)
- **High** dietary calcium intake from either nondairy or dairy sources (NOT in between meals calcium supplements) is protective against stones.
- Avoid excess animal protein intake
- Increase fruit and vegetable intake → increase citrate excretion
- Dietary oxalate restriction if calcium oxalate stones *and continue only if* urine excretion of oxalate is effectively reduced (e.g., avoid dark green leafy vegetables such as spinach, rhubarb, nuts, chocolate). If not effective, discontinue dietary oxalate restriction.
- Medications:
  - Consider medical therapy if dietary trial × 3 to 6 months does not improve urine chemical profile or evidence of increasing stone formation (increase in size/number)
  - If hypercalciuria is present:
    - Thiazide (watch for hypokalemia and treat as needed) ± low-dose K^+-sparing amiloride to increase Ca^{2+} reabsorption. Avoid triamterene due to possible crystallization and precipitation of the drug.
      - If thiazide/amiloride intolerance:
        - 40 to 60 mmol of $K-HCO_3$ or K-citrate daily. Alkalinization may both improve citrate excretion and reduce Ca^{2+} excretion. Avoid alkalinization with $NaHCO_3$ as Na^+ load increases urinary Ca^{2+} excretion. Must monitor urine pH and serum K^+ with K-salt alkalinization. NOTE: pH > 6.5 may facilitate calcium phosphate precipitation.
        - Administration of orthophosphate: reduce Ca^{2+} excretion and increase excretion of calcium stone inhibitors (pyrophosphate). Clinical effectiveness not clear.
- If hyperoxaluria is present:
  - Dietary restriction of fat and oxalate is effective in reduction of oxaluria
  - Consider pyrophosphate
  - Pyridoxine (vitamin B_6), particularly if primary hyperoxaluria type 1: Vitamin B_6 may reduce oxalate production and urinary oxalate excretion. It has been suggested to reduce risk of stone formation in women, not men.
  - For enteric hyperoxaluria, consider oral calcium carbonate or citrate (1 to 4 g daily) **WITH** meals to bind oxalate in intestinal lumen.
  - Cholestyramine binds both bile acids and oxalate, but side effects may be limiting factor.
- If hypocitraturia is present:
  - Consider adding 4 oz of lemon juice to 2 L of water daily (without added sugar)
  - Urine alkalinization to increase urinary citrate levels:
    - Lumen $Citrate^{2-} + HCO_3^-$ (from alkalinization) → $Citrate^{3-} + CO_2 + H_2O$. Reabsorption of $citrate^{3-}$ at proximal tubules (via Na-citrate cotransporter in luminal membrane) is lower than that of $citrate^{2-}$, hence higher luminal citrate availability.
    - Alkalinization also reduces intracellular citrate metabolism, resulting in higher intracellular citrate concentration. The higher intracellular citrate concentration leads to less favorable chemical gradient for tubular citrate reabsorption, hence higher luminal citrate availability. NOTE: hypokalemia

induces intracellular acidosis, hence increased intracellular citrate metabolism, lower intracellular citrate levels, and more favorable chemical gradient for tubular citrate reabsorption.

- If hypermagnesuria is present: magnesium supplement only if serum magnesium is also low. NOTE: treatment with magnesium has not been shown to reduce stone recurrence.
- If hyperuricosuria is present: consider allopurinol if there is hyperuricosuria in the absence of hypercalciuria or hyperoxaluria (ongoing study with the xanthine oxidase inhibitor febuxostat versus allopurinol versus placebo). NOTE: uric acid is no longer thought to act as nidus for calcium stones. Nonetheless, the use of allopurinol in calcium stone formers with hyperuricemia has been shown to reduce the likelihood of calcium oxalate stone recurrence.

Uric Acid Stones

Metabolic factors for uric acid stones:
- Low urine pH
- Defect in ammoniagenesis: NH_3 buffers urine pH. The lack of NH_3 results in low urine pH.
- Conditions associated with hyperuricosuria:
  - Gout, purine overproduction: myeloproliferative disorder, acute leukemia, glycogen storage disease, malignancy
  - Metabolic syndrome, obesity, diabetes mellitus, insulin resistant:
    - Excessive dietary acid intake and/or increased endogenous acid production
    - Defective NH_4^+ excretion
    - Absence of inhibitors or presence of promoters of uric acid precipitation

Management of Uric Acid Stones

- Urine alkalinization:
  - K-citrate 10 to 20 mmol bid-tid. This is the MOST important intervention for uric acid stones. Urinary alkalinization with citrate is thought to be more important than reducing uricosuria.
  - For uric acid stone formers who do not respond to alkali therapy, increase a morning or add a mid-day dose of alkali to correct the urinary pH fall that may occur late afternoon and evening.
  - K-citrate is more effective at reducing calcium oxalate supersaturation than sodium bicarbonate. Sodium bicarbonate increases urine sodium excretion and associated urine calcium.
- Reduction in uricosuria:
  - Xanthine oxidase inhibitors (allopurinol or febuxostat): reduce urinary uric acid excretion
  - Reduction of purine dietary intake
- Control or modify risk factors for metabolic syndrome

Struvite Stones a.k.a. Triple Phosphate Stones

- Composition: magnesium ammonium phosphate (struvite) and calcium carbonate-apatite. Also known as "triple phosphate": phosphate is present in its trivalent form and combines with three cations: NH_4^+, Mg^{2+}, Ca^{2+}
- Associated with anatomical abnormalities, obstruction of pelviureteric junction, calyceal diverticulum, horseshoe kidney, tubular ectasia (medullary sponge kidney), ureterocele, vesicoureteral reflux, ureteral stricture

- Urinary infection with urea splitting organisms (urease-producing organisms): *Proteus, Hemophilus, Yersinia, Klebsiella, Serratia, Citrobacter, Staphylococcus, Mycoplasma, Pseudomonas*

Management of Struvite Stones

- Treatment of underlying infections (culture specific)
- Stone removal: percutaneous nephrolithotomy > combination shock wave lithotripsy and percutaneous lithotomy > open surgery
- 4 to 6 months of suppressive low-dose antibiotics (: cephalexin, quinolones, sulfamethoxazole-trimethoprim, or nitrofurantoin (contraindicated for CrCl < 60 mL/min)
- Medical therapy: urease inhibitor acetohydroxamic acid (Lithostat) 250 mg three to four times daily
  - Reserve for patients who cannot or refuse to undergo stone removal.
  - Inadequate urinary drug level if SCr > 2 mg/dL
  - Significant side effects (40% to 60%): headaches, hemolytic anemia (15% to 20%), depression, dyspepsia, diarrhea, hallucination, palpitations, sweating, deep vein thrombosis, pulmonary embolism
- Mandatory follow-up of stone size in 3 to 4 months
- Correction of anatomical abnormality whenever possible

Cystine Stones

- Autosomal recessive (may be autosomal dominant with incomplete penetrance)
- Mutations of renal epithelial cell transporters resulting in reduced reabsorption and increased urine excretion of dibasic amino acids including cystine, ornithine, lysine, arginine (COLA). Of all these amino acids, cystine is the only crystal that is highly insoluble and forms stones.
- Renal tubular immaturity in infants, Wilson disease, and Fanconi syndrome are other causes of elevated urinary cystine levels.
- ~20% to 40% are mixed stones
- Homozygous cystinuria:
  - Lifelong, recurrent urolithiasis that is difficult to manage surgically or medically.
  - >50% of asymptomatic homozygotes develop kidney stones.
  - 75% present with bilateral calculi.
  - Typical age of onset is in the second or third decade of life; 25% in first decade; 30% to 40% in teenage years

Management of Cystine Stones

- High fluid intake 3.5 to 5.0 L/d. Note this is much higher than other types of stones. Watch for hyponatremia.
- Alkalinization of urine 40 to 80 mmol of K-citrate/day (urine pH > 7.0)
- Reduction of sodium and protein intake to reduce urinary cystine excretion
- If all else failed, use drugs that form heterodimers with cysteine, thus competing for cysteine–cysteine disulfide bond formation, the insoluble cystine.
  - D-penicillamine
  - α-mercaptopropionylglycine (tiopronin); (Both D-penicillamine and tiopronin have significant side effects: loss of taste, fever, proteinuria, serum sickness-type reactions, nephrotic syndrome)
  - Captopril (side effect: hypotension)

Drug-Associated Stones

- Calcium stone formation: loop diuretics (enhance urinary calcium excretion); vitamin D; glucocorticoids (bone resorption); calcium-containing antacids; theophylline (interferes with pyridoxine metabolism and worsens oxaluria in primary oxaluria type 1); acetazolamide, topirate (both agents alkalinize urine via inhibition of carbonic anhydrase and thereby increase risk of calcium phosphate stones); amphotericin B (alkalinize urine due to H^+-back leak); high dose (i.e., $>>$500 mg/d) vitamin C (metabolized to oxalate)
- Uric acid stone formation: probenecid
- Common medications that may crystallize into stones: triamterene, acyclovir (high intravenous dose, e.g., treatment dose for encephalitis), indinavir, allopurinol (xanthine stones)

Stone Diagnosis

- Imaging studies:
  - Ultrasound versus noncontrast helical computed tomography (CT):
    - Ultrasound may miss ureteral stones < 3 mm
    - Cost, availability
    - Radiation exposure with CT
    - Contrast-enhanced CT may be required to diagnose indinavir stones.
  - Plain film (Kidney–Ureter–Bladder, KUB):
    - Detects calcium stones > 5 mm
    - Low dose of radiation
    - Inexpensive
  - Magnetic resonance imaging: poor tool for visualizing stones
  - Intravenous pyelogram: contrast dye exposure
  NOTE: Radiologic trivia:
- Radiolucent "stones" on KUB:
  - Uric acid and xanthine stones
  - Case report of pseudoephedrine/guaifenesin stone
  - Cystine and struvite stones are often but not always radiopaque.
- Staghorn-appearing stones are typically associated with struvite, but may be seen in other stone types: struvite (triple phosphate, magnesium ammonium phosphate) $>>$ calcium carbonate apatite $>$ cystine, uric acid stones
- Biochemical evaluation:
  - First-time uncomplicated stone presentation: Minimal evaluation:
    - Basic chemistry, SCa, phosphorus, uric acid
    - Routine urinalysis; consider 24-hour urine for volume, creatinine, pH, calcium, oxalate, citrate, uric acid
    - Complete metabolic profile evaluation outlined below is optional.
  - Indications for complete metabolic profile evaluation:
    - Recurrent stone or bilateral stone disease
    - Family history of stones
    - Presence of inflammatory bowel disease, malabsorption
    - Past medical history with any of gout, RTA, primary hPTH, osteoporosis or pathologic skeletal fractures, nephrocalcinosis, or bariatric surgery
    - Struvite, cystine, uric acid, or calcium phosphate
    - Pediatric patients.
  - Complete metabolic profile evaluation:

- Analysis of stone composition if available
- Two 24-hour urine collections (one during usual daily activities and diet, i.e., workday, and one during resting day, i.e., weekend to evaluate for work-related factors) for volume, creatinine (for estimate of collection adequacy), pH (hint to type of stone), Na^+ (relevant in calcium stones), stone substrates: Ca^{2+}, oxalate, uric acid, cystine (if young age or strong family history of cystine stones), ammonium, stone inhibitors: citrate, Mg^{2+}, K^+, dietary protein intake: SO_4^{2-} (high content of sulfate-containing amino acids reflects animal protein intake), urea nitrogen
- Laboratory calculations of urinary supersaturation of stone substrates if available
- Serum: full chemistry including calcium, phosphate, magnesium, uric acid
- If SCa is high or high–normal, obtain PTH, 1,25 vitamin D, chest X-Ray (sarcoidosis). Consider urine PCR for mycobacterium tuberculosis in endemic areas.

Management of Kidney Stones: General Considerations

Stone passage depends on stone location and stone size:
- Stone location: Proximal stones are less likely than distal stones to pass spontaneously.
- Stone size:
  - <5 mm, spontaneous passing rate up to 95%
  - 5 to 8 mm, spontaneous passing rate 60% to 70%
  - ≥8 mm, spontaneous passing rate ~10% to 20%
Pain control:
- NSAIDS if no volume depletion, kidney disease, gastrointestinal bleed, or contraindications:
  - Low cost
  - Inhibit prostaglandin mediated pain pathways
  - Decrease ureteral contractility
  - Stop NSAIDS at least 3 days prior to shock-wave lithotripsy to minimize bleeding risks.
- Otherwise use opioids: faster onset of pain relief compared with NSAIDS but concerns for abuse potential
- Combination of NSAIDS and opioids may be considered.

UROLOGIC MANAGEMENT OPTIONS
(AMERICAN UROLOGICAL ASSOCIATION: EVIDENCE-BASED RECOMMENDATIONS TO GUIDE CHOICE OF MODALITY)

- <10 mm: Observation if pain is controlled and no evidence of obstruction or infection. Initiate medical expulsion therapy below.
- Medical expulsion therapy (MET):
  - 4 to 6 week trial of α-blockers (e.g., tamsulosin) or CCB, (e.g., nifedipine only if hypertensive, watch for reflex tachycardia) ± low-dose glucocorticoid (e.g., prednisone 20 to 25 mg daily × 10 days)
  - Rationale for α-blockers:
    - Inhibit basal ureteral tone and peristaltic frequency and decrease intensity of ureteral contractions, thereby facilitating stone passage
    - Slightly faster stone passage compared with CCB

- Urology consult if MET fails:
  - Symptomatic smaller stones that do not pass: ESWL/ureteroscopy
  - Larger or more complex stones, impacted stones in proximal ureter: percutaneous nephrolithotomy
  - Altered anatomy (previous surgeries, malignancy, etc.): open/laparoscopic surgery

Indications for urgent urologic consult:

- Presence of infection with urinary tract obstruction
- Urosepsis
- Intractable pain or vomiting, or both
- Acute kidney failure
- Obstruction in solitary or transplanted kidney
- Bilateral obstructing stones

MONITORING RESPONSE

- 24-hour urine collection after 6 to 8 weeks for chemical profile, pH, and volume. Note that follow-up measurement of urine calcium level may *not* be a reliable predictor of treatment effectiveness for reducing stone recurrence risk. Increased fluid intake, however, has been shown to significantly reduce risk of stone recurrence over 5 year follow-up.
- Imaging studies: helical CT or ultrasound at 1 year. If negative, repeat in 2 to 4 years depending on findings.

Access the eBook for self-assessment questions.

4

Chronic Kidney Disease

Golriz Jafari, Phuong-Thu T. Pham, and Phuong-Chi T. Pham

ASSESSMENT

Chronic kidney disease (CKD) is classified based on (1) cause, (2) glomerular filtration rate (GFR) category, and (3) albuminuria category.

Glomerular Filtration Rate (GFR)

- GFR is traditionally estimated based on clearance of a solute that is 100% freely filtered.
- GFR is used to define CKD, guide routine care, evaluate and manage expected complications of CKD, assess CKD progression, determine drug dosing, and assess prognosis.
- Traditionally, creatinine has been used as the "solute" of choice because creatinine is relatively freely filtered. Recall that clearance of any solute is UV/P, where U and P are the concentrations of the solute in the urine and plasma respectively, and V is the urine volume per unit time. Clearance of creatinine is traditionally used to approximate GFR, that is creatinine clearance ~ GFR, or

$$GFR = [\text{urine creatinine concentration}] \times \text{urine volume}/ [\text{plasma creatinine concentration}]$$

- The ideal solute for calculation of GFR should be
  - Naturally made (endogenous) in the plasma
  - 100% freely filtered by the glomerulus
  - Not secreted by renal tubules
  - Not reabsorbed by renal tubules

Limitations of using creatinine as a marker of GFR:
- Creatinine level may reflect muscle mass and dietary intake independent of glomerular filtration.
- Creatinine levels are typically in the low-normal range for elderly patients or patients with malnutrition, limb amputation(s), or cirrhosis (reduced hepatic creatine synthesis, volume overload/dilutional). Creatinine in the high-normal range may be normal in muscular young individuals.

> **NOTE**
> - A solute that is both filtered by the glomerulus and secreted by the tubules (e.g., creatinine) will overestimate the GFR, since there will be more solute in the urine than if the solute comes from filtration alone. Additionally, tubular creatinine secretion is upregulated in advanced CKD which can further overestimate GFR in this patient population.
> - A solute that is both filtered by the glomerulus and reabsorbed by the tubules (e.g., urea) will underestimate the GFR, since less solute will be seen in the urine than if the solute comes from filtration alone.
> - For reasons above, GFR estimates from 24-hour urine collection in advanced CKD are typically calculated as the average of creatinine and urea clearances.
> - Alternatively, drugs that competitively inhibit tubular secretion of creatinine may be used prior to and during the 24-hour urine collection for a better assessment of GFR. Cimetidine may be used for this purpose.

- Creatinine and urea clearances require a 24-hour urine collection and can be cumbersome.

Other Methods to Estimate GFR

- Use of exogenous filtration markers (in lieu of SCr): inulin, iothalamate, iohexol, ethylenediaminetetraacetic acid, and diethylenetriainepentaacetic acid. These markers are chelated to radioisotopes for easy detection with nuclear scanning. In clinical settings where determination of exact kidney function is necessary (i.e., evaluation of potential kidney donor's kidney function), GFR as measured by inulin or iothalamate may be obtained.
- Equations to estimate GFR (eGFR):
  - Cockcroft–Gault (CG) formula (dependent variables: age, gender, weight, SCr):
    - Male: CrCl (mL/min) = [(140 − age) × weight (kg)]/[72 × SCr (mg/dL)]
    - Female: same as formula for male above × 0.85 (empirical correction factor for presumed lower muscle mass in females)
    - Note CG formula is in mL/min. To normalize to 1.73 m^2 body surface area (BSA), multiply CrCl above by the ratio (1.73 m^2/patient's BSA).
    - Limitations of CG formula:
      - CrCl is overestimated in patients with overweight or volume overload (because the weight term is in the numerator).
      - eGFR is likely overestimated because it is based on creatinine clearance, not true GFR. Tubular creatinine secretion is not accounted for.
      - CG formula is based on old methods of SCr measurement and may not be accurate with modern SCr measurements.
      - Traditionally, CG formula has been used for drug-dosing. However, it is now controversial whether CG would be accurate for drug-dosing purposes with modern SCr measurements.
  - Modification of Diet in Renal Disease (MDRD) Study:
    - Derived from patients with CKD
    - MDRD equations were derived based on urinary clearance of ^{125}I-iothalamate.
    - MDRD-4 variables (age, gender, race [African American vs. non-African American], calibrated standardized SCr). The latter (SCr) should be measured by specific assay traceable to the international standard reference materials and minimal bias compared to isotope-dilution mass spectrometry (IDMS) reference methodology.

- MDRD-6 variables (age, gender, race [African American vs. non-African American], calibrated standardized Scr, albumin, blood urea nitrogen [BUN])

$$eGFR = 170 \times SCr^{-0.999} \times age^{-0.176} \times [0.762 \text{ if female}] \times [1.180 \text{ if black}] \times BUN^{-0.17} \times Albumin^{0.318}$$

- Limitations of MDRD equations:
  - *Underestimate* GFR in patients with GFR > 60 mL/min/1.73 m^2 which over-report incidence of CKD. Many laboratories report eGFR greater than 60 as ">60 mL/min/1.73 m^2" rather than an actual calculated value due to inaccurate estimates in patients with higher GFR range.
  - Not validated in geriatric patients, children, and pregnant women
  - Not validated in nonsteady states such as acute kidney injury
  - Not derived for races other than "White" or "African American"
  - Both MDRD-4 and CG overestimate true GFR in sick hospitalized patients. Incorporation of BUN and albumin (MDRD-6) partially improves GFR estimates.
- Chronic Kidney Disease Epidemiology Collaboration (CKD-EPI):
  - Derived from large database of research studies' participants with diverse characteristics including those with and without CKD, diabetes mellitus (DM), and known organ transplantation.
  - Dependent variables are similar to those used in MDRD-4 and include: age, gender, White or Black race, SCr
  - Derived based on either serum creatinine alone CKD-EPI(creat), cystatin C alone CKD-EPI(cys), or both SCr and cystatin C CKD-EPI(creat-cys)
    - Compared to CKD-EPI(creat), CKD-EPI(cys) is not more accurate in estimating measured GFR, but is more accurate for estimating GFR in patients with low BMI and more accurate for risk predictions.
    - Compared to either CKD-EPI(creat) or CKD-EPI(cys) alone, combined CKD-EPI(creat-cys) is more accurate for estimating GFR.
  - CKD-EPI(creat) equation:

$$eGFR = 141 \times min(SCr/k,1)^a \times max(SCr/k,1)^{-1.209} \times 0.993^{age} \times [1.018 \text{ if female} \times [1.159 \text{ if black}],$$

where SCr is serum creatinine (mg/dL), k is 0.7 for females and 0.9 for males, a is -0.329 for females and -0.411 for males, min indicates the minimum of SCr/k or 1, and max indicates the maximum of SCr/k or 1.

- Advantages of CKD-EPI over MDRD:
  - Similar accuracy as MRDR for GFR < 60 mL/min/1.73 m^2
  - Better accuracy for eGFR > 60 mL/min/1.73 m^2
  - Lower CKD prevalence (since CKD-EPI(SCr) is better at estimating higher GFR)
  - Better accuracy for risk predictions
  - Applicable across more diverse population
- Advantages of MDRD over CKD-EPI: MDRD performs better and provides better accuracy in estimating GFR in severely obese individuals.
- The use of Cystatin C in lieu of SCr:
  - Cystatin is a cationic low-molecular-weight cysteine proteinase inhibitor that is produced at a constant rate by all nucleated cells. It is 99% filtered by glomerulus and metabolized by proximal tubular cells.

- Serum cystatin C level may thus reflect GFR.
- Normal range:
  - Both males and females: age 20 to 50: 0.70 to 1.21 mg/L; age > 50: 0.84 to 1.55 mg/L
  - Young healthy individuals: 0.53 to 0.95 mg/L
- Advantages of using cystatin C over creatinine:
  - Cystatin C may more accurately estimate GFR than SCr in patients with reduced muscle mass (e.g., liver disease, neuromuscular disease).
  - Cystatin C may detect acute kidney injury (AKI) earlier than SCr.
  - Cystatin C has been reported to be a better predictor of deaths from cardiovascular causes and CKD complications.
  - Whereas cystatin C correlates linearly with cardiovascular risk (e.g., heart failure), SCr correlates in a J-curve relationship.
- Limitations:
  - There is evidence of tubular secretion of cystatin and extrarenal elimination (15% to 20%); thus, GFR may be overestimated.
  - Cystatin production and metabolism may be altered by various clinical conditions. Higher cystatin levels may be seen in patients with older age, male gender, white race, obesity, DM, inflammatory state, lower serum albumin level. Other factors that may alter cystatin levels: thyroid disease, malignancy, steroids.
  - Cystatin measurement is expensive and not yet widely available.
  - Standardization of cystatin measurement is still lacking.
  - Unless combined with SCr, eGFR formulas with cystatin C alone are not more accurate in estimating GFR or predicting ESRD.
  - While cystatin-C-alone–based eGFR appears to be a better biomarker for mortality and CKD complications, SCr-based eGFR serves as a better predictor of ESRD. This is thought to be non-GFR determinants of cystatin C level, such as inflammation and vascular remodeling.

KDIGO Recommendations

- Use SCr *and* a GFR-estimating equation for initial assessment (rather than using SCr alone).
- Clinical laboratories should measure SCr using a specific assay with calibration traceable to the international standard reference materials and minimal bias compared to IDMS reference methodology.
- Clinical laboratories should report eGFR in adults using the CKD-EPI equation.
- Racial–ethnic and regional modifications to CKD-EPI creatinine equations are required.
- Additional testing (e.g., cystatin C) or clearance measurement is suggested for confirmation when SCr-based eGFR is less accurate (e.g., patients with low muscle mass).
- In adults with eGFR(Cr) of 45 to 59 mL/min/1.73 m^2 who have no other markers of kidney damage and confirmation is required, cystatin C measurement is suggested. If eGFR(cys) or eGFR(Cr-cys) is also <60 mL/min/1.73 m^2, the diagnosis of CKD is confirmed.
- GFR measurement using an exogenous filtration marker is suggested under circumstances where more accurate ascertainment of GFR will impact on treatment decisions (e.g., kidney donation).

- Limitations of eGFR formulas:
  - Less accurate in nonsteady state
  - Accuracy may be compromised in presence of factors other than GFR that alter SCr levels (e.g., extremes of muscle mass, presence of inhibitors of tubular secretion of creatinine, dietary intake) or factors that interfere with creatinine assay.

GFR Categories

- G1: eGFR $\geq$ 90 mL/min/1.73 m^2
- G2: eGFR 60 to 89
- G3a: eGFR 45 to 59
- G3b: eGFR 30 to 44
- G4: eGFR 15 to 29
- G5: eGFR < 15

> **NOTE** GFR estimates for drug dosing should be obtained by the same method/equation used by the drug company.

Assessment of Proteinuria

Albuminuria Categories

- A1: Normal to mildly increased albuminuria: albumin excretion rate (AER) < 30 mg/24 h or albumin-to-creatinine ratio (ACR) < 30 mg/g
- A2: Moderately increased: AER 30 to 300 mg/24 h or ACR 30 to 300 mg/g (3 to 30 mg/mEq)
- A3: Severely increased: AER > 300 mg/24 h or ACR > 300 mg/g

Total Proteinuria

- Normal degree of proteinuria is generally <150 to 200 mg/d.
- Methods to assess proteinuria:
  - Routine urinalysis dipstick (RUA) detects predominantly albuminuria based on its ability to change pH.
    - RUA does not detect tubular proteins or light-chain immunoglobulins well.
    - The degree of proteinuria based on RUA must be correlated to hydration status.
  - 24-hour urine proteinuria detects all types of proteins but is cumbersome to collect. Interpretation of proteinuria from a 24-hour collection requires confirmation of collection adequacy, that is 15 to 20 mg/kg/d of creatinine for females, 20 to 25 mg/kg/d for males.

> **NOTE**
> - Proteinuria comprised of <25% albuminuria suggests either the presence of low molecular weight proteins due to tubular injury and/or overflow proteinuria from monoclonal gammopathy.
> - Significant proteinuria mismatch (i.e., high degree of proteinuria from either PCR or 24-hour urine collection in association with minimal proteinuria from RUA) suggests presence of free light chains (Bence Jones protein).
> - "Selectivity of proteinuria" refers to the ratio of clearance of IgG (molecular weight of 160,000 Da) to that of transferrin (88,000 Da). A value < 0.1 indicates highly selective proteinuria, suggests the diagnosis of minimal change disease in children, and predicts corticosteroid responsiveness.

- Protein-to-creatinine ratio (PCR) detects all types of proteins and reduces variations due to hydration status. It is typically expressed as mg/mg Cr or mg/g Cr. For newly diagnosed CKD, obtain either urine PCR or 24-hour urine collection for proteinuria.
- Microalbumin dipstick detects albuminuria, a marker of glomerular basement membrane defect.

CKD Epidemiology

- CKD definition (KDOQI):
  - Kidney damage ≥ 3 months, as defined by *structural or functional abnormalities* of the kidney, with or without a decrease in GFR, manifest by either pathologic abnormalities or markers of kidney damage, including abnormalities in the composition of the blood or urine, or abnormalities in imaging tests, or having
  - GFR < 60 mL/min/1.73 m^2 for ≥3 months with or without underlying kidney damage (e.g., hepatorenal or cardiorenal syndrome)
- Overall lifetime risks for CKD stages 3a, 3b, 4, and ESRD in the United States have been reported to be 59.1%, 33.6%, 11.5%, and 3.6% respectively.
- Women had greater CKD risk but lower ESRD risk.
- Lifetime risks of CKD stages 4 and 5 and ESRD were higher in blacks and developed 10 to 15 years earlier than in whites.
- While the prevalence of CKD stages 1 to 4 remain relatively stable over the years, the prevalence for ESRD (stage 5) has increased at a much greater rate. The difference in the prevalence increase is referred to as the "CKD and ESRD paradox."
- Theories for CKD and ESRD paradox:
  - Improved survival of CKD patients from cardiovascular events over the years
  - More rapid loss of kidney function over the years—unlikely, due to more aggressive BP control and more use of ACEI/ARB.
  - Earlier RRT initiation in more recent years compared to past years
- DM is the leading cause of CKD in developed and many developing countries.

Predictors of CKD Progression

KDIGO 2012: In predicting risk for outcome of CKD, identify (1) cause of CKD, (2) GFR category, (3) albuminuria category, (4) other risk factors and comorbid conditions.

- CKD progression (KDIGO):
  - Progression of CKD is defined as having a drop in CKD category accompanied by ≥25% decline from baseline eGFR.
  - Rapid progression of CKD is defined as a sustained eGFR decline > 5 mL/min/1.73 m^2/y.
- Key predictors of CKD progression:
  - Hypertension (HTN): MDRD participants assigned to lower MAP target < 92 mm Hg were 32% less likely to develop ESRD compared with those assigned to "usual" BP target MAP of <107 mm Hg.
  - Proteinuria:
    - Proteins in tubular lumen (albumin, complement factors, e.g., C3, membrane attack complex (C5b-9), growth factors, and other nonselective inflammatory proteins) are endocytosed and metabolized by proximal tubular cells which can lead to direct tubular injury and/or complement activation with resultant tubulointerstitial inflammation.

- Of interest, statins have been shown to reduce proximal tubular endocytosis of albumin.
- Exposure of tubular epithelial cells to high protein concentration has been shown to increase the synthesis of endothelin 1, a potent vasoconstrictor and a stimulator of renal cell proliferation and extracellular matrix and TGF-β synthesis. TGF-β is known to increase collagen and fibronectin production which play a role of tissue fibrosis.
- Angiotensin II:
  - Increases plasma protein filtration via both hemodynamic effect and direct podocyte effect, the latter via stimulation of AT_1R.
  - Increases oxidative stress–associated injury, synthesis of cytokines, chemokines, TGF-β, connective tissue growth factor, chemotactic and cell adhesion molecules, all leading to increased plasma mesangial cell proliferation, extracellular matrix synthesis, and macrophage activation and infiltration.
  - Increases aldosterone synthesis. Aldosterone increases plasminogen activator–*inhibiting* factor I (PAI-I). Plasminogen activator normally induces proteolysis. Plasminogen activator *inhibitor* PAI-I reduces mesangiolysis and fibrinolysis, thus favoring mesangial expansion and fibrosis.
- APOL1 gene variants: Blacks (with or without diabetes) with two APOL1 risk alleles develop more rapid CKD progression and increased risk of ESRD.
- Other possible predictors of CKD progression:
  - Presence of risk factors for cardiovascular disease: metabolic syndrome, elevated homocysteine, dyslipidemia, inflammatory prothrombotic and/or oxidative stress markers
  - Both cardio- and peripheral vascular diseases
  - High body mass index (BMI):
    - U-shaped association with clinical outcomes for all-cause mortality, incidence of ESRD, doubling of SCr, and eGFR decline. Outcomes are worse for those with BMIs < 25 kg/m^2 and >35 kg/m^2, and best for those with BMI between 25 and 29.9 kg/m^2.
    - Accumulation of lipids in tissues such as that seen with nonalcoholic fatty liver disease is thought to induce worse outcomes via the release of inflammatory, profibrotic, coagulant, oxidative mediators.
  - Hyperuricemia
  - Smoking
  - Apolipoprotein E (APOE) genetic variation
  - Increased pulse pressure > 10 mm Hg
  - Hypomagnesemia
  - Fluid overload has been suggested to be a more important factor than DM for rapid progression and initiation of renal-replacement therapy in CKD stages 4 and 5. More studies are needed.
  - Recent myocardial infarction

Slowing Progression of CKD

- Use of Renin–Angiotensin–Aldosterone System (RAAS) inhibitors:
  - Renoprotective effects of ACEI and ARB are beyond those of BP control
  - Reduces glomerular HTN, hyperfiltration, protein filtration
  - Inhibits aldosterone-induced increase in PAI-I, the major inhibitor of fibrinolysis and proteolysis, thus reduction in extracellular proteins/collagen accumulation

- Reduces TGF-β production
- Increases hepatocyte growth factor, a factor with antifibrotic potential
- Reduces albuminuria. Albuminuria has been shown to stimulate inflammatory response, vasoactive peptide production/release (endothelin), and fibrotic processes.
- Combination RAAS (ACEI and ARB) inhibition therapy:
  - There may be synergistic reduction in proteinuria and BP control, but endpoints of renoprotection and cardiovascular mortality have not been proven.
  - ONTARGET trial involving patients with established cardiovascular disease, not kidney disease: increased hyperkalemia and AKI
  - ALTITUDE trial involving diabetic patients with both high cardiovascular and renal risks: the addition of a direct renin inhibitor (aliskiren) to either ACEI or ARB led to worse kidney function deterioration, hyperkalemia, and stroke. Trial stopped early.
  - Nephron-VA-D trial involving patients with DM2, microalbuminuria, and moderate to severe renal impairment (eGFR 30 to 90 mL/min/1.73 m^2): the use of combination ACEI and ARB synergistically lowered proteinuria but was stopped early due to severe hyperkalemia and AKI.
- Mineralocorticoid-receptor antagonists (MRA):
  - Spironolactone decreases proteinuria (albuminuria) in CKD subjects and also theoretically reduces tissue fibrosis.
  - Problem: hyperkalemia; Potential solution: concurrent use with gut potassium binder (patiromer)
- Combination ACEI and MRA may reduce proteinuria more than combination ACEI and ARB. Hyperkalemia, however, has been shown to be worse with the former combination.
- Blood pressure control:
  - KDIGO 2012 suggests the following treatment goals:
    - Treat BP to <140/90 mm Hg for either diabetic or nondiabetic adults with CKD *and* albuminuria < 30 mg/24 h or equivalent.
    - Treat BP to <130/80 mm Hg for either diabetic or nondiabetic adults with CDK *and* albuminuria > 30 mg/24 h (or equivalent).
    - Use an ACEI or ARB in diabetic adults with CKD *and* urine albumin excretion (UAE) ≥ 30 mg/24 h (or equivalent).
    - Use an ACEI or ARB in nondiabetic adults with CKD and UAE > 300 mg/24 h (or equivalent).
  - Clinical trials involving BP control versus GFR decline:
    - MDRD study involving patients with nondiabetic proteinuric renal disease: strict BP control to target 125/75 mm Hg in patients with proteinuria > 1 g/d reduced GFR decline more than target 140/90 mm Hg. However, 48% of lower target BP group received ACEI compared with 28% in higher BP group.
    - African American Study of Kidney Disease and Hypertension (AASK) trial: Strict BP control to MAP 92 mm Hg (equivalent to 125/75 mm Hg) did not result in reduced GFR decline compared to higher MAP group of 102 to 107 mm Hg (equivalent to 135/85 to 140/90 mm Hg), unless significant proteinuria was present.
    - Ramipril Efficacy in Nephropathy 2 (REIN-2) trial involving patients with chronic, nondiabetic, proteinuric nephropathies: Addition of other agents to baseline ramipril to achieve tight BP control < 130/80 mm Hg did not confer additional benefits in terms of reduction in proteinuria or GFR rate of decline.

- Keeping BP > 128/85 mm Hg may be advisable due to concerns for possible "J-curve" phenomenon of worse cardiovascular outcomes.
  - J-curve phenomenon observed (Farnett et al.): Literature review of 13 studies noted that lower DBP control was associated with worse cardiac events but not stroke. The beneficial DBP was thought to be 85 mm Hg.
  - Irbesartan Diabetic Nephropathy Trial (IDNT): DBP < 85 mm Hg was associated with a trend for increase in all-cause mortality, a significant increase in myocardial infarction, but decreased risk for strokes. Goal BP 120/85 mm Hg was recommended.
- J curve not observed:
  - Hypertension Optimal Treatment (HOT) trial: Patients assigned to DBP goal < 80 mm Hg had fewer cardiovascular outcomes than other group. No J-curve effect was noted.
- Appropriate Blood Pressure Control in Diabetes (ABCD) trial: no difference in cardiovascular outcome or benefit with BP target of 132/75 versus 138/85 mm Hg
- Reduction of proteinuria:
  - REIN study (Ramipril): baseline proteinuria correlated significantly with GFR decline.
  - ARB was shown to be renoprotective (time to doubling of SCr, progression to ESRD, death): Reduction of End points in Non-Insulin Dependent Diabetes Mellitus with Angiotensin II Antagonist Losartan (RENAAL), IDNT (irbesartan 150 mg/300 mg vs. amlodipine).
- Glycemia control in patients with DM:
  - KDOQI guideline: target hemoglobin A1C ~7% if safely tolerated to prevent or delay progression of microvascular complications of diabetes including DKD. Tighter control is not indicated.
  - ADVANCE, ACCORD, VADT: glycemic control reduced albuminuria, but no change in GFR.
  - DCCT, EDIC, UKPDS: glycemic control reduced both albuminuria and GFR decline
  - Intensive glycemic control led to increased hypoglycemic episodes.
- Correction of metabolic acidosis:
  - Metabolic acidosis usually occurs by eGFR < 30 mL/min/1.73 m^2.
  - Adverse associated clinical effects:
    - Increased oxidation of branched chain amino acids (valine, leucine, isoleucine)
    - Increased protein degradation, catabolic rate, muscle breakdown
    - Decreased albumin synthesis
    - Impaired vitamin D synthesis
    - Impaired bone metabolism, increased bone lysis
    - Accelerated CKD progression
    - Upregulation of ammonia, endothelin, and aldosterone production to promote tubular acid excretion
  - KDIGO 2012: oral bicarbonate supplement to keep serum HCO_3^- ≥ 22 mEq/L.
  - Alkalinization does not worsen BP but may reduce CKD progression rate.
  - Of note, HCO_3^- > 24 mEq/L may be associated with higher rate of heart failure independent of alkali supplementation. Mechanism not known (unclear if this could be due to underlying respiratory acidosis).

Other considerations to slow CKD progression:
- Endothelin antagonists:
  - Endothelin 1 mediates secretion of proinflammatory cytokines, growth factors, TGF-β.

- Type A receptor (ET_AR) mediates vasoconstriction, sodium retention, podocyte dysfunction.
- Type B receptor (ET_BR) mediates vasodilatation, sodium excretion.
- Avosentan (nonselective ET-1 inhibitor) was associated with increased CHF.
- Clinical studies on ET_AR-selective antagonism are pending (RADAR trial).
- Albuminuria reduction:
  - BP Control
  - RAAS inhibition
  - DPP4-inhibitors (sitagliptin, linagliptin)
    - Sitagliptin: decreases albuminuria by 20% in a prospective observation study
    - Linagliptin
      - Mainly metabolized and eliminated by liver, no renal dose adjustment needed
      - Meta-analysis of 13 randomized controlled trials (RCT) involving 5,500 patients: Linagliptin confers a 16% reduction in a composite renal end point consisting of micro- and macroalbuminuria, loss of eGFR > 50% from baseline, AKI, or death.
  - Sodium–glucose cotransporter 2 (SGLT2) inhibitors:
    - SGLT2 is located apically in proximal tubules and is responsible for the reabsorption of filtered glucose.
    - SGLT2 inhibitor reduces urinary glucose excretion, thus decreases fasting glucose, and HbA1C.
    - SGLT2 inhibitors block renal glucose reabsorption, induce weight loss, and reduce albuminuria. Long-term safety and renal and cardiovascular protective efficacy are pending.
  - Pentoxifylline (PTF):
    - Methylxanthine derivative that acts as a phosphodiesterase inhibitor with antiinflammatory, antiproliferative, antifibrotic properties.
    - Meta-analysis of 10 RCTs ($n = 476$) involving patients with DM2 and proteinuria/albuminuria revealed significant albuminuria reduction by 300 mg/d.
    - Effect of Pentoxifylline (PTF) on Renal Function and Albuminuria in DKD: PREDIAN Trial 2014:
      - Open-label, prospective, randomized: Would adding PTF to RAAS blockade slow progression in DM2 and CKD 3-4?
      - PTF (1,200 mg/d) ($n = 82$) versus control ($n = 87$) × 2 years. All received similar doses of RAAS inhibitors.
      - eGFR had decreased by 2.1 ± 0.4 in PTF versus 6.5 ± 0.4 mL/min/1.73 m^2 in control ($p < 0.001$). Albuminuria was +5.7% in control versus −14.9% in PTF ($p = 0.001$).
      - PTF plus RAAS inhibitors led to smaller decline in eGFR and greater reduction of albuminuria.
  - Statins:
    - ASCOT trial: 10,305 subjects with HTN and >3 cardiovascular risk factors: Atorvastatin significantly improved eGFR compared to placebo.
    - SHARP trial:
      - Combination simvastatin and ezetimibe conferred a 17% cardiovascular risk reduction in patients with CKD.
      - Renoprotective effect not proven
    - PLANET trial: Atorvastatin versus rosuvastatin in patients with diabetic and nondiabetic CKD:
      - Atorvastatin improved proteinuria, not eGFR.
      - Rosuvastatin was associated with a fall in eGFR.

- Fluvastatin RCT: no improvement in proteinuria
- Recent meta-analysis revealed that statin ameliorated eGFR decline but not reduction in proteinuria via unclear mechanisms. The renoprotective effects were thought to be dependent on greater dosage and duration of statin use.
- KDIGO general lipid guidelines for *nondialysis, nontransplant* CKD patients (2013):
  - Initial assessment of lipid status with a lipid profile is recommended for adults with CKD, but follow-up measurements are not required for the majority of patients.
  - In adults ≥ 50 years old with CKD and eGFR > 60 mL/min/1.73 m^2, treatment with a statin is recommended (regardless of lipid profile).
  - In adults ≥ 50 years old with eGFR < 60 mL/min/1.73 m^2, treatment with a statin or statin/ezetimibe combination is recommended.
  - In adults aged 18 to 49 with CKD, treatment with a statin is suggested for those with one or more of the following: known coronary artery disease, DM, prior ischemic stroke, or estimated 10-year incidence of coronary death or nonfatal myocardial infarction > 10%.
- Uric acid lowering therapy:
  - Pathogenesis of kidney injury with elevated serum uric acid levels:
    - RAAS activation, oxidative stress, mitochondrial dysfunction, epithelial–mesenchymal transition, endothelial dysfunction, vascular smooth muscle proliferation
  - Clinical complications attributed to hyperuricemia: arteriosclerosis, glomerular HTN, glomerulosclerosis, interstitial disease, AKI, metabolic syndrome, nonalcoholic fatty liver disease, HTN, DM
  - Clinical impact of uric acid–lowering therapy:
    - Meta-analysis (Wang et al.): 11 papers, total $n = 753$: Uric acid lowering is associated with significant lowering of SCr and increase of eGFR.
    - Japanese HTN Evaluation with ARB Losartan Therapy (J-HEALTH) study: $n = 7,629$ hypertensive patients: Change in serum UA inversely correlated with change in eGFR and associated with lower cardiovascular events.
    - Bottom line for uric acid–lowering therapy: larger clinical trials are still needed.
      - KDIGO 2012: "There is INSUFFICIENT EVIDENCE to support or refute the use of UA lowering agents in CKD and either symptomatic or asymptomatic hyperuricemia in order to delay progression of CKD."
      - Treatment of hyperuricemia is "not benign."
        - Stevens Johnson syndrome may occur with allopurinol therapy.
        - Both allopurinol and febuxostat (xanthine oxidase inhibitors) can increase urinary xanthine levels which can be nephrotoxic.
- Antifibrotic agents: Pirfenidone
  - Oral agent that can inhibit various cytokines including TGF-β, tumor necrosis factor-α, platelet derived growth factor and epithelial growth factor.
  - Proved effective in reducing injury in cyclosporine and tacrolimus nephrotoxicity, antiglomerular basement membrane glomerulonephritis, doxorubicin toxicity in experimental models
  - Awaiting results from clinical trials for renoprotective effects
- KDIGO 2012 dietary suggestions:
  - Lower protein intake to 0.8 g/kg/d in adults with eGFR < 30 mL/min/1.73 m^2 (with or without DM) with appropriate education
  - Avoid high protein intake > 1.3 g/kg/d in adults with CKD at risk of progression.
  - Lower salt intake < 2 g elemental sodium per day (<90 mmol/d). Lower salt intake is associated with decreased proteinuria independent of BP lowering effect.

- Recently, however, there are concerns for low-sodium diet–induced activation of RAAS and SNS, higher risks for CKD progression and odds of death. Two to 3 g daily sodium intake may be a more prudent approach. Lower sodium intake in patients with proteinuria > 1 g/d may be associated with increased AKI events and excessive stimulation of RAAS.

Nonrenal biomarkers in CKD:
- Troponin:
  - Increased troponin level is associated with a twofold to fourfold increased risk of all-cause mortality and major cardiovascular events.
  - In asymptomatic CKD patients, elevated troponin levels may indicate chronic structural heart disease (e.g., left ventricular hypertrophy, diastolic dysfunction, reduced ejection fraction) rather than ACS.
- Brain natriuretic peptide (BNP):
  - BNP is a less reliable marker of volume overload in CKD patients. Interpret with caution in patients with eGFR < 60 mL/min/1.73 m^2.
  - However, BNP levels provide a good index for left ventricular mass and dysfunction.
- D-dimer level can be elevated in CKD. A higher cutoff value may be needed in patients with advanced CKD to rule out pulmonary embolism.
- Acute phase reactants associated with cardiovascular risk that may be elevated in CKD: fibrinogen, ceruloplasmin

Reversal of CKD:
- Is reversal of CKD possible?
- Pancreas transplant in eight type 1 diabetic patients with diabetic kidney disease revealed regression of glomerular lesions. However, full functional recovery was not achieved.
- Targets to consider for possible reversal: PAI-I, Angiotensin II, TGF-β.

DIABETIC KIDNEY DISEASE

(See Chapter 6)

NONDIABETIC KIDNEY DISEASE

(Also see Chapters 6 and 7)

Nephrosclerosis with Aging

- Structural changes with aging:
  - Reduction in kidney mass: 250 to 270 g kidney mass in 40 to 50 years old becomes 180 to 200 g by the age of 70 to 90.
  - Cortical thinning with relative medullary sparing (likely due to increased glomerulosclerosis)
- Histologic changes with aging:
  - Global glomerulosclerosis: It has been suggested that the percentage of glomerulosclerosis on kidney biopsy from aging alone should be less than [age/2 - 10]. Anything greater should raise suspicion for pathologic changes.
  - Ischemic changes with segmental adhesion to Bowman capsule
  - Tubular atrophy with cystic formation
  - Interstitial fibrosis
  - Arteriolar intimal fibrosis—may be associated with thinning of media; hyaline arteriosclerosis seen in smaller vessels

- Functional changes with aging:
  - GFR reduction of 0.8 mL/min/1.73 m^2 per year after age 40
  - GFR decline of 7 to 8 mL/min/1.73 m^2 per year in those with underlying CKD
  - Albuminuria in 30% among patients $\geq$ 70 years old
  - Reduced concentrating and diluting capacity which explains the propensity for increased nocturia and hyponatremia respectively in the elderly.

CKD and Pregnancy

- Effects of pregnancy on volume homeostasis and the kidneys in women with *normal* kidney function:
  - Total Na$^+$ retention 950 mmol = 22 g
  - Water retention 6 to 8 L
  - Plasma volume increases by 30% to 45% (up to 1.25 L) by second trimester.
  - Kidney length increases by 1 cm.
  - Renal plasma flow and GFR increase by 50% by the second trimester: creatinine clearance < 110 mL/min is abnormal. Accordingly, a midterm SCr is expected to be as low as 0.4 to 0.6 mg/dL. A SCr $\geq$ 1.0 mg/dL is most likely abnormal.
  - Increased loss of water-soluble vitamins, hence the need for prenatal vitamins.
  - Increased proteinuria up to 300 mg/d is normal (predominantly tubular [non-albumin, low molecular weight] proteinuria).
  - Glucosuria is considered physiologic for later stages of pregnancy which may be due to reduced tubular reabsorption or hyperfiltration overflow. However, early glucosuria requires testing for glucose intolerance, undiagnosed DM.
  - Neurohormonal and other changes:
    - Systemic arterial vasodilation mediated by nitric oxide (NO) and relaxin
    - Increased compensatory ADH, RAAS
    - Increased cardiac output, increased thirst
  - Electrolyte changes: lower serum osmolality (270 to 275 mOsm/kg vs. nonpregnancy range of 280 to 290), lower S[Na$^+$] (132 to 135 vs. nonpregnancy range of 138 to 142 mEq/L)
- Hemodynamic changes made by the kidneys during pregnancy are essential for normal fetal growth and development. Reduced renal function can adversely affect fetal outcomes.
- Hyperdynamic changes and glomerular hyperfiltration in pregnancy accelerates progression of CKD.
- Baseline creatinine in patients with CKD predicts poor outcomes:
  - Creatinine < 1.5 mg/dL:
    - Permanent loss of GFR in <10% of women
    - Live births in >90% of women
  - Creatinine 1.5 to 2.5 mg/dL:
    - Maternal HTN and proteinuria in 50%
    - Decline or permanent loss of GFR in 30% of women
    - 10% incidence of ESRD soon after pregnancy
    - 60% risk of preterm delivery, 37% intrauterine growth retardation and 7% fetal loss
  - Creatinine > 2.5 mg/dL:
    - Progression to ESRD highly likely during or soon after pregnancy
    - High rate of fetal loss

NOTE Poorly controlled HTN exaggerates kidney injury and GFR decline in pregnancy.

- Management of CKD patients during pregnancy:
  - Discontinue ACEI/ARB and statins.
  - Monitor creatinine and proteinuria (urine protein/creatinine ratio).
  - For chronic HTN BP goals in pregnancy, see Hypertension chapter.
  - Start low-dose aspirin 75 to 150 mg daily before 16 weeks if SCr > 1.5 mg/dL to prevent preeclampsia.
  - Renal-replacement therapy (RRT):
    - RRT initiation is generally recommended at eGFR < 20 mL/min/1.73 m^2 or BUN > 50 mg/dL.
    - Increasing dialysis dose improves gestational age, live birth rates, birth weight and lower rates of maternal HTN, polyhydramnios.
      - HD: increase weekly sessions to achieve >24 to 28 h/wk.
      - PD: low volume/highly frequent dwells
      - BUN goal < 45 mg/dL.
    - Tight control of maternal weight and optimize ultrafiltration to keep constant maternal/fetal hemodynamics to avoid growth retardation or poor outcomes. Consider intradialytic fetal monitoring.
    - Nutritional support (avoid protein restriction), vitamins, folate supplements
    - Iron supplement to keep serum ferritin levels of 200 to 300 µg/mL
    - Maintain hemoglobin 10 to 11 g/dL with erythropoiesis stimulating agent.
    - Supplement calcium 1.5 to 2.0 g/d.

CHRONIC KIDNEY DISEASE COMPLICATIONS

- Hypertension:
  - Prevalence of HTN reaches ~80% to 90% in patients with CKD stage ≥ 3.
  - Pathogenesis: sodium retention, increased peripheral resistance due to increased activities of the sympathetic and RAAS
- Fluid overload:
  - Impaired pressure natriuresis
  - Increased renal sodium reabsorption due to increased angiotensin II and aldosterone
- Cardiovascular complications:
  - Hyperlipidemia:
    - Statin therapy has been shown to have little or no effect on all-cause mortality or cardiovascular outcome in dialysis patients, unlike that observed in the general population.
    - The difference in statin effect is thought to be due to nontraditional mechanisms of disease of coronary artery disease in dialysis patients.
    - Initiation of statin therapy is not recommended in patients being started on dialysis. Continuation of existing statin therapy may be reasonable. Risks/benefits discussion should be done with patients.
  - Sudden cardiac deaths:
    - Account for 25% to 30% of all deaths in prevalent dialysis patients in the United States. This is 20 times higher than that observed in the general population.
    - Potential contributing factors: low levels of long-chain n-3 fatty acids, low dialysate concentrations of potassium (<2 mEq/L), calcium (<2.5 mEq/L), inadequate dialysis, higher ultrafiltration volumes

- Atrial fibrillation:
  - Increased incidence of both atrial fibrillation and stroke in ESRD patients
  - Swedish registry: Within each CKD stage, those treated with warfarin had ~25% reduced risk of composite end point of mortality, stroke, and MI. Although bleeding was increased with advanced CKD, there was no increased bleeding risk within CKD strata, suggesting that CKD per se (and not necessarily warfarin) increases bleeding risk.
  - Specific data regarding anticoagulation in ESRD patients are lacking.
  - Anticoagulation is suggested to be "individualized" based on risks and benefits.
- Coronary artery disease:
  - High prevalence in CKD and ESRD patients
  - Nontraditional risks (serum phosphate, albumin, C-reactive protein, dialysis vintage) may predict major cardiovascular events in HD patients.
  - Traditional risks (hyperlipidemia, BP, pulse pressure) may not predict outcomes.
  - CKD patients are less likely than non-CKD counterparts to receive cardiovascular intervention, cardiovascular diagnostic studies, and treatment including aspirin and β-blockers.
  - Routine management of cardiovascular risks per KDIGO:
    - Level of care for ischemic heart disease should not be "prejudiced" by their CKD.
    - Adults at risk for atherosclerotic disease should be offered antiplatelet therapy if benefit outweighs bleeding risk.
    - In patients with GFR < 60 mL/min/1.73 m^2, BNP/N-terminal-proBNP and troponin levels should be interpreted with caution.
  - Invasive interventions: coronary artery bypass grafting has been shown to be associated with a lower risk of death compared with percutaneous coronary intervention at 5-year follow-up for multivessel disease (USRDS data 1997 to 2009).
  - The use of drug eluting stent improves revascularization of blood vessels compared with a bare metal stent in patients with CKD stage 3.
  - Addition of spironolactone to ACEI or ARB therapy in patients receiving RRT: if safely tolerated (i.e., hyperkalemia), may reduce left ventricular hypertrophy and improve survival
  - Other interventions:
    - Fish oil (e.g., 4 g daily) has been suggested to lower risk for cardiovascular events.
    - Smoking cessation
- Anemia/iron deficiency:
  - Hypoproliferative normochromic normocytic anemia, where anemia is defined as having hemoglobin < 13.0 g/dL in males and <12.0 g/dL in females.
  - Onset:
    - Typically occurs at CKD stage IIIa for males and IIIb for females
    - Patients with DM tend to have anemia at earlier CKD stage.
    - PCKD patients tend to have anemia at later stage and less severe anemia.
    - Patients with chronic tubulointerstitial disease tend to have earlier and more severe anemia.
  - Complications of anemia:
    - Fatigue, poor quality of life, difficulty with concentration, impaired judgment, sleep disturbance
    - Left ventricular hypertrophy

- Sexual dysfunction
- Impaired immune response
- Platelet dysfunction
- Anemia is a "risk multiplier" for mortality in patients with CKD
- Pathogenesis of anemia in CKD:
  - Reduced renal erythropoietin production due to loss of kidney mass. Erythropoietin is made by peritubular interstitial fibroblasts in the kidneys.
  - Inflammatory state in CKD reduces erythropoietin production and increases hepatic synthesis of hepcidin.
    - Hepcidin reduces gastrointestinal absorption of iron and enhances iron sequestration in macrophages and hepatocytes.
    - Ferroportin is a transmembrane protein on macrophages and enterocytes that normally exports intracellular iron into circulation for use in erythropoiesis. Hepcidin binds to and internalizes ferroportin. In effect, hepcidin reduces cellular iron export into circulation for effective erythropoiesis.
  - Red blood cell half-life is shortened in uremia.
  - Severe secondary hyperparathyroidism can induce bone marrow fibrosis and results in ineffective erythropoiesis.
- KDIGO 2012 suggestions:
  - Monitor hemoglobin at least yearly for patients with CKD stage 3, twice yearly for stage 4 CKD, every 3 months for stage 5.
  - Evaluation of anemia: complete blood count with differential, absolute reticulocyte count, serum ferritin, serum transferrin saturation (TSAT), B_{12}, folate levels
  - Iron deficiency:
    - For CKD 3 and 4: Ferritin < 100 ng/mL and TSAT < 20% usually indicate absolute iron deficiency.
    - For dialysis patients: Ferritin < 200 ng/mL and TSAT < 20% usually indicates absolute iron deficiency.
  - Erythropoietin level is not generally checked because "normal" level may still be inadequate for patients with CKD when there may be some degree of bone marrow resistance to erythropoietin.
  - Exclude other common causes of anemia
  - Iron supplement trial (1 to 3 months) in CKD patients with anemia if ferritin ≤ 500 μg/L and total iron saturation ≤ 30%. NOTE: risks associated with intravenous iron include increased oxidative stress, endothelial injury, vascular calcifications, and plaque formation, and impaired leukocyte function and facilitated bacterial growth.
    - Avoid use of IV iron in patients with systemic infections.
    - Hold intravenous iron if ferritin > 500 ng/mL. Note, however, that even when KDOQI iron parameters have been reached, anemia may still respond iron therapy in some patients. This is referred to as "functional iron deficiency."
  - Monitor iron status (TSAT and ferritin) ≥ 3 months during ESA therapy
  - Use of ESA:
    - Avoid in patients with active malignancy particularly when cure is anticipated, history of stroke, or history of malignancy (increased thromboembolic risk and survival in some cancers).
    - Initiate when Hb values trend downward and reach levels < 9 to 10 g/dL after iron store has been repleted. Monitor Hb ≥ 1 month while on ESA.
    - Goal Hb 10 to 11 g/dL. Avoid ESA when Hb > 10 g/dL.
    - ESA is not recommended to maintain Hb > 11.5 g/dL.
    - Monitor Hb every 3 months when on stable ESA doses.

- Empirical use of adjuvant therapies including androgens, vitamin C, D, E, folic acid, L-carnitine, and PTF is not suggested. Although carnitine is involved in RBC plasma membrane remodeling, hence improved RBC survival, routine carnitine replacement has *not* been shown to improve responsiveness to ESA.
- ESA hyporesponsiveness:
  - Initial ESA hyporesponsiveness is defined as having no increase in Hb levels from baseline after one month of appropriate ESA weight-based dosing.
  - ESA dose escalation greater than doubling of initial weight-based dose should be avoided.
  - Initial hyporesponsiveness despite appropriate weight–based dosing:
    - Evaluate for common deficiencies: iron, vitamin B_{12}/folate/carnitine
    - Other possible causes: inflammatory or infectious state, underdialysis, severe secondary hyperparathyroidism, aluminum toxicity, use of RAAS inhibitors, underlying bone marrow disorders, hemoglobinopathies, blood loss/hemolysis
  - Subsequent ESA hyporesponsiveness:
    - This is defined as having two increases in ESA doses up to 50% beyond initial stable maintenance dose for desired Hb.
    - Evaluation for hyporesponsiveness:
      - Routine evaluation similar to initial hyporesponsiveness above
      - Also consider pure red cell aplasia (PRCA): antibody-mediated destruction of ESA that may occur in patients on ESA for >8 weeks. Very rare
      - Suspect PRCA if there is a sudden and rapid drop of Hb, normal white blood cell (WBC) and platelet count, and low reticulocyte count.
  - Red blood cell transfusions:
    - Avoid if possible, particularly in kidney transplant candidates due to risk of allosensitization.
    - Consider RBC transfusions if refractory or contraindicated to ESA.
- CKD-mineral bone disease (CKD-MBD):
  - CKD-MBD refers to disorders of systemic mineral metabolism involving abnormalities in biochemical profile, bone turnover, mineralization and volume, and/or vascular and soft tissue calcifications. Biochemical profile refers to serum calcium, phosphate, PTH, and vitamin D metabolism.
  - Bone "TMV" terminology:
    - **T**urnover: low, normal, high
    - **M**ineralization: normal, abnormal
    - **V**olume (reflects net bone formation and resorption rates and is related to bone porosity, strength, and fragility): low, normal, high
  - Renal osteodystrophy refers to various bone histomorphologic abnormalities due to disturbances in bone turnover, mineralization, and volume as a consequence of CKD-MBD. All bone disorders are associated with increased fracture risks.
    - Osteitis fibrosa cystica:
      - High bone turnover disease: high rates of bone formation and resorption
      - Condition seen with secondary hPTH
      - Most common bone disorder observed in patients receiving hemodialysis
      - Bone histomorphology: increased osteoblastic and osteoclastic activity with a high fraction of trabecular surface covered by osteoid seams, osteoid–osteoblast interface, abnormal collagen deposition, marrow fibrosis

- Turnover: High (increased osteoblastic and osteoclastic activity, may be evidenced by increased tetracycline uptake)
  - Mineralization: Normal or defective
  - Volume: Variable
- Adynamic bone disease (ABD):
  - Low rates of bone formation and resorption, may be evidenced by low tetracycline uptake
  - Associated with over suppression of secondary hPTH with overzealous administration of active vitamin D and calcium in patients with relative PTH resistance
  - Most common bone disorder observed in patients receiving peritoneal dialysis
  - Bone histomorphology:
    - Turnover: low (absence of active bone resorption and bone formation)
    - Mineralization: abnormal (no osteoid, no mineralization)
    - Volume: normal
  - Risks for ABD:
    - Over suppression of PTH
    - Advanced age
    - DM
    - Aluminum deposition (e.g., previously observed in patients receiving aluminum-based phosphate binders)
  - Clinical clues:
    - Relatively low serum intact PTH level
    - Hypercalcemia (serum calcium not taken up by bone due to low bone formation)
    - Hypophosphatemia (low bone resorption)
- Osteomalacia:
  - Low bone formation and low bone density, poor bone mineralization
  - May be seen with aluminum toxicity
  - Turnover: normal
  - Mineralization: abnormal
  - Volume: increased
- Mixed uremic osteodystrophy: mixed findings of above conditions
  - Most common bone disorder in patients with CKD stages 3 to 5
  - Turnover: high
  - Mineralization: abnormal
  - Volume: low
- Other bone conditions:
  - Osteoporosis:
    - Increased bone breakdown relative to bone production
    - Bone density (or mass) is at least 2.5 standard deviation less than peak bone mass
    - Management of osteoporosis in patients with CKD:
      - Poorly defined
      - Problems with diagnosis per routine dual-energy X-ray absorptiometry (DEXA) (See Diagnostic Testing)
      - Strict phosphorus/protein restriction improves renal osteodystrophy, but thought to worsen osteoporosis
      - Problems with bisphosphonates:
        - Concerns for over suppression of bone formation with long-term use

- Bone biopsy is recommended to exclude low-bone turnover disease prior to bisphosphonate therapy.
- Severe hypocalcemia may occur in those with vitamin D deficiency.
- Safety issue: FDA warnings against use of bisphosphonates in patients with GFR < 30 mL/min/1.73 m^2.
  - Rapid administration in rats has been shown to lead to AKI.
  - Human studies, likely safe renal-wise in patients with age associated reduced GFR (GFR > 30)
  - KDIGO suggests *not* to prescribe bisphosphonate to patients with GFR < 30 mL/min/1.73 m^2 without a strong clinical rationale.
- Treatment of known CKD-MBD has priority over treatment of osteoporosis.
- Other therapeutic options:
  - Assess adequacy of protein intake (low protein intake is associated with lower BMD).
  - Correction of metabolic acidosis
  - Maintain muscle mass as it provides an increased load for stimulation of bone turnover
  - Nitric oxide supplementation (use of nitrates) may be considered. Canadian multicenter osteoporosis study showed significant positive association between nitrate use and higher bone mass density. Although similar study in CKD patients is lacking, consideration for use of nitrates is worthwhile as they also benefit endothelial dysfunction, a common problem in CKD patients.
- Osteopenia:
  - Similar to osteoporosis, but milder condition. Bone density is 1 to 2.5 standard deviation less than peak bone mass.
- Diagnostic testing:
  - Imaging:
    - DEXA:
      - Determines both mineral content and bone area
      - Limitations: DEXA may overestimate BMD in CKD patients, likely due to vascular calcifications and/or hPTH-induced increased trabecular to cortical bone ratio. KDIGO does *not* recommend routine BMD testing in CKD 3-5.
    - Quantitative CT: measures 3D bone volume and can differentiate cortical and trabecular bone geometry and morphology.
    - Micro-MRI: high resolution MRI
    - Quantitative ultrasound: Measures appendicular skeletal density (most often calcaneal bone) may be better than DEXA. Limited data in CKD.
  - Bone biopsy:
    - Gold standard
    - Bone biopsy is obtained from anterior iliac crest after tetracycline labeling at two different times separated by 11 to 14 days. Tetracycline binds to newly formed bone at unmineralized bone interface. Measuring the distance between the two lines allows for calculation of bone formation rate during that interval.
    - Indications for bone biopsy:
      - Unexplained fractures
      - Persistent bone pain
      - Unexplained hypophosphatemia

- Possible aluminum toxicity
- Prior to therapy with bisphosphonates (CKD 3 with abnormalities of CKD-MBD and low BMD)
- Extraosseous and vascular calcifications:
  - Basic arterial layers starting from outside to lumen: adventitia > media > intima.
  - Medial artery calcifications (MAC):
    - Concentric calcifications that can lead to arterial stiffening.
    - MAC is associated with better survival than those with intimal calcifications (seen with classic CAD risks), but worse survival compared to those with no calcifications.
  - KDIGO recommendations on screening for vascular calcifications:
    - Routine screening is not suggested.
    - If indicated, consider lateral X-ray for lumbar spine and echocardiogram for valvular calcifications.

Other Complications
Immune Dysfunction

- Contributing factors:
  - Diabetes, malnutrition, peripheral vascular disease, skin breaks (e.g., dialysis access, diabetic foot ulcers)
  - Impaired host defense mechanisms affecting all cell lines (neutrophils, monocytes, lymphocytes, dendritic cells, macrophages)
- Increased infection risks for *Staphylococcus sp.*, *Pseudomonas sp.*, other gram-negative bacteria, atypical bacteria including *Mycobacterium tuberculosis*, viruses (herpes simplex)
  - ESRD patients are estimated to have a 50-fold increased risk in developing active tuberculosis infection.
  - Interferon release assays (e.g., QuantiFERON or T-SPOT.TB testing), which measures the response of sensitized T cells to mycobacterial antigens correlates with past TB radiologic evidence better than traditional skin testing.
- Increased malignancy risks reported in patients receiving renal replacement therapy (RRT):
  - Increased risks reported in kidney, bladder, cervix, multiple myeloma, thyroid and other endocrine glands.
  - No increased risks reported in breast, prostate, stomach, intestine, lungs
- Management: malignancy screening guidelines for CKD are not well established. Screen at least per routine for age, gender, personal risk factors, family history, and pretransplant evaluation.

Acquired cystic kidney disease (ACKD) and renal cell carcinoma (RCC):
- Definition: Presence of >3 to 5 macroscopic cysts in individuals without a hereditary cause of cystic disease
- Prevalence:
  - May occur prior to dialysis
  - At dialysis initiation: 5% to 20%;
  - By 10 years on dialysis: 80% to 100%
- Pathogenesis of ACKD is likely multifactorial and may be related to:
  - Loss of nephrons followed by tubular cell hypertrophy, hyperplasia, and epithelial cyst formation.
  - Activation of proto-oncogenes and accumulation of mutagens in a uremic milieu
  - Genetic susceptibility

- Malignant transformation to RCC:
  - Cumulative incidence < 1% up to 7% among ACKD.
  - Up to 40-fold increased risk of RCC in ACKD compared with the general population.
  - Risk factors associated with RCC transformation: male gender (7:1 compared to females), African American, prolonged dialysis, severe ACKD with marked kidney enlargement.
  - Management: surveillance imaging studies per symptoms and patient life expectancy:
    - Low life expectancy: no screening
    - Good life expectancy: yearly kidney ultrasound
    - Presence of hematuria, flank pain, unexplained fevers, erythrocytosis, worsening BP: immediate kidney ultrasound, consider CT urogram
  - See Renal Cystic Diseases in Tubular, Interstitial, and Cystic Diseases chapter for interpretation of imaging studies.
- ACKD may regress to some degree with a successful kidney transplant.

Malnutrition:
- Malnutrition adversely affects survival in ESRD
- Global assessment of malnutrition:
  - Physical characteristics:
    - BMI:
      - Better survival with higher BMI (i.e., >25 kg/m^2) compared with counterpart with normal or low BMI
      - Survival advantage of higher BMI may more specifically pertain to patients > 65 years of age and not necessarily younger patients.
      - Cause of death is more commonly due to cardiovascular events in patients with higher BMI and noncardiovascular etiology in those with lower BMI.
      - Anthropometric measurements (e.g., skin-fold thickness, limb circumference)
    - Biomarkers for both nutritional and inflammatory status:
      - Serum albumin (accuracy may be reduced with dilutional hypervolemia, severe albuminuria). Lower albumin level is a strong predictor of mortality in dialysis patients.
      - Total iron binding capacity is reduced in inflammatory states
      - C-reactive protein level is increased in inflammatory states
- Malnutrition–inflammation complex syndrome (a.k.a. protein–energy wasting syndrome):
  - Concurrent malnutrition and inflammation
  - Prevalence is up to 70% in dialysis patients
  - May arise from poor dietary intake, coexisting illnesses, genetic susceptibility, dialysis procedures, infections
  - Management:
    - Protein supplements (e.g., 14 to 20 g three times weekly) given to patients with serum albumin concentration < 3.5 g/dL has been shown to improve hospitalization and survival rates.
    - Other interventions that have been suggested to be beneficial: anabolic steroids, ω-3 polyunsaturated fatty acids, folic acid, selenium.
    - PTF 400 mg daily has been suggested to reduce inflammatory cytokines in ESRD patients. Hard-outcome data are needed.
- Nutritional recommendations per KDOQI (Table 4.1):

Neurologic complications:
- Mood swings, agitation, delirium

Table 4.1	Nutritional recommendations per KDOQI guidelines		
Daily Intake	**Pre-ESRD**	**Hemodialysis**	**Peritoneal Dialysis**
Protein (g/kg dry BW)	0.6–1.0	1.1–1.2	1.0–1.3
Energy (kcal/kg)	35 (<60 y)	35 (<60 y)	35 (<60 y)
	30–35 (>60 y)	30–35 (>60 y)	30–35 (>60 y)[a]
Sodium (mEq)	<100	<100	<100
Calcium (mg)	<2,000	<2,000	<2,000

BW, body weight; y, year of age.

[a]Including calories provided from dialysate (e.g., dextrose).

- Impaired cognition, perception, concentration, loss of recent memory, visual hallucinations
- Hyperreflexia, tremors, asterixis
- Dysarthria, altered gait, clumsiness, convulsions
- Depression:
  - Most common psychiatric disorder in chronic dialysis patients.
  - Most common psychiatric disorder requiring hospitalization in dialysis patients.
  - Correlates with a ≥30% increase in mortality.
  - Risk for increased cardiovascular disease and mortality
  - Risks: younger age, patients with lower serum creatinine and albumin
  - Routine screening recommended at first dialysis, biannually or more as needed
  - Treatment: antidepressants +/− psychiatric referral. Most antidepressants are hepatically metabolized and do not require dose adjustment with the exceptions of paroxetine and venlafaxine.
- Sleep disorders:
  - Poor sleeping score is associated with increased relative risk of death ~1.3 (DOPPS).
  - Insomnia:
    - Most common sleep disorder in dialysis patients (prevalence up to 70%).
    - Insomnia is associated with restless leg syndrome, depression, and pain, and *vice versa*.
  - Sleep apnea:
    - Prevalence up to 50% compared to <5% in general population.
    - Pathogenesis: fluid overload leading to upper airway congestion "rostral fluid shift" during sleep, uremia induced alteration in central ventilator control, presence of comorbid conditions.
    - Nocturnal episodes of arterial oxygen desaturation is associated with higher cardiovascular events and worse survival in hemodialysis patients.
    - Compared to conventional hemodialysis, daily nocturnal hemodialysis reduces the apnea–hyponea index (episodes of apnea per hour of sleep).
    - Treatment of sleep apnea improves survival.
- Restless leg syndrome:
  - Unpleasant sensation in lower extremities with compulsive need to move legs, worse in the evening, improves with walking.
  - Incidence reported to be up to 60%.
  - Associated with higher risk for cardiovascular events *and* mortality

- Contributing factors:
  - Reduced dopaminergic modulation of intracortical excitability, with reduced supraspinal inhibition and resultant spinal cord excitability
  - Iron (Fe) deficiency: Fe is cofactor for tyrosine hydroxylase, the rate-limiting step in the synthesis of dopamine.
  - Others: Altered calcium/phosphate metabolism, hyperhomocystenemia, anemia, sympathetic nervous system activation, peripheral neuropathy.
- Treatment options: Adequate dialysis; Fe supplemention if deficient; Dopamine receptor agonists such as pramipexole or ropinirole, levodopa plus decarboxylase inhibitors (Sinemet); Others: gabapentin (renal dose adjustment is required), opioids, benzodiazepines, aerobic exercise, avoidance of caffeine, alcohol, and nicotine at bedtime
- Bleeding diathesis:
  - Contributing factors:
    - Platelet dysfunction
    - Uremic toxins (e.g., urea, guanidosuccinic acid, phenolic acid, methylguanidine) may interfere with ADP-induced platelet aggregation and thromboxane A_2 (thromboxane A_2 increases platelet aggregation).
    - Anemia:
      - Dilutional effect of platelets with reduced red blood cell mass
      - Red blood cells bind NO. With anemia, increased free NO stimulates cGMP production with subsequent suppression of thromboxane A_2 and ADP production. RBCs also release thromboxane A_2 and ADP.
      - EPO deficiency: EPO increases platelet production.
    - von Willebrand factor (vWF) abnormalities
    - Vessel abnormalities resulting in ineffective vasoconstriction
  - Corrective measures:
    - Dialysis: rapid onset of action with dialysis removal of uremic toxins
    - ESA administration: requires ~7 days to increase platelet count and function.
    - DDAVP:
      - Rapid (within an hour) onset of action with endothelial release of factors VIII and vWF
      - Therapeutic effect of DDAVP is ~24 hours and becomes refractory within 48 hours due to depletion of stored factors
      - Use with great caution (if at all) in patients with increased risks for cardiovascular diseases due to potential rapid BP changes (i.e., HTN, hypotension and reflex tachycardia).
    - Cryoprecipitate:
      - Immediate onset of action, duration of action 4 to 12 hours
      - Contains factors VIII, XIII, vWF, fibrinogen, and other clotting factors
    - Conjugated estrogen:
      - Onset of action 6 h to 5 to 7 days, duration of action 2 to 3 weeks
      - Mechanism of action: decrease L-arginine production (NO precursor), decrease antithrombin III and protein S levels, increase factor VII.

Other CKD-Related Issues

- Intravenous contrast media with imaging studies:
  - Iodinated radiocontrast media used with CT: See Acute Kidney Injury in Acute Kidney Injury/ICU Nephrology chapter
  - Gadolinium:
    - KDIGO recommends against its use in those with GFR < 15 mL/min/1.73 m^2.

- For patients with GFR < 30 mL/min/1.73 m^2 who require the use of an MRI contrast agent, a macrocyclic chelate preparation should be offered.
- KDIGO immunization recommendations for CKD patients:
  - Annual influenza vaccine if not contraindicated
  - Polyvalent pneumococcal vaccine for all adult CKD patients regardless of stage if no contraindication. The vaccine is to be given in the following order: 1. PCV13, 2. first dose of PSV23 8 weeks after PCV13, 3. second dose of PSV23 5 years later. Additionally, those who receive PSV23 before age 65 should receive another dose at age 65 or later if 5 years or more have elapsed since the previous PSV23 dose.
  - Hepatitis B vaccine for all adults with eGFR < 30 mL/min/1.73 m^2 and those with high risk of CKD progression. Confirm response serology.
  - Others per routine: tetanus, diphtheria, pertussis (Td/Tdap), varicella, human papillomavirus, zoster, measles, mumps, rubella (MMR)
  - Vaccines that are contraindicated in immunocompromising conditions (e.g. transplant recipients, patients receiving immunosuppressive therapy) excluding HIV: varicella, zoster, MMR
- Others: Phosphate-containing bowel preparation is not recommended in patients with GFR < 60 mL/min/1.73 m^2 due to risk of acute phosphate nephropathy.

STAGE IV AND V CHRONIC KIDNEY DISEASE

- Advanced uremic symptoms: see CKD complications and associated symptoms.
- Preparation for end-stage renal disease and RRT.
- Initiation of maintenance dialysis:
  - Time of initiation per KDOQI: "When patients reach stage 5 CKD (estimated GFR < 15 mL/min/1.73 m^2), nephrologists should evaluate the benefits, risks, and disadvantages of beginning kidney replacement therapy. Particular clinical considerations and certain characteristic complications of kidney failure may prompt initiation of therapy before stage 5."
  - "Particular considerations" for earlier initiation:
    - Recurring hyperkalemia despite corrections of all contributing factors
    - Volume overload leading to pulmonary edema or refractory to diuretics
    - Uremic pericarditis, unexplained pericardial effusion
    - Nausea/vomiting
    - Severe metabolic acidosis, particularly if cannot tolerate oral alkalinization
    - Declining health
    - Malnutrition:
      - General indicators: decline in serum albumin, weight loss
      - Patients with <90% of standard body weight (SBW) are considered to be mildly to moderately malnourished, and those who are <70% of SBW are considered severely malnourished. It is recommended that a target body weight for maintenance dialysis patients is between 90% and 110% of SBW (NHANES III).
  - Criteria for dialysis initiation for those with a failed transplant are similar to those for those with ESRD of native kidneys.
  - IDEAL trial:
    - $n = 828$ adults with progressive CKD and eGFR 10 to 15 mL/min/1.73 m^2 randomized to start dialysis at eGFR 10 to 15 versus 5.0 to 7.0 mL/min/1.73 m^2 (CG equation).

- At a median follow-up of 3.59 years, there was no difference in mortality or adverse events (cardiovascular events, infection, or dialysis complications).
- However, 75.9% of patients in the late-start group initiated dialysis prior to reaching target eGFR of 7.0 mL/min/1.73 m^2 due to uremic symptoms, volume overload, etc.
- Of interest, early dialysis start, defined as initiation at eGFR $\geq$ 10 mL/min/1.73 m^2 increased from 19% to 54% between 1996 and 2009, but stable at 54% from 2009 to 2011. Reasons for shift are unclear, but thought to be partially due to eGFR application.
- Planning for end-of-life care or withdrawal of RRT (The Renal Association 2014):
  - Estimate and discuss with patients prognosis and quality of life both with and without RRT.
  - Patients with deteriorating condition/comorbidities despite dialysis should be given consideration for end-of-life care.
  - For patients with poor life expectancy, maintain a supportive care registry to ensure care needs are met and provide opportunity for advance care planning.
  - Dialysis withdrawal should include end-of-life care planning by patient and all involved healthcare professionals. Assessment for competence and evaluation for depression should be performed.

END-STAGE RENAL DISEASE

Epidemiology of ESRD
- The most common etiologies leading to ESRD in the United States are DM and HTN.
- Dialysis initiation for a failed kidney transplant comprises ~5% of all incident dialysis patients in the United States over the past two decades.
- Regional differences are likely due to population differences: Network 16 (Pacific Northwest) has the lowest rate of ESRD, whereas Network 8 (Southeastern United States) has the highest rate of ESRD.

U.S. Prospective Payment System for ESRD
- In 2011, the US Centers for Medicare and Medicaid Services launched the prospective payment system (PPS) for ESRD care, when the "bundled" payment system was created. This policy
  - Limits the use of some medications and services in ESRD patients and
  - Increases monthly margin payment per PD compared with HD patient. Prior to this policy, payments favored adding an HD over PD patient.
  - The Study to Evaluate the Prospective Payment System Impact on Small Dialysis Organizations (STEPPS) revealed:
    - A decline in ESA doses and mean hemoglobin levels which coincided with the transition to PPS.
    - African American patients who tend to have higher ESA requirement to achieve target Hb were noted to have greater reductions in ESA doses in association with a greater proportion of patients with Hb < 10 g/dL, and

greater need for transfusions, compared to other groups. Long-term patient outcomes of PPS are needed.
* Decrease in intravenous vitamin D analogues and an increase in oral therapies
* Increase in serum parathyroid levels from 273 to 324 pg/dL

Factors Associated with Worse Survival in the Dialysis Patient

* Patient factors: Black worse than White which is worse than Asians, poor nutritional status (lower serum albumin, lower cholesterol levels, lower BMI), presence of inflammation or high inflammatory markers (higher C-reactive peptide levels), troponin leaks, lower predialysis serum potassium levels, loss of residual kidney function, poor control of bone mineral disease, depression, sleep apnea, restless leg syndrome
* Dialysis factors: (Highest death rates on) Mondays for Monday/Wednesday/Friday hemodialysis patients and Tuesdays for Tuesday/Thursday/Saturday dialysis patients (presumably due to cardiovascular complications/volume overload/electrolyte abnormalities), use of dialysate $K^+ < 2$ mEq/L, lower dialysis duration, higher ultrafiltration (UF) rate (i.e., >13 mL/kg/h), intradialytic myocardial stunning (measured as intradialytic regional wall motion abnormalities; higher risk of myocardial stunning with higher UF and intradialytic hypotensive episodes)

Principles of Dialysis

* Solute clearance by dialysis occurs via diffusion, convection, or both.
  * Diffusion is determined by concentration difference between blood and dialysate.
  * Convection, a.k.a. "solvent drag," occurs with ultrafiltration where smaller solutes are "dragged" by the movement of water across the dialysis membrane.

Forms of Dialysis

* Peritoneal dialysis relies on both diffusion and convection across peritoneal membrane for solute clearance. Water clearance relies on the osmolality of the dialysate.
* Hemodialysis relies mostly on diffusion for solute clearance.
* Continuous dialysis (Also see ICU Nephrology in Acute Kidney Injury/ICU Nephrology chapter):
  * Continuous venovenous hemodialysis refers to diffusion driven dialysis with the use of a dialysate solution performed over 24 hours.
  * Continuous venovenous hemo**filtration** refers to treatment where large ultrafiltration volume is coupled with replacement fluid to increase removal of larger and less diffusible solutes (middle molecules) via convection. Replacement fluid may be administered pre-, mid-, or postfiltration.
  * Continuous venovenous hemo**dia**filtration refers to the combination of the above two forms which include both hemofiltration and hemodialysis. Hemodiafiltration is good for clearance of both low- and middle-molecular-weight uremic toxins compared to mostly small molecules with conventional HD.
Dialysis membrane characteristics:
* Hemodialysis membrane:
  * Membrane used for dialysis is made of substituted cellulose, cellulosynthetics, or synthetics.
  * Resistance for solute movement across membrane depends on membrane thickness, unstirred fluid layers next to the membrane.
  * Type/size of solute removal depends on pore size of membrane.

- Peritoneal membrane:
  - Membrane used is the peritoneal membrane.
  - Resistance for solute movement from circulation across the membrane into the abdominal cavity depends on stagnant capillary fluid film, capillary endothelium, endothelial basement membrane, interstitium, mesothelium, and stagnant peritoneal membrane fluid film.
  - The natural peritoneal membrane has pores of various sizes that allow the removal of solutes of different sizes. In general, these pores are classified into three-pore sizes, known as the "three-pore size model":
    - Large pores, 20 to 40 nm, responsible for solute removal by convection and protein loss.
    - Small pores, 4 to 6 nm, correspond to interendothelial clefts, allows for diffusion of smaller molecules across the membrane, including urea, Cr, Na^+, K^+.
    - Ultrapores, <0.8 nm, correspond to aquaporins which are responsible for H_2O removal without concurrent solute/sodium removal, a process known as "H_2O transport sieving" or "sodium sieving" since solutes/sodium are "left behind."
- Optimization of dialysis membrane:
  - Hemodialysis:
    - Membrane material: the frequency of complement activation occurs in the following order: cellulose > substituted cellulose, cellulosynthetic, > synthetic. Membranes with high degree of complement activation induce more problems with anaphylactic shock or nonspecific allergic reactions to patients. Cellulose membranes are no longer used.
    - Sterilization techniques: gamma radiation; electron (E)-beam (risk of thrombocytopenia); ethylene oxide (risk of anaphylactoid reactions)
    - UF coefficient: K_{uf}: 3.3 to 83 mL/h/mm Hg
      - Higher K_{uf} provides greater dialysis efficiency and flux. The former, due to increased "solvent drag" from convection.
      - Use lower transmembrane pressure for membranes with higher Kuf to achieve the same volume of ultrafiltration.
      - Example: What should the transmembrane pressure (TMP) be to remove 500 mL/h for membranes with the following Kuf: (NOTE: Know how to calculate TMP or UF volume from Kuf)
        - Kuf 50 mL/h/mm Hg: TMP = 500 mL/h ÷ 50 mL/h/mm Hg = 10 mm Hg
    - Membranes with larger pore size provide "higher flux" dialysis.
    - Mass transfer coefficient for urea: KoA urea (maximum theoretical clearance): 245 to 1000$^+$ mL/min (<500 "low efficiency," 500 to 700 "moderate efficiency," >700 "high efficiency")
    - Surface area of dialysis membrane: 1 to 2.1 m^2. The larger the surface area, the greater the dialysis efficiency.
  - Peritoneal dialysis:
    - The peritoneal surface area may be increased by using a high dialysate volume for greater dialysis efficiency. The higher the volume, the higher the contact surface for dialysis. The maximum peritoneal dialysate volume tolerated is typically 2 to 3 L.
    - Unlike hemodialysis membranes, the intrinsic characteristics of the peritoneal membrane cannot be "changed" to optimize dialysis efficiency:
      - Intrinsic peritoneal membrane resistance

- Hydraulic conductance (density of small pores and ultrapores, distance of capillaries from mesothelium)
- Inflammatory versus sclerotic state (increased peritoneal vascularity with acute inflammation leads to higher solute transport into dialysate, but lower UF with prolonged dwell due to more rapid achievement of osmotic equilibrium between blood and dialysate)
- Factors that determine dialysis efficiency:
  - Hemodialysis: the greater the following factors, the greater the "dialysis efficiency."
    - Membrane surface area
    - KoA and K_{uf} of membrane
    - Duration of dialysis
    - Dialysate flow rate (Q_d)
    - Blood flow rate (Q_b)
    - Vascular access flow (Q_a)
    - Concentration gradient difference of solute between dialysate and blood

> **NOTE**
> - Understand the difference between "high efficiency" and "high flux."
> - Dialysis efficiency is *not* dependent on dialyzer membrane type, but rather the membrane's KoA, Kuf, and surface area.
> - Access recirculation reduces dialysis efficiency.
> - For central venous catheter, cardiopulmonary recirculation is higher in patients with lower cardiac output, thus lower dialysis efficiency.

- Peritoneal dialysis:
  - Peritoneal membrane characteristics
  - Patient mobility: poor dialysis in immobilized patient due to stagnant dialysate
  - Concentration gradient between blood and dialysate which depends on dwell time and number of exchanges
  - Ultrafiltration:
    - Concentration of osmotically active agent in dialysate (e.g., glucose, icodextrin)
    - Hydrostatic pressure gradient (patient's blood pressure)
  - Fluid absorption back into circulation
  - Capillary vasodilatory versus vasoconstrictive state
  - Oncotic pressure gradient, which depends on:
    - Sieving property of solute: the higher the sieving coefficient (solute crosses membrane more easily) the greater convective transport for the solute
    - Reflection coefficient of osmotic agent in dialysate (high value suggests agent does not cross the membrane easily, but "reflects" back into peritoneal fluid). Maintenance of osmotic gradient depends on the reflection coefficient for the osmotic agent (i.e., glucose: 0.03, polyglucose icodextrin ~1.0). The agent with a high reflection coefficient (icodextrin) is able to maintain the osmotic difference between the blood and dialysate better, hence better osmotic force favoring ultrafiltration into peritoneum.

NOTE Icodextrin versus dextrose:
- Icodextrin solution may be considered in patients with DM (or high transporters) who have lost adequate UF with dextrose solutions.
- The metabolites of icodextrin, maltose and polysaccharides, can lead to falsely high glucose level readings with regular finger glucose check devices, thus *masking life-threatening hypoglycemia*.
- Icodextrin can also lead to falsely low levels of amylase.
- Difference between dextrose and icodextrin with regard to water transport:
  - Water transport with dextrose can occur via two routes:
    - Water and concurrent solute (i.e., Na^+) transport through interendothelial cell pores
    - Dextrose can also open aquaporins (AQ1) and allow *water-only* transport which results in "sodium sieving."
    - Effect of sodium sieving:
      - Early dwell: dialysate is diluted by ultrafiltrate from H_2O transport across AQ1 without concurrent Na^+ movement across peritoneal membrane. Hypernatremia is possible in this phase.
      - Longer dwell: concentration gradient (lower $[Na^+]$ in dialysate compared to that of blood) favors Na^+ loss into dialysate via smaller peritoneal membrane pores.
      - Na^+ loss with a 4-hour, 1.5% dextrose, 2 L exchange is minimal, but a 4-hour 4.25% dextrose, 2 L dwell can be up to 70 mEq.
  - Icodextrin does not open up aquaporins. Water transport with icodextrin only occurs concurrently with solute transport through interendothelial cell pores. There is no sodium sieving with icodextrin.
- Cautions with icodextrin: contraindicated in patients with known allergy to cornstarch or icodextrin, maltose or isomaltose intolerance, glycogen storage disease, and preexisting severe lactic acidosis. Blistering and exfoliative skin eruptions have been reported with icodextrin.

Selection of RRT Modality: HD versus PD

- PD provides greater independence and patient satisfaction.
- Lower cost with PD
- Similar outcomes (hospitalizations, mortality) compared to HD during the first 4 to 5 years.
- Current national trend favors PD program expansion, with goal of 30% to 40% of all RRT.
- Dialysis education: Treatment options education program (TOPS): attendees have an adjusted odds ratio of 5.13 to choose PD over HD compared with nonattendees. Of interest, mortality adjusted hazard ratio was 0.61 for TOPS attendees.
- HD, but *not* PD, is associated with intradialytic "myocardial stunning" presumably due to myocardial ischemia.
  - Myocardial stunning is measured as intradialytic regional wall motion abnormalities
  - Myocardial stunning is associated with poor prognosis and worse survival
  - Risks: higher UF and intradialytic hypotensive episodes
- Australia and New Zealand Dialysis and Transplant Registry (ANZDATA):
  - In-center HD < 3 times per week had increased risk for cardiac mortality on Mondays compared to all other days of the week. This is thought to be due to hyperkalemia and/or myocardial infarction.

- Patients on PD, home HD, and in-center HD $\geq$ 3 times per week had no significant variation in cardiac death across all days of the week. This suggests more frequent dialysis treatments, and not dialysis modality, contributed to survival benefits.

HEMODIALYSIS

- Absolute contraindications: exhausted sites for vascular access
- Relative contraindications:
  - End-stage heart/liver/lung disease (most common reasons to withhold hemodialysis)
  - Difficult vascular access
  - Needle phobia
  - Coagulopathy
- Considerations for home hemodialysis
  - Relatively young and relatively "healthy" individual
  - Must have an independent devoted partner
- Hemodialysis apparatus
  - Arterial pressure monitor
  - Blood pump
  - Dialyzer a.k.a. "Kidney"
  - Venous pressure monitor
  - Air trap and air detector

Water Treatment for Hemodialysis

- On average, weekly hemodialysis requires ~500 L of H_2O (assuming an average dialysate flow of 800 mL/min, 3 to 4 h/dialysis treatment, three treatments per week).
- Water purification steps: required steps (carbon filtration and reverse osmosis)
  - Carbon filtration:
    - Removes chlorine and chloramine (added from municipal water) and organic contaminants. NOTE: chloramine can cause hemolysis.
    - Carbon filtration is done prior to reverse osmosis (see below) because chlorine and chloramine can damage the membrane used in reverse osmosis.
  - Softeners (optional if hard water to protect reverse osmosis membrane):
    - Exchanges calcium and magnesium ions for sodium ions.
    - This step may be added prior to reverse osmosis to protect the reverse osmosis membrane. Accumulation of calcium and magnesium can cause fouling of osmosis membrane.
  - Reverse osmosis:
    - A process whereby water is forced across a semipermeable membrane by high-pressure system
    - Reverse osmosis removes dissolved inorganic elements including metal ions (i.e., zinc, fluoride, copper, aluminum, arsenic), salts, chemicals, organic elements, bacteria, viruses, and endotoxins.
  - Deionization:
    - Further removes residual ions by exchange resins made up of both cations and anions (e.g., hydrogen and hydroxyl ions respectively) to exchange for

negatively and positively charged ionic contaminants respectively following reverse osmosis.
  - Close monitoring of the product water-specific resistivity or conductivity is required to detect changes consistent with depletion of resins. NOTE: Depletion of resins can cause release of previously removed ions such as *fluoride and may result in acute toxicity and death*. Chronic fluoride exposure can contribute to osteodystrophy.
  - Note that the deionizer provides a good milieu for bacterial proliferation. Extra step for bacterial control is needed.
 - Ultrafilter/endotoxin filter: extra and optional step used to remove any residual bacteria and endotoxins.
- Routine microbiologic testing must be performed for both bacterial count (<100 CFU/mL) and endotoxins (<0.5 EU/mL). Corrective measures must be done at half of maximal allowable levels. Water purification for dialysis does not produce "sterile" water.
- Hospital bedside and home hemodialysis water purification:
  - Water treatment approach is similar as outpatient fixed-station systems.
  - Mobile units similarly require a carbon filtration, reverse osmosis system, and point-of-use ultrafiltration, with or without a softener prior to carbon filtration.
  - Bacterial proliferation is a major concern for mobile units.
  - Steps to minimize bacterial proliferation:
    - Use a direct-(H_2O) feed system instead of storage tank.
    - Use a point-of-use ultrafilter.
    - Use a backflow prevention device in case the mobile system is connected directly to the hospital potable water supply.

Hemodialysis Vascular Access

- Type of vascular access goal for chronic hemodialysis: arteriovenous fistula (AVF) 60%, arteriovenous graft (AVG) 30%, temporary catheter $< 10\%$
- Acute temporary catheters or cuffed, tunneled catheter (Permacath)
  - Low flow rates (300 mL/min for temporary catheters, 400 mL/min for Permacath)
  - Access dysfunction frequencies: left internal jugular catheters $>$ right internal jugular catheters $=$ femoral catheters
  - Access infections:
    - Higher rates for infections compared to AVG and AVF
    - Femoral lines are not at increased risk for infections unless patient has markedly elevated BMI.
  - Clearance (urea reduction ratio):
    - Femoral $=$ jugular catheters in terms of clearance if femoral catheters are >20 cm. Shorter femoral catheters have lower URR compared with jugular catheters.
    - For blood flow > 200 mL/min, URR is lower in femoral compared with jugular.
  - Bottom line:
    - Femoral access placement is an acceptable alternative to right jugular vein access placement in critically ill patients.
    - Femoral catheters should be longer than 20 cm to reach the inferior vena cava for better clearance.
    - Femoral catheters may have a higher rate of infection in patients with markedly elevated BMI.

- Catheter dysfunction:
  - Signs of access dysfunction or thrombosis: reduced HD blood flow or reduced Kt/V
  - Management: trial of a thrombolytic agent (e.g., t-PA 2 mg per port for 30 to 60 minutes)
  - Central vein stenosis, particularly with subclavian catheters
- AVF:
  - Preferred access due to lower risk of infectious and thrombotic complications
  - High rate of primary failure (nonmaturation), but better long-term patency compared to grafts
  - Preoperative vascular mapping increases fistula placement but fails to improve primary failure (nonmaturation). Optimal venous mapping findings:
    - Arterial diameter ≥ 2.0 mm, vein diameter ≥ 2.5 mm
    - Brachial artery flow > 80 mL/min
    - Absence of stenosis or thrombosis of draining vein up to shoulder and central vein
  - Clinical risks for AVF nonmaturation: older age, females, peripheral vascular disease, peripheral vascular disease, prior peripheral-inserted central catheter (PICC) line, forearm AVF compared to upper arm AVF
  - Optimizing AVF maturation success: 6-week postoperative ultrasound: vein depth < 5.0 mm, vein diameter > 4.0 mm, length of fistula thrill/bruit > 5.0 cm, access flow > 500 mL/min.
  - Early surgical repair:
    - Vein is too deep: repair by superficialization
    - Low access flow:
      - Due to stenosis at anastomosis or draining vein: repair by angioplasty or surgical revision
      - Due to large accessory veins: repair by surgical ligation
  - Risks for secondary AVF failure: intradialytic hypotension, high cannulation rate (i.e., daily hemodialysis)
- AVG:
  - May be considered in patients with suboptimal venous mapping parameters, failed AVF, or low expected patient survival
  - Synthetic conduit (e.g., polytetrafluoroethylene) created between an artery and vein
  - AVG maturation typically requires 2 to 3 weeks. However, vectra or flexine grafts may be used in 12 hours.
  - Risks for graft thrombosis: stenosis at anastomotic site, draining vein, or central veins
  - AVG has higher infection risks compared to AVF. Infectious lesions that involve the underlying AVG require complete surgical resection.
  - Pseudoaneurysms caused by repeated cannulations at the same site of the AVG may result in life-threatening bleeding and must be repaired surgically or with covered stent placement.
  - Improving graft patency:
    - Routine surveillance with static dialysis venous pressure or Doppler of access. For the latter, reduced blood flow, defined as <600 mL/min or fall by >25% from baseline, likely indicates significant stenosis.
    - Clinical clues for graft stenosis: prolonged bleeding, unexpected fall in Kt/V, distal edema, abnormal bruits or reduced thrill
    - Anticoagulation for protection against graft thrombosis and survival:
      - Not helpful: warfarin, clopidogrel plus aspirin combination

- Minimally helpful: dipyridamole + aspirin
- Fish oil reduces risk of thrombosis, but not long-term graft event.

Hemodialysis Complications

- Infections: most commonly, access related
- Headaches, nausea, vomiting:
  - Dialysis disequilibrium due to rapid solute removal, resultant acute fall in extracellular osmolality and subsequent cerebral edema.
    - Risks: patients with high BUN level who are aggressively dialyzed, younger age, existing neurologic disorders; use of low sodium dialysate
    - Other symptoms: blurred vision, altered mental status, muscle twitching, seizures, coma
    - Prevention is key:
      - BUN reduction should not exceed 30%.
      - Use mannitol in patients with BUN levels > 100 mg/dL (e.g., 25 g at start of dialysis, followed by 12.5 g/h.
  - Large volume removal, hypotension
  - Acute fall in caffeine level during dialysis in those with habitual high caffeine intake
  - Other electrolyte changes: rapid change in serum sodium concentrations, hypoglycemia
  - Others: subdural hematoma, increased intraocular pressure with dialysis (rare), psychological factors
  - Unlikely contributing factors: dialyzer membrane composition, biocompatibility
  - Fluoride contaminants from water system (headaches, nausea, chest pain, hypotension, neuromuscular symptoms, cardiac arrhythmias)
- Chest pain:
  - Angina:
    - Underlying coronary artery disease
    - Management: aspirin, oxygen supplement, nitrates, morphine as indicated if safely tolerated
    - If patient is on a β-blocker, make sure it is nondialyzable (carvedilol, labetalol). NOTE: Atenolol and metoprolol are dialyzable. There is evidence to suggest worse cardiovascular mortality with the use of dialyzable compared with nondialyzable β-blockers in dialysis patients.
- Hypotension (intradialytic hypotension):
  - Contributing factors:
    - Excessive fluid and/or rapid solute removal
    - Gastrointestinal blood pooling if eating during dialysis for some patients
    - Cardiovascular diseases: poor underlying cardiac function, clinically significant pericardial effusion, ischemic heart disease
    - Dialysate factors: use of acetate or low calcium concentrations
    - Dialyzer reaction (very rare with current synthetic dialyzer use)
    - Air embolism
  - Management:
    - Dialysis procedure: low dialysate temperature, avoid low calcium dialysate, slow UF (i.e., <0.35 mL/min/kg)
    - Others: Hold BP medications prior to dialysis, avoid intradialytic eating, avoid large interdialytic weight gain (IDWG), evaluate cardiac function/pericardial effusion, correct anemia and hypoalbuminemia if applicable, consider predialytic administration of low-dose midodrine.

- Hemolysis (dialysis-induced):
  - This is a potentially rapid fatal condition if not recognized immediately
    - Hemolysis differential diagnoses: problems with dialysate (e.g., overheating, erroneous electrolyte mixing leading to hypotonic dialysate, faulty water treatments with residual contaminants (e.g., metal ions [copper, nitrates], disinfectants [bleach], chloramine from municipal water), kinking of dialysis lines, problems with arterial cannulation or flow limiting blood inflow (may be seen as flattening of line)

> **NOTE** If intradialytic hemolysis occurs, stop HD but do not return hemolyzed blood back to patient. Monitor patient for hyperkalemia.

  - Clinical signs/symptoms suggestive of hemolysis: chest pain, dyspnea, back pain, bradycardia if significant hyperkalemia, port-wine appearance of blood in venous line, pink plasma in centrifuged blood specimens
  - Immediate chest pain and dyspnea are likely due to anaphylactic reaction to dialyzer membrane. In the past, this was seen in patients on ACEI/ARB with polyacrylonitrile (PAN) membrane. This is no longer used.
- Air embolism: rare with current use of air detectors, but may occur with removal of connecting caps or blood lines in patients dialyzed via central venous catheters. Management: stop HD, clamp venous return, place patient in left Trendelenburg position to get air bubbles float up away from brain and lungs
- Pulmonary embolism (thrombus migration from vascular access)
- Arrhythmias:
  - Risks likely associated with underlying ischemic or structural heart disease, left ventricular hypertrophy, mitral valve calcifications.
  - Rapid change in potassium with dialysis is a concern, but yet to be a proven risk
  - Low calcium dialysate
- Dyspnea:
  - Prior to dialysis: volume overload, pneumonia, subacute bacterial infections
  - Intra- or postdialysis: angina, allergic reaction to dialysis membrane, pericardial effusion, aspiration, pneumonia, bacteremia, reaction to any intravenous drugs given during dialysis (e.g., iron)
- Hypertension:
  - Dialyzable antihypertensive medications
  - High dialysate sodium
  - Renin angiotensin and sympathetic nervous systems activation
  - Imbalance between vasodilating NO and vasoconstricting endothelin
- Dialyzer reactions (reactions due to blood exposure to dialyzer):
  - Two major types: Type A (anaphylactoid reaction) and type B (mild reaction)
  - Type A:
    - Rare: Anaphylactoid response mediated by bradykin and/or histamine
    - Increased risk in patients with a history of allergic reactions during dialysis
    - Onset within 20 minutes of starting dialysis:
      - Major symptoms: dyspnea, burning sensation at access site or systemically, and angioedema

- Minor symptoms: reproducible symptoms with dialysis, rhinorrhea or lacrimation, abdominal cramping, itching
    - Etiologies: use of ethylene oxide for dialyzer sterilization; intravenous iron; PAN membranes in patients receiving ACE inhibitors (obsolete)
    - Management: stop dialysis and discard blood, supportive therapy with oxygen, antihistamines, epinephrine, and corticosteroid.
  - Type B:
    - Occurs within 20 to 40 minutes of starting dialysis
    - Dissipation of symptoms with subsequent dialysis treatments
    - Thought to be complement mediated
    - Previously thought to be due to membrane biocompatibility. Current data do not support this.
  - Other reactions:
    - Water-related reactions
    - Fevers/chills: consider bacterial or endotoxin contamination, possibly via back filtration at zero net UF pressure.
- Thrombocytopenia: likely due to heparin-induced thrombocytopenia ± thrombosis (HITT), particularly if seen 4 to 10 days following heparin administration. This condition is due to the production of antibodies that bind to complexes of heparin and platelet factor 4, leading to platelet activation and promotion of a prothrombotic state. Thrombocytopenia may occur with E-beam sterilization.
- Vascular access issues:
  - Access recirculation (i.e., uptake of dialyzed blood occurs when dialyzer blood flow is greater than access blood flow)
    - Causes of access recirculation:
      - Downstream stenosis or thrombosis
      - Arterial stenosis
      - Close needle placement or reversal of lines
    - Screening options:
      - Doppler ultrasound
      - Transonic access blood flow: flow < 600 mL/min or reduced by ≥25% from baseline flow suggests increased risk for access recirculation
      - Ultrasound dilution: reverse lines and saline dilution
      - Static venous pressure
      - Arterial versus venous urea to assess percentage of recirculation:

        % recirculation = [(plasma urea − arterial urea)/(plasma urea − venous urea)] × 100%; Remember: (P − A)/(P − V) × 100%.
        A value > 25% suggests significant access recirculation.

Peritoneal Dialysis

- Indications:
  - Patients who prefer PD or refuse HD
  - Patients who cannot tolerate HD due to poor cardiovascular function or who have no vascular access (e.g., severe congestive heart disease, extensive vascular disease)
  - Patients who prefer home dialysis modality and cannot perform home HD
  - No HD availability
- Absolute contraindications for PD:
  - Loss of peritoneal function, ultrafiltration failure

- Intra-abdominal adhesions blocking dialysate flow
- Surgically uncorrectable abdominal hernia
- Abdominal wall stoma
- Diaphragmatic fluid leak
- Inability to perform exchanges in absence of suitable assistant
- Poor hygiene, inability to safely perform PD for any reasons (e.g., severe physical or mental disabilities)
- Active abdominal inflammatory diseases (e.g., diverticulitis, ischemic bowel disease, intra-abdominal abscess)
- Relative contraindications for PD:
  - Recent abdominal aortic graft
  - Large kidneys due to polycystic kidney disease
  - Hernias
  - Ostomy
  - Abdominal adhesions
  - Ventriculoperitoneal shunt
  - Intolerance of intra-abdominal fluid in patients with morbid obesity
  - Severe malnutrition
  - Uncontrolled skin infection
  - Bowel disease
  - *Staphylococcus aureus* carrier
  - Homelessness

Dialysis Adequacy

KDOQI Recommendations

- Hemodialysis, given 3 times per week:
- For patients with residual kidney urea clearance $K_r < 2$ mL/min/1.73 m^2:
  - Minimally adequate dose of HD:
    - Single pool Kt/V, (spKt/V) ≥ 1.2 per dialysis (not including K_r), or
    - Urea reduction ratio URR $\geq 65\%$
  - Target dialysis dose:
    - spKt/V ≥ 1.4 (~ equilibrated Kt/V eKt/V ≥ 1.2) per dialysis (not including K_r), or
    - URR $\geq 70\%$
- For patients with residual kidney urea clearance $K_r \geq 2$ mL/min/1.73 m^2:
  - Minimally adequate dose of HD: spKt/V may be reduced
  - Target dialysis dose: $\geq 15\%$ of minimum dose

> **NOTE**
> - Optimal dialysis time and frequency are undefined: ≥ 3.5 hours? Frequent HD has been suggested for patients with problems with nutrition or volume overload, but current data show no benefit in terms of nutrition or anemia control. Additionally, for patients with residual kidney function with >100 mL/d urine output, frequent HD provides no benefit in terms of left ventricular hypertrophy.
> - UF rate > 13 mL/kg/h is associated with increased mortality. Optimal UF rate not established.
> - Current Kt/V target dosing may not be adequate in women or small patients.

- Peritoneal dialysis (PD):
  - There is increasing evidence to indicate the importance of residual kidney function in small-solute clearance in addition to PD in terms of benefiting patient survival.
  - For patients with residual kidney function (defined as urine volume > 100 mL/d):
    - Minimal "delivered" dose of total small-solute clearance should be a total (PD and kidney) $Kt/V_{urea} \geq 1.7/wk$.
    - Total (PD plus residual kidney function) Kt/V_{urea} should be measured within the first month following dialysis initiation and ≥4 months thereafter.
    - In patients with urine volume > 100 mL/d, where residual kidney function is added to PD Kt/V_{urea} to achieve goal, a repeat 24 hour urine collection for K_r must be done at least every 2 months.
  - For patients without residual kidney function (defined as urine volume ≤ 100 mL/d): Minimal "delivered" dose of total small-solute clearance should be a PD $Kt/V_{urea} \geq 1.7/wk$. This is measured within the first month following PD initiation and at least every 4 months thereafter.
- NOTE: Kt/V_{urea} as a measure for dialysis adequacy in PD is being questioned:
- PD does not have good small solute clearance, (e.g. urea clearance) which explains why PD patients have higher blood urea nitrogen and creatinine than HD patients. However, PD clears many other clinically significant uremic toxins that are not captured with Kt/V_{urea}.
- Lack of data to show that Kt/V_{urea} predicts outcome in PD.
- Optimal molecule (middle molecule) to assess Kt/V in PD is not defined.
- Current expert opinions suggest a comprehensive evaluation for PD adequacy based on multiple markers rather than just focusing on Kt/V_{urea} (Kt/V_{urea} is only a marker for small molecule clearance). Other markers to consider include preservation of residual kidney function, mineral metabolism (phosphorus) control, β-2 microglobulins and p-cresol.
- Maintenance of residual renal function: even preservation of 1 mL/min reduces annual mortality by 15% to 25%.
  - Use of RAAS inhibitors (can also slow deterioration of residual kidney function)
  - Avoid contrast dye, NSAIDS, COX-2 inhibitors, nephrotoxic agents.
  - Use of diuretics for volume control has not been shown to accelerate progression of residual kidney function loss.

SPECIAL TOPICS IN CHRONIC KIDNEY DISEASE

Dermatology

Nonspecific manifestations:
- Pallor (40%): likely due to anemia.
- Hyperpigmentation (20%): Thought to be due to increased concentrations of melanocyte-stimulating hormone. Treatment: sunscreen
- Half-and-half nails (a.k.a. Lindsay nails) (20%): proximal half of nail is white, distal half of nail is normal or brown in color. Thought to be due to increased tissue concentration of melanocyte-stimulating hormone. Benign, no treatment
- Xerosis, dry scaly skin (50% to 85%): Thought to be due to dehydration of stratum corneum and reduced sebum and sweat production. Treatment: routine skin emollient application, avoid excessive washing.

- Uremic pruritis:
  - Likely multifactorial, suggested contributing factors: hypervitaminosis A, secondary hyperparathyroidism, high levels of calcium, phosphorus, magnesium, iron deficiency anemia, xerosis, increased inflammatory cytokines, abnormal neurologic signaling, imbalance of endogenous CNS opioid peptides, down-regulation of κ-opioid receptors
  - Treatment options: correction of electrolyte abnormalities, skin emollient application, small doses of gabapentin (100 mg daily) or pregabalin (25 mg daily), the κ-receptor agonist nalfurafine (5 μg daily)
- Acquired perforating dermatosis (up to 10%):
  - Unclear etiology, mostly affect African Americans, strongly associated with CKD and DM, characterized by transepidermal absence of dermal structures (i.e., collagen, keratin, elastic fibers).
  - Clinically manifested as localized pruritis, presence of firm, dome-shaped papules or nodules with central keratotic plugs on extensor surfaces of extremities and trunk. New lesions with trauma/scratching may form (Koebnerization).
  - Treatment options:
    - Topicals: steroid creams (clobetasol or β-methasone) and/or a keratolytic agent (salicylic acid, urea, or ammonium lactate); retinoid; catharidin
    - Oral therapies: antihistamines, low-dose allopurinol, acitretin, doxycline or minocycline
    - Others: cryotherapy, phototherapy
- Bullous diseases:
  - Porphyria cutanea tarda (PCT) is due to uroporphyrinogen–decarboxylase (URO-D) deficiency and is exaggerated by alcohol abuse, hepatitis C, HIV, and iron supplementation. HD patients may develop PCT due to decreased URO-D activity and poor clearance of plasma porphyrins. PD patients are less susceptible to PCT due to better porphyrin clearance. Management: avoidance of triggers (e.g., alcohol, hepatotoxic medications, sun exposure, iron overload) and use of high flux dialyzers for effective porphyrin removal.
  - Pseudoporphyria is clinically and histologically similar to PCT, but without serum and urine porphyrin abnormalities. Management: avoidance of triggers (e.g., diuretics, antibiotics, antifungals) and sun exposure. Consider N-acetylcysteine.
- Calcific uremic arteriolopathy:
  - Condition characterized by systemic medial calcification of arterioles, ischemic necrosis of skin and subcutaneous tissues
  - Associated with high morbidity and mortality (up to 45% to 80% mortality within 1 year)
  - Potential therapy:
    - Intravenous sodium thiosulfate 25 g thrice weekly followed by oral maintenance therapy if good clinical response. Efficacy is variable and duration of therapy undefined. (Poor efficacy in authors' opinion)
    - Other concurrent therapies: wound care, control of secondary hyperparathyroidism and hyperphosphatemia, optimize dialysis, use of lower calcium dialysate (only if safely tolerated due to hypotension associated with lower calcium dialysate), debridement only when absolutely necessary due to increased risk of infections
    - Avoid: warfarin, vitamin D analogues, calcium-based phosphate binders
    - Consider intensive dialysis

- Patient-related risk factors: female gender, obesity (associated with truncal lesions rather than distal lesions), dialysis vintage, skin trauma (i.e., repeated injections), hypoalbuminemia, underlying autoimmune disease, DM
- Medication-related risk factors: steroids, warfarin, vitamin D analogs, calcium-based phosphate binders, iron therapy
- Nephrogenic systemic fibrosis (NSF):
  - Scleroderma-like disorder seen in patients with severely impaired kidney function (i.e., GFR < 15 to 30 mL/min) who receive gadolinium-based contrast agents (mostly reported with Omniscan).
  - Clinical manifestations: painful, symmetric erythema and edema that become firm papules/plaques and nodules resembling burn scars. Internal organ fibrosis may occur.
  - Pathogenesis: increased production and migration of circulating fibrocytes to susceptible tissues with ongoing inflammation or injury
  - Increased risks: PD compared to HD, elevated serum phosphate levels, exposure to high dose or repeated exposures
  - Triggering factors: underlying ischemic or thrombotic vascular injury, infection, high-dose erythropoietin therapy
  - Management:
    - KEY: avoidance of linear and ionic gadolinium in patients with GFR < 30 mL/min or AKI
    - Initiate HD as soon as possible *only if* ESRD. Note, however, that even with immediate postexposure dialysis, patient may not be protected from developing NSF due to first-pass effect.
    - Beneficial medical therapies reported: corticosteroids, sirolimus, PTF, methotrexate, high-dose intravenous Ig, imatinib mesylate, alefacept, sodium thiosulfate
    - Other reported beneficial interventions: successful renal transplant, ultraviolet A phototherapy, plasmapheresis
- Dialysis β2-microglobulin amyloidosis:
  - Increased risk: long-term hemodialysis or continuous ambulatory peritoneal dialysis
  - β2-microglobulin is a major constituent of amyloid fibrils that can deposit in synovial membranes and osteoarticular sites leading to destructive osteoarthropathies or major solid organs such as heart and GI tract.
  - Incidence > 95% with >15 years of hemodialysis vintage in the past, but likely lower at present due to greater removal of β2-microglobulin with high flux dialysis.
  - Clinical manifestations: carpal tunnel syndrome, flexor tenosynovitis, subchondral bone cysts/erosions, fractures, heart failure, pulmonary HTN, GI bleed
  - Pathogenesis: poor clearance without residual kidney function, inflammatory state, prolonged uremic exposure, advanced glycation end products of β2-microglobulin
  - Management: supportive, physical and/or occupational therapy, surgical repair

SPECIAL HEMODIALYSIS ISSUES

- High-flux dialysis may confer improved cardiovascular mortality over low-flux in multicenter analyses, but questioned at facility-level analysis.
- Reuse of dialyzers: no significant harm or benefit has been shown with dialyzer reuse compared with single-use dialyzers.
- Kt/V, problem with V:
  - Single pool Kt/V > 1.7, where V is based on the volume of distribution of urea or total body volume, is not associated with improved survival, whereas higher Kt/V normalized for body surface area Kt/Vs, is associated with survival benefit.
  - There are concerns that using the traditional Kt/V for dialysis dosing may result in inadequate HD, particularly for female patients and children.
  - Higher Kt/V may be associated with higher hypotensive episodes.
- Dialysis duration:
  - Ideal duration unknown
  - DOPPS: increasing dialysis treatment time was associated with a reduction in all-cause mortality, increased hemoglobin, albumin, decreased WBC count and phosphate levels.
  - Nocturnal HD:
    - Associated with lower interdialytic weight gain, better serum albumin levels, systolic blood pressure, serum phosphorus, and WBC count compared with matched control from in-center HD patients
    - 25% reduction in risk for death after adjustment for age, BMI, and dialysis vintage
    - Potential problems: high dropout rate, higher vascular access complications compared to in-center HD
- Target body dry weight, body volume:
  - Higher interdialytic weight gain is associated with increased mortality.
  - Measurements of body volume: B-natriuretic peptides, blood volume monitoring, bioimpedance
    - Blood volume monitoring (BVM): a method whereby blood volume changes is detected by changes in intravascular hematocrit. Theoretically, when the UF rate is the same as the rate of interstitial fluid mobilizing into the intravascular volume, there is no change in Hct. When UFR is higher than the rate of interstitial fluid moving into the intravascular space, Hct will be expected to increase. BVM is designed to reduce hypotension episodes during ultrafiltration with HD, but it does not detect the excess volume in interstitial space and cannot determine dry weights in HD patients.
    - Bioimpedance: a method whereby current frequencies ranging from 5 to 1,000 kHz are passed through the skin. While low-frequency currents preferentially pass through the extracellular fluid space due to its inability to penetrate cell membranes, high-frequency current can penetrate the extracellular and intracellular space. Comparisons of these values to those of nonuremic patients can help quantify total body water volume, intracellular and extracellular volumes in dialysis patients.
- Dialysate electrolyte concentrations:
  - Sodium:
    - Sodium modeling: Using dialysate [Na^+] greater than that of patient's plasma minimizes intradialytic hypotension and symptoms of disequilibrium at the expense of sodium gain, increased thirst, IDGW, and predialysis BP.

- Using dialysate [Na$^+$] lower (e.g., 5%) than that of patient's plasma can improve UF to achieve dry weight (temporary measure only). See DOPPS study.
  - DOPPS: patients with serum [Na$^+$] < 137 mEq/L appear to have survival benefits when higher dialysate [Na$^+$] (>140 mEq/L) was used. Similar finding was not appreciated in patients with higher S[Na$^+$].
- Potassium:
  - There is a theoretical concern that rapid change plasma potassium (i.e., use of much lower dialysate [K+] compared to patient's plasma level) may induce arrhythmias.
  - This concern remains to be proven. Nonetheless, there are data to suggest increased risk of sudden cardiac death with the use of dialysate [K$^+$] < 2 mEq/L for patients with S[K$^+$] < 6.5 mEq/L.
- Calcium:
  - Ideal dialysate calcium concentration is 2.5 to 2.75 mEq/L.
  - Lower dialysate calcium concentration is associated with increased risk for cardiac arrest, intradialytic hypotension, and secondary hyperparathyroidism.
  - Higher dialysate calcium concentration may lead to increased vascular and soft tissue calcifications.
- Bicarbonate:
  - HD patients with serum bicarbonate concentration < 22 mEq/L have an increased risk of all-cause and cardiovascular mortality compared to those with levels 24 to 25 mEq/L.
  - Predialysis serum bicarbonate concentration > 27 mEq/L is also associated with higher risk of death! Bottom line: Keep goal serum bicarbonate between 22 and 27 mEq/L.

Special Peritoneal Dialysis Issues

- Both lower (<3.5 mEq/L) and higher (>5.5 mEq/L) serum potassium concentration ranges are associated with higher risk for all-cause mortality.
- Unplanned PD (acute PD initiation) does not appear to increase infectious complications compared with planned PD as opposed to unplanned HD compared with planned HD.
- Mortality data regarding the use of PD versus HD for AKI are conflicting. Nonetheless, it must be noted that PD may be the only available option in developing countries.
- Risks for early switch to HD (i.e., by 6 months on PD):
  - HD initiation prior to PD
  - Development of peritonitis within 6 months on PD
  - PD following a failed kidney transplant
  - Poor PD expertise by dialysis staff
- PD access issues:
  - May be done surgically via laparoscopic approach or with interventional radiology under fluoroscopic guidance
  - Surgically placed catheter should have folding of omentum to avoid catheter tip migration and malfunction.
  - A surgically inserted catheter with a straight intraperitoneal segment has been shown to improve catheter survival, not the number of cuffs or configuration of subcutaneous segment.

- PD blood pressure and volume control:
  - BP in PD tends to improve over the first 2 years, but subsequently worsens.
  - Similar to HD, BP control in PD may be achieved with salt restriction and optimal fluid removal via UF.
  - Inadequate UF is a predictor of worse survival
  - Excessive salt restriction and ultrafiltration, however, are associated with reduced urine volume, possibly loss of residual kidney function, and ultimately reduced survival. CANUSA study revealed reduction of relative mortality risk to 0.64 for every 250 mL of daily urine output and 0.88 for every 5 L/wk of residual renal GFR.
  - RAAS inhibitors should be considered first-line antihypertensive therapy:
    - Has been shown to preserve residual kidney function
    - Has been shown to preserve peritoneal membrane function, evidenced by slower conversion to rapid transporters. Protective effect is presumed to be via antifibrotic properties of RAAS inhibitors.
    - Known to be cardioprotective

PD Complications

- Exit site infections:
  - Typical organisms: *Staphylococcus epidermidis* or *aureus* > gram-negative organisms (e.g., *Pseudomonas aeruginosa*)
  - *Seasonal variations in causative pathogens:* Staphylococcal epidermidis and gram-negative species in warmer seasons; *Corynebacterium* and fungal species in cold seasons.
  - Prophylaxis: mupirocin or gentamicin cream. NOTE: Polysporin cream may be associated with increased fungal infections.
- Peritonitis:
  - May contribute up to 15% of deaths in PD
  - Risks:
    - Exit site or tunnel infection
    - Summer greater than colder months (presumably due to increased sweating, moisture with summer months).
    - Low dialysate $[Ca^{2+}] < 1.75$ mEq/L
    - Of note, with the use of Y-set tubing system and proper flushing prior to filling, the risk for peritonitis is similar for CAPD and CCPD.
  - Prophylactic measures:
    - Patient education for proper PD techniques
    - Routine use of topical exit site antibiotic creams (mupirocin)
  - Diagnosis:
    - PD cell count with >100 WBC consisting of >50% polymorphonuclear leukocytes (PMN). >50% PMN is likely a better indicator for peritonitis than having >100 WBC. False negatives may be seen if cell count is obtained early in the course of peritonitis or during short exchanges.
    - Most common organism: gram-positive cocci, for example, staphylococcal epidermidis, culture negative, gram negative organisms, polymicrobials, much less commonly, fungi (*Candida* is most common), and rarely, tuberculosis
    - Of interest, streptococcal peritonitis is associated with severe abdominal pain.
    - If gram-negative organisms (e.g., *Escherichia coli* or *Enterobacter*), polymicrobials, consider bowel perforation or diverticulitis. NOTE: use of prophylactic antibiotic is not necessary for colonoscopy if the sole reason for antibiotic use is PD.

- Risks for fungal infections: immunosuppressive state, DM, malnutrition, recurrent use of multiple antibiotics
- Empirical therapy per International Society for PD: vancomycin or first-generation cephalosporins for gram-positive organisms *plus* third-generation cephalosporin or gentamicin for gram-negative organisms.
- Antibiotic administration:
  - Intraperitoneal route is generally preferred over intravenous route.
  - If residual kidney function > 100 mL/d increase antibiotic dose by 25%.
  - Duration of treatment is generally 2 weeks for *S. epidermidis* and 3 weeks for *S. aureus* and gram-negative organisms.
- The fear for gentamicin-induced loss of residual kidney function (with use up to three courses) is likely unwarranted based on data from ANZDATA registry.
- Definitions of relapsing, recurrent, repeat, and refractory peritonitis:
  - Relapsing: same organism within 4 weeks of treatment completion. Likely due to biofilm. Catheter replacement is indicated. If biofilm is suspected cause of relapsing peritonitis, catheter may be replaced if there is no evidence of infection.
  - Recurrent: different organisms within 4 weeks of treatment completion
  - Repeat: same organism after 4 weeks of treatment completion
  - Refractory: persistent infection after 5 days of appropriate antibiotics
- For culture negative peritonitis not responding to empirical antibiotic or monocytic/eosinophilic peritonitis, consider other causes: fungi, virus, mycobacterium, allergic response to peritoneal dialysate (e.g., icodextrin) or drugs (look for systemic signs/symptoms of allergic reactions), underlying malignancies, lymphoproliferative diseases, CO_2 infusion with laparoscopic procedures.
- The use of "biocompatible" PD solutions:
  - Solutions designed to have low glucose degradation products or use of glucose-sparing osmotic agents (e.g., icodextrin or amino acids) and relatively neutral pH with the use of lactate or bicarbonate buffer.
  - Biocompatible solutions have been suggested to reduce peritoneal membrane damage, residual renal function decline, and possibly peritonitis rate and improve metabolic profile in patients with DM. More data are needed.
  - PET testing may not be equivalent between conventional and biocompatible solutions with long-term use. While small molecule transport rates and ultrafiltration appear to be equivalent, transport of β2-microglobulin and albumin may be higher for biocompatible solutions. Longitudinal follow-up of PET should be done with the same dialysate solution.
- UF failure:
  - Evaluate for common causes of apparent UF "failure":
    - Rule out volume overload from other etiologies: loss of residual kidney function, congestive heart failure, dietary noncompliance, PD noncompliance
    - PD related causes: mechanical problems with PD procedure (migration, kinking of catheter), constipation affecting dialysate flow, fibrin plug (fibrin may be seen in drainage bags), dialysate leaks to other body cavities, peritoneal membrane failure. In the case of fibrin plugs, irrigate tubing system and add heparin to dialysate bags.
  - Peritoneal membrane failure with resultant UF failure:
    - Definition:
      - Inability to maintain euvolemia despite use of >3 hypertonic dialysate solutions per day, or

- ■ Failure to ultrafilter >400 mL with a 4.25% solution for 4 hours (Rule of 4s)
  - Peritoneal equilibration testing reveals high D/P of creatinine (i.e., >0.8)
- Causes of peritoneal membrane failure:
  - Early: acute inflammation
  - Late: alterations in peritoneal membrane (e.g., thickening, fibrosis)
- Management of high transporters:
  - Strict dietary salt and water restriction
  - Use high-dose diuretics if residual kidney function (consider bumetanide over furosemide for better bioavailability and less ototoxicity).
  - Replace one or two 1.5% exchanges with a more hypertonic dialysate (2.5% or even 4.25% dextrose) plus one exchange with icodextrin daily.
  - Shorten dwell times; consider switching from CAPD to nighttime automated PD with or without mid-day exchange depending on residual kidney function.
  - Switch to hemodialysis if all else fails.
- Peritoneal fibrosis:
  - Suggested fibrosis inducing factors: TGF-β, atrial natriuretic peptide, aldosterone
  - Encapsulating peritoneal sclerosis:
    - Severe form of peritoneal sclerosis, manifested as abdominal pain, thickened bowel walls, bowel obstruction, with possible associated weight loss
    - Risk factors: severe peritonitis, discontinuation of PD, genetic predisposition, PD vintage, younger age, high glucose load and chronic exposure to glucose degradation products
    - Diagnosis:
      - ■ Symptoms: abdominal pain, bowel obstruction, UF failure, malnutrition, weight loss, bloody dialysate
      - ■ CT findings of thickening of peritoneal membrane or encapsulation of bowel loops, bowel tethering, peritoneal calcifications
      - ■ Peritoneal biopsy (may be done during catheter surgical manipulation)
    - Treatment options:
      - ■ Medical therapy: tamoxifen (inhibitor of TGF-β production), immunosuppressive therapy (e.g., prednisone, azathioprine, mycophenolate mofetil)
      - ■ Surgical intervention in case of bowel obstruction
      - ■ Peritoneal rest, transfer to hemodialysis, consider total parenteral nutrition
    - Experimental interventions: N-acetylcysteine, eplerenone, glutamine supplementation, and the vasoactive glycosaminoglycan sulodexide
- Other problems:
  - Bloody dialysate: menstruation, ruptured ovarian cysts, bowel ischemia/infarction, intra-abdominal malignancy, trauma, early encapsulating peritoneal sclerosis, mycobacterium. Add heparin to dialysate to avoid clotting of catheter if benign cause.
  - Green dialysate: consider biliary source
  - Milky white dialysate: hyperlipidemia (triglycerides or chylomicrons), disruption of lymphatics
  - Dialysate leaks (subcutaneous or other body cavities):
    - Early leaks (usually external leak):
      - ■ Poor tissue healing due to early use of PD following catheter insertion
      - ■ Faulty catheter insertion
    - Late leaks: hernias, straining, infections

- Obtain T2-weighted MRI (dialysate can be detected without the use of gadolinium), CT with addition of contrast to dialysate, or nuclear study with addition of tracer to dialysate. NOTE: CT and nuclear study only detect current leaks, whereas MRI can detect existing leaks.
  - Perform physical examination to assess for obvious fluid collections.
  - If icodextrin dialysate is used, addition of povidone iodine to the aspirated fluid will turn bluish-black. This is thought to be due to the reaction between iodine and icodextrin starch.
- Indications for PD catheter removal:
  - Tunnel infection or severe exit site infection
  - Catheter-related sepsis
  - Fungal or mycobacterial infections (switch to hemodialysis for 2 to 3 weeks is required prior to replacement with new catheter)
  - Abdominal perforation (may be suspected if increased PD amylase)
  - Refractory peritonitis (treatment failure despite appropriate antibiotics > 5 days)
  - Presence of biofilm in patients with relapsing peritonitis.

Home Hemodialysis Issues

- Vascular access complications:
  - Increased access related events with more frequent dialysis
  - Buttonhole versus rope-ladder technique:
    - Rope-ladder technique refers to rotating cannulation sites for HD access: increased risk of hematoma and aneurysm formation compared to buttonhole
    - Buttonhole technique refers to needling at a the same site for HD access:
      - Presumed to be easier with prolonged use due to the development of a skin "tract" or buttonhole
      - Lower pain scores compared to rope-ladder technique
      - Increased rate of infections (double compared to rope ladder) presumably due to poor cleaning techniques and/or failure to remove scab prior to cannulation.

Predictors of Cardiovascular Events, Mortality in ESRD

- Residual kidney function: as measured by traditional serum creatinine or cystatin C has been suggested to improve cardiovascular events and mortality
- Hypertension:
  - Predialysis SBP > 160 mm Hg or <130 mm Hg likely has worse survival ("U" curve). NOTE: Home BP and ambulatory BP measurement better diagnose HTN than dialysis unit measured values in the hemodialysis patient.
  - Intradialytic BP variations: either significant SBP increase or fall observed with HD is associated with higher mortality regardless of absolute BP level.
  - Intradialytic HTN:
    - Mechanisms: removal of dialyzable antihypertensive medications with HD (See Strategies to achieve BP goal in the hemodialysis patient below)
    - Activation of renin angiotensin system
    - Activation of sympathetic nervous system
    - Vascular endothelial damage
    - Higher dialysate sodium compared with that of plasma with net sodium retention
    - Advantages of using carvedilol in patients with intradialytic HTN:
      - Nondialyzability, thus stable intradialytic blood level

- ■ Shown to improve endothelial function, intradialytic HTN, as well as ambulatory interdialytic BP
  - ■ May improve survival from cardiovascular complications
- Target BP:
  - Predialysis < 140/90, postdialysis < 130/80 mm Hg
  - Ambulatory BP measurements: daytime < 135/80, nighttime < 120/80 mm Hg
  - Treatment to target BP must be individualized.
  - BP treatment is associated with lower all-cause mortality and cardiovascular events and mortality.
- Strategies to achieve BP goal in the hemodialysis patient:
  - Volume control:
    - ■ Dietary sodium restriction < 2 g/d
    - ■ Maximize UF as tolerated, increase dialysis time as needed, to achieve "dry weight."
      - Dry weight is not just a nonedematous weight, but the weight at which normotension is achieved without the use (or minimal use) of antihypertensive medications without signs and symptoms of hypotension.
      - To achieve dry weight as defined, gradually withdraw antihypertensive medications as safely tolerated, followed by sequential UF as tolerated.
      - Amount of UF (L) at each session may be roughly estimated as follows: IDWG + 0.05 to 0.1 kg/10 kg body weight per dialysis session until "dry weight" is reached. Example: IDWG = 2 kg, patient's total body weight is 70 kg. Attempt UF in the range of $[2 + 0.05 \times 7]$ to $[2 + 0.1 \times 7] = 2.35$ to 2.7 L as tolerated.
    - ■ Minimize dialysate $[Na^+]$ to minimize thirst, hence IDWG and BP (e.g., consider using dialysate $[Na^+]$ that is $0.95 \times$ predialysis $S[Na^+]$ if safely tolerated and possible).
    - ■ More frequent dialysis:
      - Nocturnal or frequent (6 times/wk) dialysis reduces blood pressure, the number of antihypertensive medications, and left ventricular mass.
      - Frequent dialysis is associated with more access complications.
    - ■ Addition of antihypertensive medications: use nondialyzable medications such as carvedilol, angiotensin receptor blockers, or fosinopril. NOTE: Most ACE inhibitors are dialyzable. Atenolol and metoprolol are highly dialyzable. Other less dialyzable drugs: labetalol, amlodipine, clonidine, hydralazine, aldosterone blockers, α-blockers
- Intradialytic hypotension:
  - Defined as a symptomatic fall in SBP $\geq$ 20 mm Hg or MAP $\geq$ 10 mm Hg requiring intervention
  - Associated with increased mortality, clotted vascular access, cardiovascular events
  - Risks: age $\geq$ 65, underlying heart disease, low baseline BP, undiagnosed pericardial effusion, autonomic dysfunction (diabetes, prolonged uremia), malnutrition, severe anemia, higher IDWG
  - Management:
    - ■ Patient-related behavior: dietary sodium and water restriction, avoid eating prior to and during dialysis
    - ■ Adjust antihypertensive medications: hold antihypertensive medications prior to dialysis; avoid use of long-acting vasodilators.
    - ■ Dialysis procedure: reassess dry weight, avoid excessive and aggressive UF, consider increasing dialysis time for slower UF rate, use dialysate temperature lower than patient's body temperature, consider use of dialysate

sodium modeling (may be at the expense of higher IDWG), avoid dialysate $[Ca^{2+}] < 2.25$ mEq/L and $[Mg^{2+}] < 1.0$ mEq/L.
- Other:
  - Evaluate 2D echocardiogram for LV function and pericardial effusion
  - Consider adding midodrine 5 to 10 mg 30 minutes prior the dialysis. Note that midodrine is dialyzable, so it should not last postdialysis. Also, be aware that midodrine can cause bradycardia and should be used with great caution in patients receiving negative chronotropic agents.

Pregnancy in ESRD

- Conception prior to HD initiation is associated with higher live birth rates, but similar birth weight and gestational age when compared to those conceived after HD initiation.
- Dialysis management:
  - Intensification of HD (i.e., 6 to 7 dialysis treatments of 6 to 8 hour duration for a total of >36 hours of dialysis weekly) is recommended for better maternal and fetal outcomes.
  - Rapid fluid shifts and volume removal should be avoided.

Responsibilities of the Dialysis Unit Medical Director

While the medical directors' responsibilities for adverse outcomes from patients' comorbid conditions may be undefined, medical directors are held responsible for any complications that arise from the dialysis procedure.
- Quality assessment and performance improvement
  - Infection control
  - Water treatment quality
  - Minimization of risks for adverse outcomes associated with the dialysis procedure
- Staff education and training: ensure that all staff working at the unit have received adequate education and training and perform per standard practice.
- Patient assessment and developing plan of care
- Adherence to patient care and safety policies
- Adherence to discharge and transfer policies

> **NOTE** Self-referral and Stark Law
> - Started in 1989 barring medical directors to self-refer patients to own unit where there is a "financial relationship." It was later recognized that Stark law would prevent medical directors from practicing patient care.
> - Later amendments exempted medical directors to refer to own dialysis units.

Review of Dialysis Indices, Calculations

- Kt/V of a solute is the *proportion of volume V that has undergone clearance of that specific solute over duration of time t,* where K essentially represents the clearance capacity, t = the duration over which the clearance process takes place, and V = the volume that undergoes the clearance. The term Kt represents the solute cleared over time t.
  - Kt/V of solute A = 1 means that the total body volume V has been cleared of solute A (assuming a single pool).
  - Kt/V of solute A = 0.6 means that 60% of V has been cleared of solute A (assuming a single pool).

- Currently, creatinine and urea clearances are commonly used as surrogates for all other (toxic) metabolite clearance.
- Urea clearance: conventional indices:
  - Urea reduction ratio (URR)
    - URR = (pre − post)/pre = (1 − post/pre), which may also be expressed as %
    - Example: predialysis BUN 100 mg/dL, postdialysis BUN 66 mg/dL, URR = (100 − 66)/100 = 0.34 or 34%.
  - Single pool Kt/V (SpKt/V) of urea
    - This is a dimensionless ratio which represents the fractional clearance of urea from a single pool, where
      - K = dialyzer blood water urea clearance (L/h)
      - t = dialysis duration (h)
      - V = volume of distribution of urea (L). Since we cannot "drain" the entire patient's body volume V to pass through the dialyzer at any single time point, the volume that passes through the dialyzer is from a continuous mixture of dialyzed and nondialyzed volumes. Clearance of any solute thus follows a natural logarithmic (decay) pattern, hence
      - spKt/V = −ln (1 − URR)
  - What would URR be when spKt/V = 1 (i.e., the whole tank volume has gone through dialysis)?
    - 1 = −ln (1 − URR), solving for URR:

$$-1 = \ln (1 - URR)$$

$$e^{(-1)} = (1 - URR)$$

$$URR = 1 - e^{(-1)} = 0.63$$

With the continuous remixing of dialyzed to nondialyzed volumes, the *maximum portion of the body volume V* that can be cleared of solutes after running the entire body volume sequentially through the dialyzer is 0.63.

- Note the spKt/V equation above does not take other factors into account:
  - Continuing urea generation (while dialysis is going on)
  - UF alters the volume V, thus Kt/V.
  - With corrections for above factors, spKt/V becomes
    - spKt/V = −ln (R − 0.008 × t) + (4 − 3.5 × R) × 0.55 × UF/V, where
      - 0.008 × t takes into account the continuing urea generation, and
      - (4 − 3.5 × R) × 0.55 × UF/V takes into account UF, and
      - R = 1 − URR
- Inbound versus rebound (multipool model):
  - A solute such as urea is sequestered into other compartments (not just single pool).
  - Inbound refers to the sequestration/movement of urea (solutes) into other compartments during dialysis.
  - Rebound refers to the release of urea (solutes) from other compartments into the blood volume that is accessible to dialysis.
  - These occurrences lead to the concept of equilibrated Kt/V, or eKt/V. This is measured 30 to 60 minutes postdialysis.
  - In general, eKt/V = spKt/V − rebound. To measure rebound, blood sampling is measured 30 to 60 minutes postdialysis. To avoid waiting, eKt/V may be estimated to be ~0.8 × Kt/V. (i.e., eKt/V is typically 20% less than Kt/V).
  - Rebound may also be estimated as (without waiting for 30 to 60 minutes):
    - Rebound = 0.6 × rate of dialysis − 0.03 (arterial access)

- Rebound $= 0.47 \times$ rate of dialysis $- 0.02$ (venous access) [measured 15 sec $-$ 2 min postdialysis], where rate of dialysis is (spKt/V)/t
- How does UF affect clearance? Again, spKt/V $= -\ln(1 - \text{URR})$
  - Given the same URR, increasing UF volume, hence smaller V, would result in a higher Kt/V.
  - Given the same Kt/V, increasing UF volume would reduce URR
- What is the difference between whole blood versus plasma clearance? Solute clearance per whole blood volume is lower than that of equivalent plasma volume. Whereas solutes dissolved in plasma are accessible to dialysis, solutes inside red blood cells are not accessible to dialysis.
- How does increasing hemoglobin level affect dialysis clearance? Correction of anemia does lead to reduced solute clearance. More dialysis may be needed to achieve goal Kt/V.

Other Terms in Dialysis

- Ultrafiltration coefficient, K_{UF}:
  - Characteristic of membrane, expressed as mL/hour/mm Hg of TMP applied
  - Example: K_{UF} of 10 mL/h/mm Hg implies that in order to ultrafiltrate 500 mL/h, a TMP of 50 mm Hg would have to be applied.
  - TMP $=$ Desired UF/K_{UF}
- Dialyzer clearance, KoA:
  - KoA is the maximum theoretical clearance of any dialyzer. True solute removal is typically 5% to 30% less than published KoA.
  - Choosing a dialysis KoA for a patient depends on blood flow, dialysate flow, and desired urea clearance to meet a specified Kt/V.
- Standardized Kt/V (Std Kt/V) is a continuous clearance equivalent that takes into account the continuing generation of the solute being cleared. Std Kt/V may be used to compare any form of dialysis (home, daily, conventional, peritoneal dialyses).
- Membrane efficiency versus flux:
  - Efficiency implies amount of solute removed. High efficiency may be obtained with large surface area membranes. A high-efficiency dialysis membrane may have either small or large pores and can remove small and/or large molecules.
  - High flux implies ability to remove larger molecules such as β2-microglobulins. High flux dialyzer membranes have larger pores.
- Calculations:
  - Be able to calculate the time required to dialyze a patient to achieve a Kt/V of 1.4, given a volume of 42 L, blood flow of 450 mL/min, dialysate flow of 500 mL/min, KoA of 600. Hint: K can be obtained from the dialyzer nomogram if given blood flow, dialysate flow, and KoA.
  - K (residual kidney function), denoted as K_{ru}
  - $K_{ru} = \text{UUN/BUN}_{mean} \times$ urine flow rate, where UUN $=$ urine urea nitrogen, BUN $=$ blood urea nitrogen, $\text{BUN}_{mean} = 0.9 \times$ BUN measured immediately prior to hemodialysis.
  - Adding K_{ru} to Kt/V_{urea}:
    - Peritoneal dialysis (PD), Kt/V for PD is denoted as K_{pu}:
      - $K_{ru} + K_{pu}$ are additive because both are operative during steady state situation (i.e., nonchanging, nonfluctuating BUN during PD)
    - Hemodialysis (HD):
      - In HD, K_{ru} and $K_{total\ water}$ are *not* additive.

- ■ $K_{total\ water}$ from the dialyzer is operative during a period of changing BUN, and hence is less efficient in terms of urea removal than K_{ru}.
- ■ $K_{total\ water}$ from HD can be estimated as an equivalent urea clearance, denoted as eK_{ru}, as follow:
  - • $eK_{ru} = g/TAC$, where
  - • g = urea nitrogen generation rate, and
  - • TAC = time-average urea nitrogen level
- • Calculate weekly Kt/V from eK_{ru}:
  - • Example, eKru = 9 mL/min, V = 35 L
  - • Kt/V = [9 mL/min × 1,440 min/d × 7 d/wk]/35,000 mL = 2.6
- • Determining hemodialysis prescription based on K, t, or Kt/V:
  - • K is based on dialyzer KoA, blood flow rate, dialysate flow rate (information obtained from dialyzer nomogram).
  - • T = dialysis duration
  - • V ~55% total body weight
- • Calculate clearance in peritoneal dialysis:

> **NOTE**   By convention, CrCl is normalized to 1.73 m² body surface area, whereas urea clearance is normalized to volume.

- • Continuous ambulatory peritoneal dialysis (CAPD):
  - ■ Recall clearance = [U]V/[P]
  - ■ In CAPD, urine = dialysate, and
    - • Clearance = K
    - • [U] = concentration of urea in dialysate drained
    - • V = total dialysate volume *drained*, may be denoted as V_d. Example for a four times exchange using 2.5 L exchanges, with UF of 2 L, V_d = 4 × 2.5 + 2 = 12 L.
    - • [P] = blood urea concentration
  - ■ **Example:** 50-year-old man, weight 75 kg, body surface area of 1.7 m², total body volume 35 L, performs CAPD four times a day using 2.5 L exchanges daily, net UF 2.0 L. Laboratory findings: BUN = 67 mg/dL, dialysate urea nitrogen = 58 mg/dL, serum creatinine 10.2 mg/dL, dialysate creatinine 5.7 mg/dL.
- • What is his weekly Kt/V?
  - • Kt/V = ([U]V_d/[P]) × 7 days)/V

$$= (58 × (4 × 2.5 + 2.0)/67) × 7)/35$$

$$= 2.1$$

- • What is his daily creatinine clearance?
  - • K (clearance) = ([U]V_d/[P])

$$= 5.7 × (4 × 2.5 + 2.0)/10.2 = 6.7\ L/d$$

- • By convention, CrCl is expressed as clearance per minute and normalized to body surface area of 1.73 m². Thus, his CrCl is = 6.7 L × 1.73/1.7

$$= 6.8\ L/d,\ or\ 6,800\ mL/1,440\ min/1.73\ m^2$$

$$= 4.7\ mL/min/1.73\ m^2$$

- Automated peritoneal dialysis (APD):
  - **Example:** A 49-year-old female, 58 kg, APD five exchanges $\times$ 2.2 L each nightly, plus 6 hour 2 L day dwell. V = 32 L, BSA = 1.8 m^2, 24-hour dialysate drain volume = 15 L. Pooled dialysate drain chemistries: urea 44 mg/dL, creatinine 4.5 mg/dL. Mid-afternoon BUN 68 mg/dL, serum creatinine 8.9 mg/dL. Residual kidney function: creatinine clearance 3 mL/min, urea clearance 2 mL/min

> **NOTE** For APD (mostly night PD), BUN will vary significantly between morning and at night. The preferred "steady state" value is mid-afternoon.

  - Calculate total weekly Kt/V:
    - Kt/V (PD) + (daily urea clearance $\times$ 7 days)/V

    $$= (([U]V_d/[P]) \times 7 \text{ days})/V + \text{Urea clearance} \times 7 \text{ days}/V$$

    $$= (44 \times 15/68) \times 7/32 + (0.002 \times 1{,}440) \times 7 \text{ days}/32$$

    $$= 2.12 + 0.63 = 2.75$$

  - Calculate total weekly creatinine clearance:
    - [daily K (PD) + daily creatinine clearance] $\times$ 7 days $\times$ 1.73/patient's BSA

    $$= [([U]V_d/[P]) + \text{daily creatinine clearance}] \times 7 \times 1.73/1.5$$

    $$= ([4.5 \times 15/8.9 + (0.003 \times 1{,}440)] \times 7) \times 1.73/1.5$$

    $$= (7.58 + 4.32) \times 7 \times 1.73/1.8$$

    $$= 80 \text{ L/wk}/1.73 \text{ m}^2$$

    $$= 7.9 \text{ mL/min}/1.73 \text{ m}^2$$

- Calculation of Kt/V for continuous renal replacement therapy (CRRT):
  - Assumption: since the dialysate inflow rate for CRRT is very slow (i.e., 15 to 20 mL/min), there is adequate time for urea from plasma to diffuse across the dialysis membrane and equilibrate with the dialysate. Hence, outflow dialysate urea concentration reaches that of plasma and dialysate urea concentration = plasma urea concentration.
  - Thus, daily urea clearance = dialysate outflow rate (mL/min) $\times$ 1,440 min/d
  - Daily Kt/V = daily urea clearance/V
  - **Example:** A patient with a V of 35 L, dialysate outflow rate of 20 mL/min has
- Daily urea clearance = 20 mL/min $\times$ 1,440 min/d = 28,800 mL = 28.8 L
- Daily Kt/V = 28.8/35 = 0.82

Access the eBook for self-assessment questions.

Hypertension

Phuong-Mai T. Pham, Cynthia C. Nast, Son V. Pham,
and Phuong-Anh T. Pham

DEFINITIONS/GENERAL CONCEPTS

Epidemiology

- World Health Organization: hypertension (HTN) ranks *first* among leading risk factors attributable to "Global Disability-Adjusted Life-Years."
- National Health and Nutrition Examination Survey (NHANES) data:
  - Improved patient awareness of their HTN diagnosis over the years: 69% in 1988 versus 81% in 2008
  - More are being treated: 54% in 1988 versus 70% in 2008
  - More treated hypertensives are at goal: 51% in 1988 versus 69% in 2008
- HTN per ambulatory blood pressure monitoring (ABPM) is an independent predictor for cardiovascular outcomes. HTN is thought to be a better predictor of cardiovascular outcomes than eGFR. Combination of both HTN and eGFR improves predictive value in an additive manner (in patients with eGFR > 60 mL/min/1.73 m^2).
- Arterial stiffness as measured by either carotid to femoral pulse wave pressure or brachial to carotid pulse pressure ratio predicts future HTN.
- Most of the following definitions and basic evaluations and management of hypertension are based on the Reports of the Joint National Committee [JNC] on Prevention, Detection, Evaluation, and Treatment of High Blood Pressure 7 and 8.

Definitions

- General HTN: BP definitions are based on the average of two or more properly measured readings at >2 visits *after initial screen*.
- Adults > 18 years of age:
  - Normal: systolic blood pressure (SBP) < 120 mm Hg *and* diastolic blood pressure (DBP) < 80 mm Hg
  - Prehypertension:
    - SBP 120 to 139 mm Hg *or* DBP 80 to 89 mm Hg
    - Seen in up to 30% of population
    - Affected individuals may have exaggerated physiologic stress responses.
    - There is a greater frequency of obesity, dyslipidemia, other cardiovascular risk factors among individuals with prehypertension.
    - Adverse effects associated with prehypertension:
      - Twofold increase in cardiovascular events compared with normotensive individuals.

- Threefold increase in likelihood for eventual HTN; Risk increased with weight gains.
- Stage 1: 140 to 159 mm Hg *or* DBP 90 to 99 mm Hg
- Stage 2: >160 mm Hg *or* >100 mm Hg
- Ambulatory definitions of HTN:
  - 24-hour average > 135/85 mm Hg
  - Daytime (awake) average > 140/90 mm Hg
  - Nighttime (asleep) average > 125/75 mm Hg
- Children < 18 years of age:
  - HTN: blood pressure at 95th percentile or greater for age and gender
  - Special notes:
    - Prepubertal HTN: predominantly due to renal etiologies
    - Postpubertal HTN: mild HTN is associated with primary HTN, whereas more severe HTN is more likely of renal origin
    - HTN may also be due to earlier growth spurt and bigger size for age.

Indications for Ambulatory BP Measurements

- Suspected white coat hypertension (WCH)
- Apparent drug resistance (BP not at goal despite being on maximal and optimal drug combination, but not yet ruled out WCH, noncompliance, proper BP measuring techniques, etc.)
- Hypotensive symptoms
- Autonomic dysfunction
- Episodic HTN
- Evaluation of nocturnal decreases in BP as prognostic factor for target organ disease (left ventricular hypertrophy, ischemic optic neuropathy)
- Evaluation of BP changes in patients with paroxysmal nocturnal dyspnea and nocturnal angina
- Carotid sinus syncope
- Pacemaker syndromes
- Safety of withdrawing antihypertensive medications
- Assess 24-hour BP control on once-daily medication
- Borderline HTN with target organ damage
- Evaluation of antihypertensive drug therapy in clinical trials

Special Types of Hypertension

- White coat hypertension (WCH):
  - Normal BP with usual activities, but higher in clinical setting (doctor's office)
  - Clinical significance unclear:
    - Some studies revealed increased left ventricular mass index compared to individuals with normal BP.
    - Affected individuals may have impaired diastolic function and higher levels of catecholamines, renin/aldosterone, low-density lipoproteins.
    - May be at increased risk for eventual sustained HTN
  - Start antihypertensive if
    - Persistently elevated clinic BP and
    - Target organ damage *or* elevated 24-hour ambulatory BP
- Masked HTN:
  - BP measured in the clinical setting is lower than that measured in the ambulatory setting (opposite of WCH).

- 10-year risks of stroke and cardiovascular mortality may be similar to those of individuals with sustained HTN.
- Start antihypertensive if
  - Persistently normal clinic BP,
  - Target organ damage, and
  - High 24-hour ambulatory BP
- Sustained HTN: HTN both in and out of clinic setting, although BP tends to be higher in the former.
- Pseudohypertension:
  - Cuff BP is higher when compared with intra-arterial pressure because of excessive atheromatosis and/or medial hypertrophy in arterial tree.
  - May be diagnosed by Osler maneuver:
    - Inflate BP cuff above SBP (detected by loss of pulse with auscultation).
    - Osler maneuver is positive when either brachial or radial artery remains palpable despite loss of pulse by auscultation.
    - Pseudohypertension is defined as having cuff-measured DBP > 10 to 15 mm Hg compared with that of intra-arterial measurement.
    - Management of BP should be based on intra-arterial value.
- Isolated systolic hypertension (ISH):
  - Occurs with stiffening of large arteries, leading to reduced vessel capacitance and acceleration of pulse wave velocity, hence widening of pulse pressure.
  - Increase in SPB continues throughout life, in contrast to DBP, which increases and peaks by age of 50 then decreases later in life.
  - After 50 years, SBP is more important than DBP.
- Isolated diastolic hypertension (IDH), DBP > 90 mm Hg with SBP < 140 mm Hg:
  - More common in young overweight/obese males.
  - More common than combined systolic and diastolic HTN (SDH) and ISH in individuals < 40 years of age. IDH is rare in individuals > 60 years old.
  - Clinical significance unclear:
    - Rate of progression or conversion to SDH noted to be 55% in 6.7 years in Framingham Heart Study.
    - Finland study involving 3,267 healthy men aged 32 to 45 with untreated IDH had *no* increase in all-cause mortality.
  - Management of IDH:
    - Focus on salt restriction and weight loss, the latter if overweight or obese.
    - Pharmacologic antihypertensive therapy if end-organ damage, (e.g. proteinuria or left ventricular HTN on ECG) or hypothyroidism. Hypothyroidism is associated with BP rise that is more pronounced with diastolic than systolic BP.
    - If no specific indication for any antihypertensive class, IDH patients tend to respond well with just one agent, typically better with an angiotensin converting enzyme inhibitor (ACEI) or angiotensin receptor blocker (ARB) than dihydropyridine calcium channel blocker (CCB).
- Drug-resistant HTN:
  - BP not at goal despite optimal doses (optimal dose, defined as >50% of maximal dose recommended for treatment of HTN) of three different antihypertensive drug classes, one of which is a diuretic.
  - Alternatively, BP is at goal with optimal doses of four appropriate antihypertensive drug classes, one of which is a diuretic.
  - Apparent (drug)-resistant HTN: Patients with *apparent* "drug-resistant HTN" are those who meet criteria above, but have *not* been ruled out for proper BP techniques, WCH, noncompliance, and improper BP medication regimens.

- Pseudoresistant HTN: Patients who initially meet criteria for "drug-resistant HTN" but later fail to meet the same criteria following proper BP measuring techniques, ambulatory BP measurements, and/or compliance with proper BP medication regimens.
- Apparent resistant HTN may be seen in 15% of the population treated for HTN in the United States. However, ~50% of the population have pseudoresistant HTN. True resistant HTN is approximated at 5% of treated hypertensives.
- Accelerated HTN:
  - Severe diastolic HTN, typically defined as having DBP > 120 mm Hg with grade III retinopathy (arteriolosclerotic changes of arteriolar narrowing and nicking plus hypertensive changes of flame-shaped hemorrhages and soft exudates). Malignant HTN is similar to accelerated HTN but with grade IV retinopathy (i.e., grade III *plus* papilledema) ± hypertensive encephalopathy. Distinction between malignant and accelerated HTN is not clinically necessary in terms of treatment.
  - Hypertensive urgency: accelerated HTN requiring *BP lowering within hours*; also defined as having DBP > 120 mm Hg in asymptomatic patients.
  - Hypertensive emergency: accelerated HTN requiring *BP lowering within minutes* (i.e., acute aortic dissection, acute left ventricular failure, intracerebral hemorrhage [ICH], pheochromocytoma [PHEO] crises, drug abuse, eclampsia).
- HTN in pregnancy:
  - BP > 140/90 mm Hg
  - SBP > 30 mm Hg or DBP > 15 mm Hg increase compared with BP prior to pregnancy, but <140/90 should be managed as high-risk patients per US National High BP Education Program)

Other Observations Regarding Blood Pressure

- Blood pressure circadian pattern:
  - BP during sleep is ~10% to 20% below daytime BP. Patients with nighttime BP fall are referred to as "dippers."
  - In CKD patients:
    - The proportion of dippers decreases with increasing CKD stage.
    - The proportion of "risers" (patients with increase nighttime BP) increases with increasing CKD stage.
- Between-arm BP differences:
  - Between-arm BP differences of 4 to 5 mm Hg occur in healthy people.
  - Values > 10 mm Hg should be considered for vascular assessment.
  - Values > 15 mm Hg is a predictor of prevalent vascular disease and death.
  - BP treatment should be based on higher BP arm.
- Geomedicine (modern study of place of dwelling and health consequences) suggests contribution of air pollution to higher BP.

General Evaluation and Management of HTN

- Assessment of target organ damage and cardiovascular risk factors: lipid panel including HDL, LDL cholesterol, and fasting triglycerides, kidney function, proteinuria, ECG, evidence of metabolic syndrome, diabetes mellitus

- Assessment of plasma renin activity (PRA) "renin profiling":
  - PRA > 0.65 ng/mL/h (typically seen in younger Caucasians) may have HTN associated with vasoconstriction and respond well to ACEI or ARB, β-blockers.
  - PRA < 0.65 ng/mL/h (typically seen in African Americans, Afro-Caribbeans, and older Caucasians) may indicate volume expansion–related HTN, and may respond well to diuretics and CCB.
- Lifestyle modifications in the management of HTN (JNC 7):
  - Weight reduction: maintain normal body weight (e.g., body mass index 18.5 to 24.9 kg/m^2) → SBP reduction ~5 to 20 mm Hg per 10-kg weight loss.
  - Adopt DASH eating plan (consume diet rich in fruits, vegetables, low-fat dairy products with reduced content of saturated and total fat) → SBP reduction ~8 to 14 mm Hg.
  - Sodium restriction (<2.4 g sodium or 6 g of NaCl daily) → SBP reduction ~2 to 8 mm Hg.
  - Physical activity: regular aerobic activity, for example, 30-minute brisk walk daily, most days of week → SBP 4 to 9 mm Hg.
  - Moderation of alcohol consumption (<2 drinks daily in most men, <1 drink daily in women and lighter-weight persons) → SBP reduction ~2 to 4 mm Hg.
  - For overall cardiovascular risk reduction, stop smoking.
- Clinical clues suggesting secondary HTN:
  - Severe (e.g., BP > 180/110 mm Hg) or drug resistant HTN
  - Acute rise in BP in a patient with previously stable values
  - Age < 30 years in nonobese, non-black patients with a negative family history of HTN and no other risk factors for HTN
  - Malignant or accelerated HTN
  - Onset of HTN age < 20 or >50

Factors to Consider in Patients with Difficult to Treat HTN

- Proper BP measurements with proper-sized cuff, in quiet environment, in relaxed patient without prior ingestion of caffeine, alcohol, or nicotine
- Volume overload or failure to add a diuretic with the use of antihypertensive medications that can induce reflex sodium retention
- Drug-induced and -related causes:
  - Prescription-related causes: inadequate dosing, inappropriate combinations, NSAIDS, cyclooxygenase-2 (COX-2) inhibitors, oral contraceptives, adrenal steroids, glucocorticosteroids calcineurin inhibitors, antidepressants (monoamine oxidase-inhibitors, venlafaxine), erythropoiesis-stimulating agents, vascular endothelial growth factor inhibitors
  - Patient-related causes: dietary and herbal supplementation (ephedra, ma huang, bitter orange), caffeine, sympathomimetics (decongestants, anorectics), licorice, recreational drugs (cocaine, amphetamines, methamphetamines), noncompliance
- Obesity
- Excess alcohol intake
- Identifiable causes (Fig. 5.1)

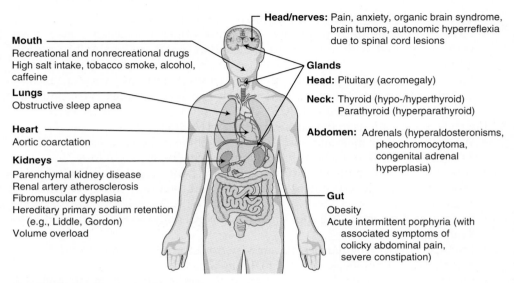

Head/nerves: Pain, anxiety, organic brain syndrome, brain tumors, autonomic hyperreflexia due to spinal cord lesions

Mouth
Recreational and nonrecreational drugs
High salt intake, tobacco smoke, alcohol, caffeine

Lungs
Obstructive sleep apnea

Heart
Aortic coarctation

Kidneys
Parenchymal kidney disease
Renal artery atherosclerosis
Fibromuscular dysplasia
Hereditary primary sodium retention
(e.g., Liddle, Gordon)
Volume overload

Glands

Head: Pituitary (acromegaly)

Neck: Thyroid (hypo-/hyperthyroid)
Parathyroid (hyperparathyroid)

Abdomen: Adrenals (hyperaldosteronisms, pheochromocytoma, congenital adrenal hyperplasia)

Gut
Obesity
Acute intermittent porphyria (with associated symptoms of colicky abdominal pain, severe constipation)

FIGURE 5.1 Secondary causes of hypertension by organ system.

PRIMARY (ESSENTIAL) HYPERTENSION

Pathogenesis of Primary HTN

- Increased sympathetic activity and responsiveness
- Increased angiotensin II (AII) activity and mineralocorticoid excess

Risks of Primary HTN

- Genetics: twofold risk if >1 parents with HTN
- Reduced nephron mass due to immature birth, intrauterine developmental (e.g., maternal drug use, malnutrition) and postnatal disturbances (e.g., malnutrition, infections)
- Black ethnicity (more common and severe compared to non-blacks)
- Lifestyle-associated: high salt intake, excess alcohol consumption, physical inactivity, vitamin D deficiency. Fructose intake, thus far, not proven to increase HTN risk.
- Metabolic: dyslipidemia, independent of obesity

Diagnosis of Primary HTN

- Rule out white coat HTN.
- Rule out ingestions of medications/substances that can cause HTN (i.e., caffeine, tobacco smoking, amphetamines, cocaine, sympathomimetics, etc.).
- Rule out secondary causes as per risks, signs/symptoms. See Secondary Causes of Hypertension.
- Routine testing:
  - Full history and physical examination
  - Laboratory studies: urinalysis, routine blood chemistries, serum creatinine, hemoglobin, fasting lipids, electrocardiogram
  - In "borderline" HTN, consider microalbuminuria and echocardiogram for determination of antihypertensive therapy initiation

Management of Primary HTN

- Lifestyle modifications
- Antihypertensive therapy:
  - Initiate if SBP is persistently >140 mm Hg (in patients < 60 years old) or >150 in patients > 60, and/or DBP persistently > 90 mm Hg despite lifestyle modifications.
  - Two-drug initiation may be necessary if >160/100 mm Hg (i.e., stage II HTN).
  - Drug selection depends on underlying conditions, "compelling indications" (e.g., ACEI/ARB for heart failure, post-myocardial infarction, α-blockers for benign prostate hypertrophy, β-blockers for essential tremors, hyperthyroidism, migraine, atrial fibrillation/flutter with rapid ventricular rates, potassium-sparing diuretics for hyperaldosteronism, thiazide diuretics for osteoporosis).
  - If no specific indication, three main classes may be considered for initial monotherapy: thiazide diuretics, long-acting CCB (typically dihydropyridine), and ACEI or ARB. In cases where there is no specific indication for a particular antihypertensive, it is the attained BP, *not* the specific antihypertensive used that is the major determinant of outcome.
  - Use of aldosterone antagonists at low dose:
    - Confers additional benefits in cardiovascular outcomes in patients with NYHA class III-IV heart failure, or decreased left ventricular ejection fraction after a myocardial infarction
    - Recommended to be used concurrently with thiazide diuretics to offset hypokalemia effect
    - May lower BP regardless of serum aldosterone levels
    - May reduce BP even in hemodialysis patients
    - Recommended to be added in resistant HTN. Anglo-Scandinavian cardiac outcomes trial involving 1,411 participants: the addition of spironolactone at median dose of 25 mg daily in addition to 2.9 other antihypertensive medications reduced by 21.9/9.5 mm Hg at 1.3 year-follow-up.
    - Obvious concern: hyperkalemia
  - Note specific drug contraindications:
    - ACEI in angioedema, β-blockers with poorly controlled bronchospasm, reserpine in depression, methyldopa in liver disease, ACEI/ARB/or renin inhibitors in pregnancy or pregnancy planning, β-blockers and nondihydropyridine CCB in second- or third-degree heart blocks
  - Goal of therapy:
    - In general, <140/90 mm Hg if younger than 60 years old, <150/90 mm Hg if 60 or older.
    - Goal BP may be lower if either known atherosclerotic cardiovascular disease or chronic kidney disease with proteinuria > 1 g/d (e.g., <125/75 mm Hg).
    - For patients > 65 years old, be cautious not to lower DBP < 65 mm Hg, as this may be associated with increased stroke risk.
    - NOTE: Systolic Blood Pressure Intervention Trial (SPRINT) trial (2015): randomized trial of intensive versus standard blood pressure control
      - 9,361 persons with SBP > 130 mm Hg with cardiovascular risks but *without* DM were enrolled and randomized to SBP control < 120 mm Hg or <140 mm Hg.
      - Primary composite outcome was myocardial infarction, other acute coronary syndromes, heart failure, or death from cardiovascular causes.

- At 3.26 mean follow-up years, the intensive group had a hazard ratio of 0.75 (95% confidence interval 0.64 to 0.89) in primary composite outcome compared to the standard group. Benefits appear to favor nonblack, males, <75-year old, and patients with no known cardiovascular disease.
- Notable concerns/criticisms: 1. A higher percentage of patients in the intensive group received ACEI or ARB compared with the standard group. 2. Patients in the study had low baseline BP (mean BP 140/78 mm Hg). 3. The higher number of antihypertensive medications (3 vs. 2) required in intensive group may be impractical.

END-ORGAN DAMAGE OF HYPERTENSION

Cardiovascular

- Major risk factor for premature cardiovascular disease
- In older patients, SBP and pulse pressure are better determinants of risk than DBP. (Recall DBP decreases after age 50.)
- Left ventricular hypertrophy and subsequent associations with heart failure, ventricular arrhythmias, death following myocardial infarction, sudden cardiac death

Cerebrovascular

- Most important risk factor for ischemic stroke and intracerebral or subarachnoid hemorrhage

Renal

- Major risk factor for chronic kidney disease and progression of kidney disease

Hypertensive Urgencies and Emergencies

- HTN (~BP > 180/120 mm Hg) complicated by end-organ dysfunction.
- Incidence: 0.2% of all visits to emergency department in 1 year
- Eye: grades III to IV retinopathy, flame hemorrhages, papilledema
- Cerebrovascular: hypertensive encephalopathy, stroke, intracerebral or subarachnoid hemorrhage (cerebral infarction is the most common presentation ~40%)
- Cardiac: acute aortic dissection, left ventricular failure, or myocardial infarction
- Pulmonary: pulmonary edema (~25%)
- Renal: microangiopathic hemolytic anemia
- Eclampsia (~2%)
- Management:
  - General recommendations:
    - *Gradual* BP reduction is *generally* recommended:
      - MAP reduction by ~10% to 20% in first hour, then by
      - An additional 5% to 15% over the next 23 hours, with
      - Total 24 hour BP reduction < 25%
    - *Exceptions* to gradual BP reduction over the first day:
      - Acute phase of ischemic stroke: BP *not* lowered unless >185/110 mm Hg in candidates for reperfusion therapy or >220/120 mm Hg for noncandidates.
      - Acute aortic dissection: SBP should be lowered to target of 100 to 120 mm Hg **within 20 minutes** and heart rate reduced to <60 beats per minute.

- Keep patient euvolemic to reduce further activation of the renin–angiotensin–aldosterone system, with caution not to worsen HTN with excess sodium load.
- Situation-specific considerations:
  - Head trauma: treat if cerebral perfusion pressure (mean arterial pressure minus intracranial pressure [ICP]) is >120 mm Hg and ICP is >20 mm Hg.
  - Acute heart failure:
    - Consider use of intravenous vasodilator such as sodium nitroprusside, nitroglycerin to reduce afterload.
    - Avoid hydralazine (can increase cardiac work) or β-blockers, for example, labetalol (can decrease cardiac contractility).
  - Acute coronary syndrome: consider use of IV nitroglycerin, clevidipine, nicardipine, or esmolol to reduce myocardial oxygen consumption/ischemia.
  - Acute hypertensive nephrosclerosis, renal emergencies:
    - Clinical manifestations: new-onset microscopic hematuria, elevated creatinine
    - Renal histopathology (Fig. 5.2): Fibrinoid necrosis of small arterioles (pink, amorphous fibrinoid materials within vessel wall due to necrosis) and "onion skinning" of small renal arteries. "Onion skinning" is used to describe hyperplastic arteriosclerosis with thickened concentric smooth muscle cell layer with thickened, duplicated basement membrane and narrowed lumen. In malignant HTN, these hyperplastic changes may be accompanied by fibrinoid necrosis of the arterial intima and media.
    - Renal ischemia activates the renin–angiotensin -aldosterone system (RAAS), thus excerbates the underlying HTN.
      - BP lowering may lead to worsening kidney function, particularly CCB due to the potential vasodilating effect on afferent arterioles leading to transmission of systemic HTN into glomeruli.

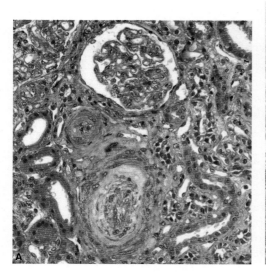 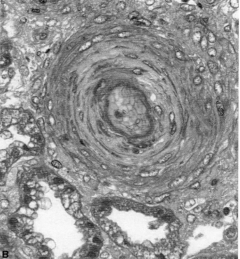

FIGURE 5.2 Accelerated/malignant hypertension (hypertensive renal emergency). **A.** Small artery and arteriole show mucoid intimal thickening, endothelial cell swelling, and severe luminal narrowing. Note fibrin (*arrow*) in the arteriolar intima and glomerular ischemic capillary wall corrugation (Masson trichrome, ×250). **B.** Small artery with "onion skin" pattern thickening of the muscularis and luminal thrombosis (Masson's trichrome, ×400).

- NOTE: Fenoldopam is associated with a temporary improvement in renal function and may be useful in renal hypertensive emergencies.
- Ingestion of sympathomimetic agents (e.g., ingestion of tyramine-containing foods in patients on chronic monoamine oxidase inhibitors, cocaine, amphetamine) or severe autonomic dysfunction (e.g., Guillain–Barré, Shy–Drager syndromes), acute spinal cord injury:
  - Treat with IV phentolamine or nitroprusside.
  - Use of β-blockers is contraindicated due to unopposed α-adrenergic vasoconstriction. NOTE: nonselective β-blockers such as labetalol and carvedilol still have predominant β-blocking activity with β-to-α blocking ratio of 7:1 or greater.

Antihypertensive Medications Used in Hypertensive Emergencies

- Nitrates: nitroglycerin, nitroprusside:
  - NO induces arteriolar and venous vasodilatation by activation of calcium sensitive potassium channels (via cGMP) in cell membranes.
  - Nitroglycerin:
    - Low antihypertensive effect
    - Consider in patients with symptomatic coronary disease or following coronary bypass.
    - Limitations: methemoglobinemia possible with prolonged use (i.e., >24 hours); *no* cyanide accumulation
  - Sodium nitroprusside:
    - Onset of action: <1 minute; activity loss within 10 minutes of discontinuation
    - Limitations: cyanide/thiocyanate toxicity: altered mental status, lactic acidosis that may occur within 4 hours
    - Risks: high dose, prolonged use >24 hours, poor kidney function
    - For high doses (i.e., 10 mcg/kg/min):
      - Do *not* use >10 minutes.
      - Add sodium thiosulfate as sulfur donor to detoxify cyanide into thiocyanate.
      - Excessive hypotension may reduce coronary, renal, and cerebral perfusion.

> **NOTE**   Sodium nitroprusside and nitroglycerin can potentially increase ICP and reduce cerebral perfusion.

- Calcium channel blockers (CCB):
  - Clevidipine: ultra-short-acting dihydropyridine CCB (half-life 1 minute)
    - Metabolizes in blood and intravascular tissues by esterases, safe for both kidney and liver failure patients.
    - Contraindicated in patients with aortic stenosis (potential severe hypotension), dyslipidemia (mixed in lipid-laden emulsion), and known allergies to soy or eggs
  - Nicardipine: longer onset of action and longer elimination half-life (3 to 6 hours)
- Selective dopamine-1 agonist: fenoldopam
  - Antihypertensive that can maintain or increase renal perfusion
  - Avoid in patients with glaucoma and sulfite sensitivity
- β-blockers:
  - Labetalol:
    - Combined β- and α-adrenergic blocker: good for patients with acute coronary syndrome. Nonetheless, prior administration of α-blockers

(e.g., phentolamine) should be done prior to using labetalol in patients with increased adrenergic states (e.g., PHEO, methamphetamine overdose, tyramine ingestion in patients on monoamine oxidase inhibitor).
- Avoid in patients with asthma, COPD, acute heart failure, 2° or 3° heart blocks and bradycardia
- Esmolol: cardioselective β-blocker with short half-life and duration of action (9 and 30 minutes respectively)
- Others:
  - Hydralazine:
    - Intravenous form (arteriolar vasodilator, with possible reflex sympathetic stimulation, i.e., tachycardia)
    - Avoid in patients with coronary artery disease or aortic dissection.
  - Enalaprilat (intravenous form of enalapril, angiotensin converting enzyme inhibitor): may cause excessive hypotension in hypovolemic patients

Suggested Medical Therapy for Specific Clinical Conditions
- Acute aortic dissection: intravenous labetalol or esmolol, followed by nicardipine or nitroprusside as needed. Goals: SBP < 100 to 120 mm Hg, heart rate < 60
- Acute pulmonary edema: nitroglycerin, enalaprilat, or nitroprusside drip. Intravenous furosemide as needed for hypervolemia. Goal BP reduction: 20% to 30%
- Acute coronary syndrome: nitroglycerin drip, β-blockers such as metoprolol or labetalol bolus therapy. Goal: limit BP reduction to 20% to 30% for SBP > 160 mm Hg
- Acute sympathetic crisis (cocaine, amphetamines): intravenous benzodiazepine and nitroglycerin or phentolamine drip, or intravenous verapamil bolus. Goal: symptomatic relief.
- Acute kidney injury (AKI): labetalol bolus or nicardipine or fenoldopam drip. Goal: BP reduction ≤ 20%
- Severe preeclampsia, eclampsia, HELLP syndrome: labetalol bolus, oral nifedipine or nicardipine. Goal: BP < 160/110 mm Hg, or <150/100 if platelet count < 100,000/mm³.
- Hypertensive encephalopathy: nicardipine, labetalol, or fenoldopam drip. Goal: decrease MAP by 15% to 20%
- Subarachnoid hemorrhage: labetalol, nicardipine, or esmolol drip. Goal: SBP < 160 mm Hg or MAP < 130 mm Hg
- Intracranial hemorrhage: labetalol, nicardipine, or esmolol drip. Goal: MAP 130 mm Hg if increased ICP to maintain cerebral perfusion pressure, otherwise MAP 110 mm Hg
- Acute ischemic stroke: labetalol or nicardipine drip. Goal: <185/110 mm Hg if fibrinolytic therapy planned
- Acute postoperative HTN: Manage pain, anxiety; evaluate acute bleed at surgical site. Nicardipine, labetalol, or esmolol drip. Goal: preoperative BP

SECONDARY CAUSES OF HYPERTENSION

Indications for Evaluation of Secondary HTN
- Drug-resistant HTN
- Refractory HTN:
  - Failure to achieve goal blood pressure (i.e., <140/90 mm Hg), despite being treated by a HTN specialist over at least three visits over a 6-month period or longer

- Refractory HTN patients tend to have higher heart rate (81 vs. 70) compared to those who are controlled, despite being on more β-blocker use. Sympathetic dysregulation is thought to play a role.

Specific Causes of Secondary HTN

- Top three causes: renal parenchymal disease, aldosteronism, renal artery disease
- Obesity:
  - Proposed contributing factors: hyperleptinemia, hyperinsulinemia, endothelial dysfunction, sympathetic nervous system (SNS) activation, kidney injury, fructose ingestion, hyperaldosteronism driven by circulating oxidized fatty acids (linoleic acid) or uric acid, concurrent obstructive sleep apnea (OSA)
    - Fructose gets phosphorylated rapidly intracellularly leading to → local adenosine triphosphate depletion and uric acid generation → uric acid–induced endothelial dysfunction, SNS activation.
    - OSA:
      - OSA occurs in 30% of patients with HTN and up to 70% to 90% of patients with drug resistant HTN.
      - The association between OSA and HTN is dependent on OSA severity and presence of obesity. Association is not significant in individuals with BMI < 25 kg/m^2 (National health and Evaluation Survey).
      - Signs and symptoms to consider OSA in hypertensive patients: snoring, gasping/choking, daytime somnolence particularly with associated functional impairment (e.g., "sleeping on the job").
      - Physical risks: older men (>50 years old), "crowded" oropharynx, large neck circumference (>50 cm or >20 inches)
      - Treatment with continuous positive airway pressure (CPAP) ventilation:
        - Improves BP control with use >4 hours in young patients (2 to 5 mm Hg reduction)
        - Recommended for symptomatic patients
      - β-blockers are most effective antihypertensive agent in OSA due to sympathetic overactivity.
      - Renal denervation improves office BP (average reduction of 34/13 mm Hg), but no significant effect on ambulatory BP (average reduction of 8 mm Hg) in small case series involving 10 patients.
  - Bariatric surgery versus lifestyle modifications/medical therapy: greater weight loss, greater BP reduction, lower antihypertensive drug requirement with bariatric surgery compared with lifestyle modifications/medical therapy alone, even in patients without morbid obesity
- Neurogenic HTN:
  - Cerebral blood flow = cerebral perfusion pressure/cerebrovascular resistance, where
  - Cerebral perfusion pressure = MAP − ICP and should be >60 mm Hg.
  - HTN after stroke:
    - Contributing factors: cushing reflex, catecholamine and cortisol release, lesion involving brain stem or hypothalamus, nonspecific response, acute stress
    - BP management per American Heart/American Stroke Associations:
      - For stroke patients receiving thrombolytic therapy:
        - Before thrombolytics: lower BP if SBP > 185 mm Hg or DBP > 110 mm Hg.
        - After thrombolytics: lower BP if SBP > 180 mm Hg or DBP > 105 mm Hg.

Table 5.1	Antihypertensive agent selection in acute cerebrovascular hypertension		
Agent	**Effect on Cerebral Blood Flow**	**Effect on Intracranial Pressure**	**Comments**
Labetalol	Neutral	Neutral	Do not affect cerebral autoregulation
Esmolol	Neutral	Neutral	May be used in the setting of cerebral ischemia or increased ICP Contraindicated if bradycardia Consensus guidelines suggest IV labetalol and nicardipine as first-line agents in acute hypertensive phase of stroke.
Nicardipine	Neutral	May increase	Long duration of action Variable effect on cerebral autoregulation May be used in patients with acute ICH and SAH Nimodipine, routinely used in patients with SAH, has been shown to improve outcome, presumably from a neuroprotective effect. Nifedipine is not recommended due to potential for hypotension.
Hydralazine	May cause both cerebral arterial and venodilation	May increase ICP May be used in patients with small to moderate-sized ICH or SAH if no increased ICP	May be used when β-blockers are contraindicated (e.g., bradycardia) Cerebral steal possible in patients with cerebral ischemia
Sodium nitroprusside			Concern for cyanide toxicity, reduced platelet aggregation Cerebral steal possible in patients with cerebral ischemia
Nitroglycerin			Cerebral steal possible in patients with cerebral ischemia
Enalaprilat	Neutral		Long duration of action

ICA, Intracranial hemorrhage; ICP, Intracranial pressure; SAH, Subarachnoid hemorrhage.

- Nonthrombolytic therapy stroke patients:
  - Antihypertensive medications should be withheld unless SBP > 220 mm Hg or DBP > 120 mm Hg.
  - When indicated, lowering BP by ~15% is reasonable.
- For acute cerebral hemorrhage:
  - If SBP > 200 mm Hg or MAP > 150 mm Hg, consider aggressive BP reduction (goal MAP 130 mm Hg if increased ICP, otherwise MAP 110 mm Hg).
  - If SBP > 180 mm Hg or MAP > 130 mm Hg *plus* evidence of or suspicion for elevated ICP, consider monitoring of ICP and reducing BP to keep cerebral perfusion pressure > 60 mm Hg.
  - If SBP > 180 mm Hg or MAP > 130 mm Hg *and* no evidence of or suspicion of elevated ICP, consider modest reduction of BP (e.g., MAP of 110 mm Hg or target BP of 160/90 mm Hg).
  - Most common agents used: IV labetalol and nicardipine
- See Table 5.1 for selection of antihypertensive agents in acute cerebrovascular HTN.
- HTN after carotid endarterectomy and endovascular procedures (e.g., angioplasty, stenting):
  - Contributing factors: carotid baroreceptor impairment after surgical manipulation, elevated catecholamine levels, activation of trigeminovascular axon reflex

- Carotid hyperperfusion syndrome following carotid endarterectomy:
  - Occurs during first week after surgery
  - Cerebral hyperperfusion is defined as having a postoperative increase in cerebral flow of >100% compared with preoperative flow on the ipsilateral side.
  - Ipsilateral symptoms: pulsatile headaches, seizures, intracranial hemorrhage, cerebral edema
  - Contralateral symptoms: neurological deficits
  - Management:
    - Continuous intra- and postoperative BP monitoring
    - Strict BP control with SBP < 120 mm Hg
    - Preferred agents: intravenous labetalol or clonidine
    - AVOID: vasodilators such as nitroglycerin, sodium nitroprusside
- HTN after spinal cord injury affecting the sixth or above the sixth thoracic spinal nerve (autonomic dysreflexia):
  - Defined as SBP > 20% *from baseline* with associated change in heart rate (brady- to tachycardia), and at least one of the following: headache, facial flushing, blurry vision, stuffy nose, sweating, piloerection. Flush sweaty skin above lesion levels is due to brain stem parasympathetic activation.
  - Occurs in up to 70% of patients with spinal injury affecting the sixth thoracic spinal nerve or higher level
  - Occurs in up to 90% of pregnant women during labor and delivery. Use of epidural or spinal anesthesia may reduce risk.
  - Pathophysiology:
    - Immediately following spinal injury: loss of supraspinal sympathetic control leading to initial period of muscle flaccidity and "spinal shock," clinically evident as bradycardia and hypotension
    - Weeks to months following injury: extrajunctional sprouting of α-receptors, denervation hypersensitivity, impaired presynaptic uptake of norepinephrine, and derangement of spinal glutamatergic neurons
    - Noxious stimuli below neurologic level of the lesion triggers a spinal reflex arc that results in increased sympathetic tone and HTN.
    - Common noxious stimuli are from urinary overdistention and fecal impaction. Others: sympathomimetic medications and sildenafil citrate used for sperm retrieval
  - Management:
    - Preventive measures: good bowel, bladder, and skin care
    - Treatment:
      - Position patient upright to precipitate orthostatic BP.
      - Remove noxious stimuli (e.g., tight clothing, devices, fecal disimpaction, bladder catheterization as applicable).
      - Medications: select fast-acting, short-lived agents for persistent SBP elevation > 150 mm Hg. Consider other noxious stimuli, hospitalization if no resolution.
- Parenchymal kidney disease is the most common cause of secondary HTN.
- Simple renal cysts and HTN:
  - Association thought to be due to cyst compression on adjacent renal parenchyma resulting in focal ischemia and activation of the renin–angiotensin–aldosterone system.

- Association with HTN is strengthened with increased number of cysts (≥2) and increased cystic size > 1.4 to 2.0 cm.
- Management:
  - Cyst decompression anecdotal reports of reducing BP.
  - Use of RAAS blockers may be beneficial.
- Proteinuria and HTN:
  - Proteinuria with loss of plasminogen in urine, leads to the formation of plasmin by tubular urokinase-like plasminogen activator. Plasmin directly stimulates the distal tubular sodium epithelial channel ENaC and sodium reabsorption (thus HTN) via the proteolytic cleavage of ENaC extracellular α- and γ-subunits.
  - Potential role of amiloride or triamterene as preferred agent in the management of edema and salt sensitivity in patients with proteinuria and HTN. More data needed.
- Renovascular HTN:
  - Clinical manifestations:
    - Activation of renin–angiotensin–aldosterone system: seen in early phase in bilateral renal artery stenosis, but sustained in unilateral disease
    - Paroxysmal symptoms due to SNS activation
    - Loss of nocturnal BP dipping
    - Accelerated end-organ damage: left ventricular hypertrophy, microvascular disease, renal fibrosis
    - Abdominal systolic–diastolic bruits, sensitivity 39% to 63%, specificity 90% to 99%
    - Slow progression of renovascular HTN is thought to be associated with an adaptive response to tissue hypoxia thereby minimizing structural damage.
  - Diagnostic studies:
    - Contrast angiography: gold standard: provides both structural and functional information; Risks: procedure-related vascular injury, contrast-induced AKI (CI-AKI).
    - Spiral computed tomographic angiography: good images of vessels; Risks: CI-AKI
    - Magnetic resonance angiography with gadolinium: good structural and functional images of vessels; Risks: nephrogenic systemic fibrosis if gadolinium is used in patients with eGFR < 30 mL/min/1.73 m^2; Other disadvantages: high interobserver variability; limited sensitivity for mid and distal vascular lesions associated with FMD. A lternative MRI contrast in patients with eGFR < 30 mL/min/1.73 m^2: Feraheme
    - Captopril renography (renal nuclear scan): provides information on renal blood flow (uptake/appearance of isotope [MAG3] phase) and filtration (excretory phase), hence information on size and excretory capacity of kidney. Delayed excretory phase following captopril administration suggests significant role of AII in maintaining GFR. Advantage: high negative predictive value, that is negative test essentially rules out clinically significant renal artery stenosis.
    - Renal arterial Doppler (ultrasonography): most effective for detection of lesions in proximal main renal artery (thus likely not great study for fibromuscular dysplasia [FMD] where lesions are typically more distal). Advantages: inexpensive, readily available; Disadvantages: no functional information.

- Renal vein renin measurements: used to predict BP response to renal revascularization: a ratio > 1.5 (stenotic kidney):1.0 (nonstenotic kidney), predicts good BP response in > 90% of patients. However, nonlateralization may also have good response in ~50%.
- HTN occurs in the presence of a critical stenosis (e.g., >70% to 80%); Stenotic lesions < 60 % typically do not lead to clinically significant reduction in renal arterial flow to induce systemic activation of vasopressors to cause HTN.
- Unilateral stenosis (one-clip, two-kidney HTN model): one stenosed (experimental clipping of one renal artery) + one normal kidney
  - *Stenosed "clipped" kidney* has reduced renal perfusion pressure → stimulation of neuronal NO synthase and cyclooxygenase 2 in macula densa → release of renin from juxtaglomerular apparatus → activation of RAAS, (i.e., increased angiotensin II (AII) and aldosterone) → systemic BP increases to restore renal perfusion pressure, increased sodium retention.
  - *Normal contralateral kidney* undergoes pressure natriuresis to restore sodium and volume balance, thus counteracts the stenosed kidney's attempt to improve its own perfusion → continued RAAS activation by stenosed kidney → angiotensin II-dependent HTN; aldosterone-induced renal K^+ and H^+ secretion in the contralateral kidney, hence hypokalemia and metabolic alkalosis.
  - Long-term HTN also attributes to activation of SNS, impairment of NO generation, endothelin release, and hypertensive microvascular injury in the normal contralateral kidney.
  - Clinical implication of RAAS activation in unilateral renal artery stenosis:
    - RAAS inhibition: reduces BP, enhances lateralization of diagnostic testing, reduces GFR in stenotic kidney.
  - Common clinical conditions equivalent to one-clip, two-kidney HTN (unilateral stenosis):
    - Unilateral FMD
    - Unilateral renal atherosclerotic disease
    - Unilateral renal artery aneurysm, dissection, embolism, thrombosis, traumatic occlusion, vasospasm
    - Unilateral renal arteriovenous fistula
    - Aortic dissection affecting renal ostium
    - "Page" kidney (perinephric compression, i.e., large capsular hematoma, perinephric fibrosis)
    - Extrinsic compression (e.g., tumor) on one renal artery
    - Aortic stent occluding origin of renal artery
- Bilateral renal artery stenosis (one-clip, one-kidney HTN) or (two-clip, two-kidney HTN model):
  - Entire kidney mass is exposed to reduced pressures from site of stenosis.
  - There is no "normal nonstenotic kidney."
  - Initial activation of SNS, RAAS leads to sodium and water retention. Since there is no "normal kidney" to excrete the sodium and volume retained, volume overload eventually develops which leads to inhibition of RAAS.
  - HTN is not RAAS-dependent, but volume-dependent.
  - Clinical implications:
    - Patients can be salt-sensitive → easy development of "flash pulmonary edema," following a high dietary salt load
    - Diuretics may be effective in lowering BP.

- Use of RAAS inhibition:
  - Only lowers BP *after* euvolemia has been achieved (i.e., RAAS activation only occurs after negative feedback from volume expansion has been removed).
  - May significantly lower GFR and cause kidney failure.
  - Since RAAS is inhibited due to volume expansion, patients with bilateral renal stenosis or equivalent (see conditions below), typically do not develop hypokalemia and metabolic alkalosis. In fact, the opposite, hyperkalemia and metabolic acidosis, may be present.
- Clinical conditions equivalent to one-clip, one-kidney HTN model:
  - Bilateral arterial stenosis or stenosis of solitary kidney
  - Significant coarctation of aorta or any flow-limiting lesions (e.g., atheroembolic disease, aneurysms, extrinsic mass compression) of suprarenal abdominal aorta
  - Renal artery vasculitis
  - Congenital vascular anomalies
- Fibromuscular dysplasia (Fig. 5.3):
  - Nonatherosclerotic arteriopathy affecting large and medium-sized arteries, typically mid to distal renal artery beyond the first 2 cm from aorta.
  - Epidemiology:
    - Prevalence of clinically significant renovascular FMD is 4/1,000, cerebrovascular involvement 1/1,000 (may present with carotid flow abnormalities, stroke); may be up to 3% to 6% in normotensive individual.
    - Familial presentation in 10%, thought to be autosomal dominant.
  - Clinical manifestations:
    - Commonly seen in young (15 to 50 years old) females with early-onset HTN.
    - Associated conditions: Marfan and Ehlers–Danlos syndromes, tuberous sclerosis, cystic medial necrosis, coarctation of aorta, Alport syndrome, renal agenesis or dysgenesis, α1-antitrypsin deficiency, medullary sponge kidney, PHEO, infantile myofibromatosis, ergotamine preparation, methysergide, cigarette smoking, collagen III glomerulopathy, atherosclerotic renovascular disease.
  - Lesions are characterized by disruptions of vascular wall components with abnormal collagen deposition in bands, ± disruption of elastic membrane.

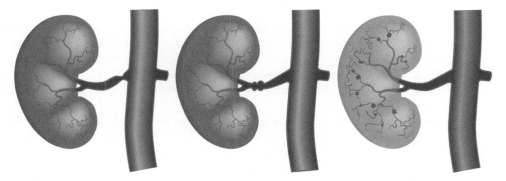

FIGURE 5.3 Renal artery stenosis, fibromuscular dysplasia, polyarteritis nodosa. Renal artery stenosis typically occurs within 2 cm from the aorta. Fibromuscular dysplasia typically occurs at the distal half to third of the renal artery. Polyarteritis nodosa occurs within the kidneys.

- FMD typically occurs in the middle or distal portions of renal artery or branch vessels and may present with aneurysms, occlusion, dissection, arteriovenous fistulas, or thrombosis.
- FMD types:
  - Medial (85% to 100%) > intimal (<10%) > adventitial (<1%)
  - Media and perimedial fibroplasia classically have "string of beads" appearance. Medial *hyperplasia* may only present as smooth stenosis of artery.
  - Initimal and adventitial fibroplasia present as smooth stenotic segments or diffuse attenuation of vessel lumen.
- Natural history:
  - Progression of disease slows down with age.
  - Rarely causes ischemic kidney failure, but associated thrombosis or dissection of affected renal vessel may lead to renal infarction.
- Management of FMD + HTN: percutaneous transluminal renal angioplasty (PTRA) versus surgical revascularization:
  - PTRA:
    - Higher chance of BP lowering following PTRA in younger patients or those with lower pre-PTRA BP, shorter duration of HTN, and positive captopril test.
    - If restenosis occurs, repeat PTRA may be performed as needed.
  - Surgical revascularization:
    - If aneurysmal dilations > 1.5 cm in diameter
    - Covered stent grafts may also be used in renal artery aneurysms.
- Atherosclerotic renal artery stenosis:
  - Atherosclerotic plaque formed from the first 1 to 2 cm of renal artery or from aorta extending into renal ostium (more proximal involvement compared with FMD).
  - Epidemiology:
    - Seen in 10% to 40% of patients undergoing coronary angiography
    - Similar prevalence in African Americans and Caucasians in one study cohort involving 870 patients > 65 years old
    - Autopsy series: prevalence of 4% to 20%; 25% to 30% in those >60 years old, 40% to 60% in those >75 years old
    - Estimated to contribute to decline in kidney function in 15% to 22% of patients with end-stage kidney disease
  - Clues to presence of ischemic renal disease due to atherosclerosis:
    - Asymmetry of kidney size
    - Recent kidney function deterioration
    - AKI following use of ACEI or ARB due to acute reduction in intraglomerular filtration pressure (due to loss of AII-dependent efferent vasoconstriction to maintain intraglomerular filtration pressure)
    - AKI following acute systemic BP reduction with any other hypertensive agents
    - Presence of flash pulmonary edema, more common in bilateral compared with unilateral stenosis
    - Consider renal stenosis in patients with known or at increased risks for atherosclerotic disease and unexplained kidney injury
    - NOTE: Most patients with renovascular HTN do not develop AKI with ACEI/ARB because
      - In unilateral renal artery stenosis, the normal contralateral kidney may still have adequate function to mask any reduced filtration pressure in the affected kidney by ACEI/ARB.

- In bilateral RAS, AII is suppressed due to sodium retention. Hence, ACEI/ARB does not directly reduce glomerular filtration pressure.
  - Those with AKI with ACEI/ARB tend to have other additional source(s) contributing to reduced renal perfusion, for example, volume depletion, cardiac decompensation.
- Management of atherosclerotic renal artery stenosis:
  - Medical therapy:
    - RAAS inhibition as safely tolerated (SCr increases less than 20% to 30% from baseline is acceptable).
    - Use of other agents as needed to control BP: CCB, diuretics, etc.
    - Daily aspirin
    - Statin as tolerated particularly if hyperlipidemia and/or CKD and >50 years old
    - Smoking cessation if applicable
  - Invasive therapy:
    - No evidence of renal or cardiovascular benefits with invasive therapy if stable kidney function and BP
    - Cardiovascular outcomes of renal atherosclerotic lesions (CORAL) trial: comparative trial for renal artery stenting versus best medical therapy involving 947 patients with uncontrolled HTN and *atherosclerotic* renal artery stenosis, BP > 155 mm Hg while on >2 BP medications
      - Average SBP was 2.3 mm Hg lower in the stent group throughout the trial (median follow-up 3.6 years).
      - No difference in incidence of cardiovascular or renal death, myocardial infarction, hospitalization for congestive heart failure, stroke, progressive CKD, or need for renal replacement therapy
    - Meta-analysis of five RCT involving 1,159 patients comparing percutaneous renal artery revascularization (with or without stenting) versus medical therapy on future occurrence of nonfatal myocardial infarction: Renal revascularization did not affect risk of nonfatal MI.
    - However, invasive therapy may be considered in younger viable (low comorbidities) patients with:
      - Rapidly progressive disease (i.e., AKI with RAAS inhibition or achievement of BP control)
      - Failure to appropriate medical therapy
      - Unexplained acute heart failure, "flash pulmonary edema"
    - Renal artery stenting versus surgical revascularization:
      - Surgical revascularization is reserved for patients with technically challenging vascular lesions or associated aortic disease.
  - Intervention being considered: concurrent renal revascularization and use of anti-inflammatory therapies or agents that can alter mitochondrial function to reduce the generation of reactive oxygen species and/or ATP depletion during reperfusion.
  - Contraindications to invasive therapy: advanced kidney disease (e.g. SCr > 3 to 4 mg/dL, kidney length < 8 cm), poor surgical candidate, or low life-expectancy.

> **NOTE** Atherosclerotic renal artery stenosis typically affects the proximal 1 to 2 cm of the renal artery from aorta, FMD involves the distal 1/2 to 1/3 of the renal artery, and polyarteritis nodosa involves multiple aneurysmal dilatations within the kidneys.

- Endocrine causes of HTN: from pituitary → thyroid → parathyroid → adrenals
  - Pituitary: acromegaly
    - Pituitary tumor producing excessive circulating growth hormone (GH). Other GH-producing tumors: pancreatic, hypothalamic, breast, bronchial malignancies
    - More common in women and older patients
    - Pathogenesis:
      - Sodium retention with inappropriately normal to only minimally low renin and aldosterone levels and normal atrial natriuretic peptide.
      - Others: GH–induced vascular hypertrophy with decreased vascular compliance, increased SNS, associated hyperthyroidism.
    - Clinical manifestations: skull, hands, feet enlargement, excessive sweating, carpal tunnel syndrome, sexual dysfunction, diabetes mellitus, thyromegaly, thyrotoxicosis, headaches, visual field defects
    - Diagnosis:
      - Elevated plasma GH, especially in response to an oral glucose tolerance test
      - Others: plasma insulin-like growth factor I, lateral skull X-ray (thickened skull vault, enlarged frontal sinuses), MRI of pituitary fossa
    - Management:
      - Tumor-specific:
        - Transphenoidal adenomectomy is treatment of choice if no contraindication
        - Tumor radiation
        - Dopaminergic agents: bromocriptine and cabergoline, octreotide
      - HTN: diuretics as primary agent, addition of others as needed
  - Pituitary: Cushing syndrome (pituitary adenoma producing excess adrenocorticotropic hormone (ACTH); other sources of excess ACTH secretion: adrenal tumors, bronchogenic carcinoma):
    - Pathogenesis:
      - Increased cardiac output and peripheral vascular resistance
      - Concurrent production of mineralocorticoids
      - Cortisol inhibition of NO
      - Increased sensitivity to catecholamines, AII, and β-adrenergic stimulation
      - Blunted response to atrial natriuretic peptide
    - Diagnosis:
      - 24-hour urine free cortisol
      - Dexamethasone suppression test
        - Low dose (1 mg) at midnight
        - High dose (partially suppresses ACTH from pituitary tumors but not with ectopic ACTH)
      - Corticotropin-releasing hormone test.
      - Imaging studies: CT or MRI of pituitary, adrenals, thorax/abdomen/pelvis
      - Simultaneous bilateral inferior petrosal sinus sampling for ACTH measurements
    - Management:
      - Cushing disease: resection of pituitary adenoma
      - Cushing syndrome:
        - Unilateral adrenalectomy if adrenal adenoma
        - Adrenal carcinoma is associated with poor survival
      - Antihypertensive medications: consider potassium-sparing diuretics

- Thyroid:
  - Hypothyroidism-associated HTN:
    - Sodium retention
    - Increased peripheral vascular resistance ; 30% of patients have diastolic HTN
    - Underdamping of swings in SNS activity
  - Hyperthyroidism-induced HTN:
    - Pathogenesis:
      - Increased cardiac output, heart rate, myocardium contractility. (Peripheral vascular resistance tends to be reduced.)
      - Expanded blood volume
      - Increased RAS activity but not SNS
    - Classic presentation: high pulse pressure HTN, ISH
- Parathyroid: Hyperparathyroidism-induced HTN is thought to be due to increased peripheral vascular resistance, presumably due to hypercalcemia.
- Adrenals:
  - PHEO:
    - 90% arise from adrenals, 10% extra-adrenal (paraganglioma, PGL).
    - Most are benign; 10% metastasize to regional lymph nodes
    - Common hormones produced: norepinephrine, epinephrine, dopamine
    - Malignant disease or large tumor mass may have very high dopamine levels.
    - Sporadic disease:
      - Often focal, unilateral involvement
      - Up to 14% have somatic mutations
    - Familial disease:
      - Typically multifocal, bilateral, extra-adrenal disease, age < 50 years old, may be associated with germ line mutations (most are autosomal dominant):
      - RET gene: multiple endocrine neoplasia type 2 (MEN 2):
        - MEN 2a: medullary thyroid carcinoma, hyperparathyroidism, cutaneous lichen amyloid
        - MEN 2b: medullary thyroid carcinoma, multiple neuromas, marfanoid habitus
        - Mostly epinephrine secretion
        - Paroxysmal symptoms
      - von Hippel–Lindau gene: von Hippel–Lindau syndrome
        - Syndrome with retinal and CNS hemangioblastomas, renal cell carcinoma, pancreatic, endolymphatic sac, epididymal tumors
        - Predominant noradrenergic secretory pattern
        - Can present primarily with asymptomatic HTN due to downregulation of α-adrenoceptors
      - Neurofibromatosis type 1 gene:
        - Neurofibromatosis type 1 (a.k.a. von Recklinghausen disease): neurofibromas, café-au-lait spots
        - Mostly epinephrine secretion
        - Paroxysmal symptoms
      - Genes encoding the B and D subunits of mitochondrial succinate dehydrogenase (SDHB, SDHB): familial PGLs (head and neck) and PHEOs; no secretory activity; no symptoms related to catecholamines, but space-occupying effect

- Hypoxia induced factor -2α (HIF-2α), somatic mutation: multiple duodenal somatostatinomas, polycythemia
- Common clinical manifestations of PHEOs:
  - Classic: paroxysmal HTN, headaches, diaphoresis, palpitations, anxiety, chest/abdominal pain, nausea/vomiting, dyspnea, pallor
  - Severe HTN with trauma, delivery, or sudden onset
  - Subclinical
- Physical examination: 2/3 labile HTN, 1/3 persistent HTN; reciprocal changes in BP and heart rate may occur with predominantly norepinephrine secreting tumors; postural hypotension; low-grade fevers, tachycardia, skin may be cool, mottled appearing.
- Diagnosis:
  - Plasma free metanephrines and normetanephrines greater than four- to fivefold of normal → positive test. High sensitivity
  - If positive plasma study, obtain urine metanephrines and normetanephrines. High sensitivity and high specificity
  - Glucagon stimulation:
    - Indicated if equivocal plasma study
    - Administer 2 mg glucagon IV bolus. Positive test: greater than threefold increase in baseline levels of catecholamines within 1 to 2 minutes
  - Clonidine suppression test:
    - Indicated if equivocal plasma study
    - Administer 0.3 mg clonidine. Positive test: failure to reduce plasma catecholamines to >50% from baseline
  - Imaging studies:
    - MRI or CT: abdomen/pelvis if no family history; neck to pelvis if family history or suspicion for genetic disease
    - If negative, consider metaiodobenzylguanidine (MIBG) scan, indium In111-labeled octreotide scan, plasma-free metanephrines coupled with vena caval sampling, or positron emission tomography (PET) scan.
    - MIBG has high sensitivity (83% to 100%) and specificity (95% to 100%) in sporadic PHEO.
    - MIBG has been suggested to be inferior to PET in the evaluation of PHEO/PGL in familial and metastatic disease.
- Management:
  - BP control:
    - α-adrenergic blockers (phenoxybenzamine [usually not well tolerated due to orthostatic hypotension]), doxazosin, terazosin
    - CCB
    - Add β-blockers if tachycardia or arrhythmias after full α-adrenergic inhibition. Consider agents with both α- and β-inhibition (e.g., carvedilol, labetalol).
  - Surgical removal:
    - Preoperative preparation: BP control weeks prior to surgery
    - Intraoperative BP management options: phentolamine, sodium nitroprusside, and magnesium sulfate
    - Postoperative management: monitor for hypoglycemia and hypotension
    - Long-term management:
      - BP control if persistent HTN
      - If malignant PHEO, use both α- and β-adrenergic blockers as needed for symptoms, radiation therapy for bone metastatic disease, and

chemotherapy (cyclophosphamide, vincristine, and dacarbazine). Median survival ~5 years.
- Follow-up (life-long):
  - Adrenal PHEO < 5 cm and no suspected hereditary syndrome: biochemical screening at 1 year, then every other year thereafter
  - PHEO > 5 cm or hereditary syndromes, multifocal PGL: biochemical evaluation after 6 months following surgery, then yearly thereafter with periodic imaging study
  - For patients with biochemically silent disease: periodic imaging study
- Adrenal incidentaloma/hyperplasia/adenoma/carcinoma:
  - Screening aldosterone/renin ratio (ARR):
    - ARR > 30 and aldosterone levels > 20 ng/dL
    - Sensitivity 90%, specificity 91%, positive predictive value 69%
    - Factors affecting ratio:
      - False negative ARR due to increased renin: dietary salt restriction, malignant or renovascular HTN, diuretics (including spironolactone, eplerenone), dihydropyridine calcium channel blockers, ACEI/ARB, selective serotonin reuptake inhibitors
      - False positive ARR due to suppressed renin: β-blockers, α-methyldopa, clonidine, NSAIDS. False positives may also occur in patients with renal dysfunction and older age.
      - Optimization of ARR measurements: normalize serum potassium levels prior to measuring ARR.
      - Avoid use of medications that can affect ARR if clinically safe.
    - Prevalence of high ARR is 16% to 20% in patients with HTN.
    - Prevalence of confirmed primary aldosteronism is 4.5% to 9.5%.
  - Confirmatory testing following positive ARR:
    - IV salt loading: 2 L NS over 4 hours (recumbent) → (+) if plasma aldosterone > 10 ng/dL (<6 ng/dL in normal subjects)
    - Oral salt loading: 2 g NaCl tablets t.i.d. × 3 days and potassium supplement → (+) if 24-hour urine aldosterone > 14 g/24-hour (U_{Na} should also be >200 mEq to assess compliance with Na load)
    - Fludrocortisone-suppression test: fludrocortisone acetate 0.1 mg q6h with high salt diet (3 mmol/kg/d) × 4 days and potassium supplement → (+) if plasma aldosterone > 5 ng/dL and PRA < 1.0 ng/mL/h.
    - Imaging studies:
      - CT/MRI imaging with adrenal cuts: Adrenal carcinoma is more likely with increasing size; 2% of masses up to 4 cm, 6% of masses from 4 to 6 cm, 25% of masses > 6 cm are malignant.
      - Adrenal venous sampling (AVS) for lateralization of aldosterone levels should be considered in good candidates for adrenalectomy (young, non-obese patients with limited end-organ damage and short duration of HTN and hypokalemia) to confirm the correct side of the hyperfunctioning gland prior to removal. NOTE: AVS for lateralization of aldosteronism should be measured along with a selectivity index (adrenal vein to inferior vena cava cortisol ratio > 5:1) to indicate successful adrenal vein catheterization. A low selectivity index may indicate erroneous blood sampling from a vein other than the adrenal vein, which may give a falsely low aldosterone level, thus falsely negative lateralization test.
  - Genetic mutations of aldosterone-producing adenomas:
    - Somatic mutation in the gene encoding the potassium channel KCNJ5 in 1/3 of adenomas (mutation in affected tissues only): Potassium selectivity

of the channel is lost, thus allowing sodium influx through channel and subsequent chronic cell depolarization. This leads to calcium influx and consequent activation of aldosterone synthase and cell proliferation. There are data to suggest better BP control following adrenalectomy of those with KCNJ5 mutations than those without these mutations.
  - Somatic mutation in gene encoding the voltage-gated calcium channel CACNA1D can lead to increased calcium influx, and subsequent activation of aldosterone synthase and cell proliferation.
  - Long-term effects of hyperaldosteronism:
    - German registry compared mortality rates of 300 patients with primary aldosteronism (either surgically or medically managed) to 600 hypertensive patients and 600 normotensive controls over a 16-year follow-up revealed:
      - No difference in mortality among the three groups.
      - Cardiovascular deaths were higher for patients with primary hyperaldosteronism (50%) compared to those with essential (38%) or normotensive controls (35%).
      - Unadjusted analyses suggested better outcomes with adrenalectomy versus medical therapy, but *not* on multivariate analyses, thought to be due to healthier patient selection for adrenalectomy.
    - In another study (Rossi et al., 2013) involving 180 patients with hyperaldosteronism: 110 adrenalectomy and 70 treated with MRA according to AVS
      - Even with BP and hypokalemia control with either medical or surgical intervention over a 3-year follow-up, the prevalence of left ventricular hypertrophy among patients with hyperaldosteronism is higher compared with that of essential HTN, 50% vs. 27%, $p < 0.001$, respectively.
      - Long-term outcomes of patients with hyperaldosteronism are likely worse than those of patients with essential HTN.
    - Most recent meta-analysis (2015), however, revealed that reduction of LV mass is not different in patients treated with adrenalectomy or mineralocorticoid receptor antagonists (MRA).
  - Management:
    - Medical intervention:
      - MRA: aldosterone antognists spironolactone or eplerenone
      - Aldosterone synthase activity blocker LC1699 versus eplerenone: eplerenone more effective in reducing BP and improving hypokalemia. LC1699, however, reduces, whereas eplerenone increases aldosterone levels. Long-term effects of elevated aldosterone levels are not known.
    - Surgical versus medical intervention:
      - Better cardiovascular mortality with surgical intervention than MRA is questioned by patient selection for surgery versus MRA.
      - Nonetheless, adrenalectomy may still be considered in younger patients with short disease duration and minimal or no evidence of end-organ damage.
  - For other conditions with the clinical triad of hypokalemia, metabolic alkalosis, and HTN triad, see Hypokalemia, in Acid-Base/Potassium chapter.
- Acute intermittent porphyria:
  - Rare autosomal dominant disorder with deficiency of porphobilinogen deaminase affecting heme production and associated with increased porphobilinogens

- Clinical manifestations:
  - Intermittent severe colicky abdominal pain, constipation, dystonic bladder with urinary retention/incontinence, dark urine, autonomic dysfunction with increased circulating catecholamine levels resulting in HTN, tachycardia, sweating, restless and tremors, peripheral neuropathy, proximal muscle weakness, neuropsychiatric disorders, SIADH with hyponatremia. Skin rash is not a typical manifestation compared to other forms of porphyria.
  - Attacks may be brought on by infections, hormonal or dietary changes, drugs.
- Diagnosis: elevated urinary porphobilinogens (urine spot test)
- Management:
  - Mild attacks: high-dose oral glucose (400 g/d) or intravenous dextrose 10% solution
  - Severe attacks, severe neurologic symptoms: hematin (hemin) 3 to 4 mg/kg/d for 4 days
  - Pain control with narcotics as needed
  - Laxatives, softeners for constipation, particularly if narcotics are used
  - Gabapentin for seizures

OTHER SPECIAL CAUSES OF HYPERTENSION

Reversible Posterior Leukoencephalopathy Syndrome

- Hypertensive syndrome associated with cerebral edema and symptoms of headaches, vomiting, confusion, seizures, cortical blindness
- Acute rise in BP results in dilatation of cerebral arteries and arterioles and increase in blood brain barrier permeability leading to brain edema.
- Underlying causes: immunosuppressive therapy, vasculitis (lupus), pregnancy (eclampsia), kidney failure, severe HTN
- Diagnosis: magnetic resonant imaging revealing cortico–subcortical areas of hyperintensity involving the occipital and parietal lobes on T2-weighted images.
- Management: BP control and treatment of underlying diseases
- Condition may be reversible, but blindness may persist.

Pregnancy

- Blood pressure in normal pregnancy:
  - DBP ↓ by 7 to 10 mm Hg in early pregnancy, by as much as 20 mm Hg in midpregnancy. DBP returns to baseline by third trimester. Nondippers may indicate risk for preeclampsia.
  - SBP only ↓ slightly due to concurrent increase in cardiac output (↑30% to 40%) and ↓ in peripheral vascular resistance.
- HTN in pregnancy:
  - BP > 140/90 mm Hg
  - NOTE: Per the US National High BP Education Program, patients with BP ≤ 140/90 mm Hg, *but* with increased SBP of >30 mm Hg or DBP > 15 mm Hg compared with prepregnancy BP, should be managed as high-risk patients.
  - Chronic HTN:
    - Occurs before 20 weeks of gestation
    - May be primary or secondary HTN
  - Gestational HTN:
    - Occurs *de novo after 20 weeks* and normalizes within 3 months postpartum

- Gestational HTN may or may not present as preeclampsia/eclampsia.
- Preeclampsia is a severe form of gestational HTN with end organ dysfunction.
- The diagnosis of preeclampsia may be made if patient has one or more of the following:
  - Urine protein to creatinine ratio > 0.3 g/g Cr.
  - SCr > 1.1 mg/dL.
  - Aspartate aminotransferase > 50 IU/L ± severe epigastric/right upper quadrant pain.
  - Neurologic symptoms
  - Thrombocytopenia and hemolysis
  - Fetal growth restriction
- NOTE: A fall in uric acid clearance is a key feature of preeclampsia. Serum uric acid levels > 5.5 mg/dL is a strong indicator of preeclampsia, and levels > 7.8 mg/dL is associated with increased maternal morbidity.
- Various forms/combinations of HTN seen during pregnancy are summarized in Table 5.2.

Preeclampsia

- Pathogenesis of preeclampsia: current understanding:
  - What happens in normal pregnancy:
    - Vascular endothelial growth factor (VEGF) and the transforming growth factor β-1 (TGFβ1) are required to maintain endothelial health in the kidney and placenta. VEGF and TGFβ1 exert their angiogenic and endothelial health-maintaining effects via binding to their respective receptors, VEGF receptor-1 and TGFβ1 receptor.
    - Vascular homeostasis is maintained by physiologic levels of VEGF and TGFβ1.

Table 5.2	Hypertension during pregnancy			
	Onset	Proteinuria	Other Abnormalities	Comments
Pre-/eclampsia	After 20 wk	Yes, after 20 wk	↑LFT, ↑LDH, ↓albumin, hemolysis, thrombocytopenia	Worst prognosis with BP > 160/110 mm Hg, oliguria, platelet count < 100 × 10^9/L, LDH > 600 IU/L, elevated LFT, pulmonary edema, neurologic symptoms
Chronic HTN	Prior to 20 wk	±Yes, prior to 20 wk	Electrocardiogram or echocardiographic evidence of left ventricular hypertrophy	Absence of BP nadir during second trimester or presence of secondary HTN increase risk of pre-/eclampsia
Chronic HTN with superimposed Pre-/eclampsia	Prior to 20 wk, worse after 20 wk	±Yes, prior to 20 wk, worse after 20 wk	↑LFT, ↑LDH, ↓albumin, hemolysis, thrombocytopenia	
Transient HTN	During or within 24 h postpartum, resolves within 3 mo	±Yes, minimal	None	May predict increased risk of permanent HTN

wk, Week; mo, month; BP, blood pressure; HTN, Hypertension; LFT, liver function tests; LDH, lactate dehydrogenase.

- What happens in preeclampsia/eclampsia:
  - There is excessive placental secretion of sFLt1 (soluble fms-like tyrosine kinase 1 which also binds to VEGF) and sEng (soluble endoglin, a truncated form of endoglin that is a cell surface receptor for TGFβ1). sFlt1 and sEng compete with endothelial receptors for VEGF and TGFβ1 for circulating VEGF and TGFβ1 respectively and deplete VEGF and TGFβ1 for endothelial cell surface binding and signaling to maintain healthy vasculature.
  - This results in endothelial cell dysfunction, decreased prostacyclin and NO production, and release of procoagulant protein.
  - Additionally, other proangiogenic factors such as placental growth factor (PlGF) and adiponectin are decreased.
  - Other antiangiogenic factors (e.g., endostatin) are increased.
  - Use of logarithmic transformed sFLT-1/PlGF ratios is being evaluated to predict preeclampsia. Higher ratio → higher risk.
  - Histopathology (Figs. 5.4 and 5.5): Glomerular tufts are described as "bloodless"; capillary lumina are narrowed due to endothelial cell swelling, referred to as "endotheliosis." In contrast, capillary loops are wide open in normal glomeruli. Foam cells with lipid vacuoles may also be seen in this condition.
- Preeclampsia and future risk of cardiovascular disease: Meta-analyses suggest an increased cardiac risk, albeit small absolute risk.
  - Association may be related to risk factors common to both preeclampsia and cardiovascular disease (e.g., obesity, glucose intolerance, high BP, kidney disease)
  - Diffuse endothelial injury occurring during preeclampsia leads to increased risk.

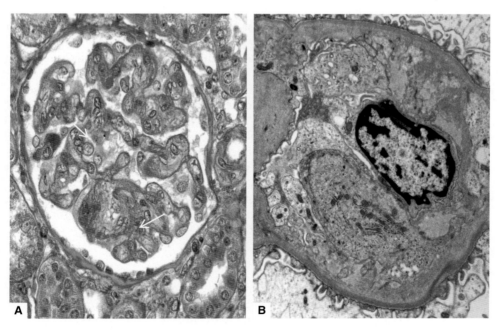

FIGURE 5.4 Histopathology of preeclampsia/eclampsia. **A.** Glomerular capillaries are filled with swollen endothelial cells and segmentally there is luminal fibrin deposition (*arrows*). There is mild podocyte hypertrophy and the adjacent arteriole is normal (Masson's trichrome, ×500). **B.** Glomerular capillary with swollen endothelial cytoplasm resulting in luminal occlusion. Podocyte foot processes are preserved, but may be effaced (×14,000).

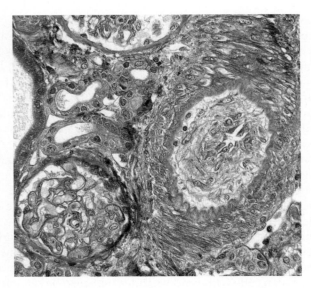

FIGURE 5.5 Large interlobular artery with marked loose mucoid intimal thickening, endothelial cell swelling and luminal narrowing (Masson's trichrome, ×250).

Eclampsia

- Same pathogenesis as preeclampsia
- Thought to be a form of posterior reversible encephalopathy syndrome (PRES)

Hemolytic anemia, elevated liver tests low platelet (HELLP syndrome of pregnancy):

- Clinical manifestations:
  - May occur in third trimester to post-partum, associated with gestational or preeclampsia/eclampsia
  - Symptoms: Midepigastric to right upper quadrant pain, malaise, nausea, vomiting
  - Maternal mortality: 1%
- Pathophysiology: Unknown; Long chain 3-hydroxyacyl-CoA-dehydrogenase deficiency of the child has been reported to be associated with both maternal HELLP and acute fatty liver of pregnancy.
- Diagnosis: hemolysis, serum lactate dehydrogenase > 600 IU/L; serum aspartate aminotransferase > 70 IU/L; and thrombocytopenia with platelet count < 100,000-150,000/µL. Twenty percent of patients may also have disseminated intravascular coagulation.
- Treatment: antihypertensive therapy similar to preeclampsia, magnesium sulfate, blood transfusion and fresh frozen plasma as needed, embolization for hepatic hemorrhage, intravenous fluid support.

Treatment of HTN in Pregnancy

- For chronic hypertensive patients:
  - Continue pre-pregnancy antihypertensive medications except ACEI/ARB /aldosterone antagonist to maintain SBP between 120 to 160 mm Hg and DBP between 80 to 105 mm Hg. For patients with chronic HTN and end organ damage, maintain BP < 140/90 mm Hg.
- For new-onset HTN:
  - Treat when SBP > 160 mm Hg or,
  - DBP > 110 mm Hg.

- Common agents to treat nonsevere HTN in pregnancy:
  - Methyldopa: 250 to 500 mg b.i.d. to q.i.d., maximum 2 g/d
  - Labetalol: 100 to 400 mg orally b.i.d. to t.i.d. (maximum 1,200 mg/d)
  - Nifedipine, extended release: 30 to 60 mg orally daily to b.i.d.
- Common agents used to treat severe HTN, that is BP > 160/110 mm Hg:
  - Labetalol (intravenous then switch or oral): avoid in asthma or heart failure. Inform neonatologist regarding possible neonatal bradycardia.
  - Nifedipine (oral): associated with reflex tachycardia
  - Hydralazine (intravenous or intramuscular): may increase risk of maternal hypotension
- Other treatment options for severe HTN:
  - Nitroglycerin
  - Diazoxide (1.5 mg IV) may be comparable to hydralazine (5 mg IV)
- For preeclampsia:
  - Control BP with agents suggested for HTN in pregnancy above.
  - NOTE: Diuretics should *not* be used in preeclampsia/eclampsia. Similarly, salt restriction is not recommended in preeclampsia/eclampsia.
  - Magnesium sulfate:
    - May lead to a transient decrease in BP at 30 minutes following 2 to 5 g IV dose
    - NOTE: Magnesium has a synergistic hypotensive effect with CCB (e.g., nifedipine): this effect may be reversed with intravenous calcium (*i.e.* 10-20 mL of 10% calcium chloride over 10 minutes, repeat up to 4 times q 20 minutes as needed).
- For eclampsia:
  - Magnesium sulfate as suggested for preeclampsia
  - Treat HTN with agents that do not cause cerebral vasodilation. Labetalol is acceptable. Nicardipine has favorable cerebral hemodynamic effects. Both hydralazine and nifedipine vasodilate cerebral vasculature. However, this should not be the sole criteria for antihypertensive medication selection.
  - Captopril may be used for severe postpartum HTN if *no* breast-feeding.
- For preeclampsia without severe features, observation and delivery at 37 weeks is suggested.

Calcineurin Inhibitor-Induced (CNI) HTN

- Cyclosporine > tacrolimus.
- CNI-induced salt-sensitive HTN in mice revealed phenotype similar to familial hyperkalemic HTN (FHH), a.k.a. pseudohypoaldosteronism type II or Gordon syndrome: renal sodium (HTN) and potassium retention (hyperkalemia), RTA, hypomagnesemia, ± hypercalciuria. See FHH below.
- Likely mechanisms: increased renal expression of the phosphorylated (active) form of the thiazide-sensitive NaCl cotransporter (NCC), along with increases in the expression of kinases that mediate activation of NCC
- Likely best treated with thiazide diuretics

Familial Hyperkalemic HTN, a.k.a. Pseudohypoaldosteronism Type II, Gordon Syndrome

- Clinical manifestations:
  - Rare autosomal-dominant, heterogeneous syndrome
  - Electrolyte abnormalities occur as early as infancy: hyperkalemia (low renal K^+ excretion), metabolic acidosis, hypercalciuria (osteoporosis)
  - HTN:
    - May not be detected until two to four decades later
    - All patients will eventually develop HTN in adulthood.

- Kidney function is normal in most cases.
  - Low plasma renin and low-to-normal serum aldosterone levels despite normal adrenal function
- Primary defects:
  - Increased sodium chloride cotransport (NCC) expression *and* activity due to mutations of its regulatory molecules:
    - Increased Na^+ reabsorption at NCC leads to reduced Na^+ delivery to collecting tubules, hence reduced K^+ excretion (hyperkalemia) and reduced H^+ excretion (metabolic acidosis). See renal tubular acidosis section for mechanisms of how low Na^+ delivery to collecting tubules can lead to hyperkalemia and metabolic acidosis.
    - Hyperkalemia also contributes to reduced H^+ excretion (via reduced ammoniagenesis).
  - Increased paracellular chloride reabsorption
  - Increased NaCl reabsorption above leads to volume expansion, HTN, and inhibition of RAAS, hence low renin ± low aldosterone levels. Low aldosterone levels can also contribute to hyperkalemia and metabolic acidosis.
  - Reported mutations of NCC regulatory molecules leading to FHH: With-no-lysine kinases 1 to 4 (WNK 1-4) 1-4, Kelch-like 3 (KLHL3) and Cullin 3 (CUL3)
    - WNK1 gain-of-function mutation enhances NCC activity
    - Loss of function mutation of WNK4:
      - Enhances NCC activity and distal convoluted tubular (DCT) hyperplasia, thus Na^+ retention.
      - Mutated WNK4 enhances ROMK endocytosis, reduces K^+ excretion, and causes hyperkalemia.
      - Mutations in WNK4 also downregulate the transient receptor potential V5 channel (TRPV5, calcium channel) and decrease Ca^{2+} reabsorption in DCT, thus hypercalciuria and osteoporosis.
    - KLHL3 and CUL3 mutations: Mutations in KLHL3 or CUL3 can lead to impaired ubiquitination of NCC, a process whereby NCC is normally internalized and degraded. Impaired removal of NCC from apical membrane leads to increased Na^+ reabsorption at DCT, hence HTN.
  - Summary of molecular mutations leading to the clinical PHAII syndrome: Mutations of WNK1-4:
    $\downarrow$ROMK $\rightarrow$ $\downarrow$$K^+$ secretion $\rightarrow$ hyperkalemia, reduced ammoniagenesis, metabolic acidosis
    $\uparrow$NCC activity $\rightarrow$ $\uparrow$$Na^+$ reabsorption $\rightarrow$ HTN, volume expansion induced hyporenin/hypoaldosteronism $\rightarrow$ hyperkalemia, metabolic acidosis
    $\uparrow$NCC activity $\rightarrow$ reduced Na^+ delivery to cortical collecting tubule (CCT) $\rightarrow$ $\downarrow$$K^+$ and H^+ secretion $\rightarrow$ hyperkalemia, metabolic acidosis
    $\uparrow$*paracellular* Cl^- reabsorption $\rightarrow$ $\downarrow$lumen electronegativity for optimal K^+ secretion $\rightarrow$ hyperkalemia
    $\downarrow$TRPV5 activity $\rightarrow$ $\downarrow$$Ca2^+$ reabsorption in DCT/CT $\rightarrow$ hypercalciuria $\rightarrow$ osteoporosis
- Treatment:
  - Chronic low salt diet
  - Thiazide diuretics

Liddle Syndrome

- Autosomal dominant, gain of function mutation in either the β- or γ-subunits of ENaC in the collecting tubules

- The mutations affect the PY motif of ENaC, which is the peptide segment necessary for Nedd4-2 to recognize ENaC for ubiquitination for internalization and degradation. This results in an increased number of functioning apical ENaC on the apical membranes and increased Na$^+$ reabsorption.
- Affected patients present with HTN due to increased Na$^+$ retention, hyporenin/hypoaldosteronism due to volume expansion, *but hypokalemia* and *metabolic alkalosis* due to facilitated renal K$^+$ and H$^+$ secretion in the collecting tubules via the favorable electrochemical gradient generated by the enhanced Na$^+$ reabsorption through ENaC.
- Treatment: low-sodium diet and direct ENaC inhibitors such as amiloride and triamterene. Spironolactone is *ineffective* since Liddle syndrome is not due to aldosterone-induced upregulation of ENaC. The increased ENaC activity is due to reduced internalization and degradation of apical ENaC.

Scleroderma Renal Crisis

- Epidemiology:
  - Scleroderma renal crisis (SRC) occurs in 2% with limited disease (skin involvement *below* elbows and knees only).
  - SRC occurs in ~5% to 10% of diffuse scleroderma (skin involvement *below and above* elbows and knees).
- Clinical manifestations:
  - Typically presents at diagnosis of scleroderma or within 3 to 4 years of disease onset.
  - Predominant presentations:
    - Acute onset of moderate to severe "accelerated" HTN and oliguric kidney failure
    - Accompanying features: hyperrenin, thrombotic microangiopathy, anemia, congestive heart failure, and/or hypertensive encephalopathy and retinopathy
    - 10% of SRC occurs with relative normotension which may reflect low baseline BP or concurrent acute illness with associated fall in BP.
- Risks:
  - Positive anti-RNA polymerase III antibodies (*not* anti-Scl70 or anti-U3RNP antibodies)
  - Early diffuse scleroderma, rapidly progressive skin disease and tendon friction rubs
  - Corticosteroid exposure
  - Others: HLA DRB1*0407, HLA-DRB1*1304, endothelin B receptor polymorphisms, soluble CD147
- Factors *not* associated with SRC:
  - Positive anticentromere antibody
  - Baseline BP, creatinine, proteinuria, hematuria
  - Gender
- Management:
  - ACEI are first-line therapy. ARB are *not* sufficient as first-line to control BP.
  - Goal: reduce SBP/DBP by 20/10 mm Hg per 24 hours.
  - Prophylaxis therapy:
    - None proven effective
    - Prophylactic ACEI may lead to *worse* outcome and higher likelihood or dialysis dependency for unclear reasons.
    - ARB are *not* effective. Reports of patients developing SRC while on ARB

- Renal transplantation:
  - Effective and improve survival
  - Patients should be on ≥2 years on dialysis before consideration for transplant due to high recovery rates. (Opinion-based)
  - Recurrence of SRC < 5% and more common in those with early native kidney loss due to SRC.

Novel Findings Related to HTN

- Nonosmotic sodium storage in the skin:
  - Tissue sodium is higher in hypertensive patients compared with controls, and highest among those with treatment-resistant HTN.
  - Tissue sodium decreases in patients with primary aldosteronism following adrenalectomy or treatment with spironolactone.
  - Patients with resistant HTN treated with spironolactone had sodium content levels similar to those of normotensive patients.
- Epithelial sodium channel (ENaC) and endothelial stiffness:
  - ENaC is expressed in several nonepithelial tissues including vascular endothelium.
  - Conditions associated with increased ENaC expression (e.g., experimental model of Liddle syndrome, aldosterone stimulation) are associated with increased endothelial cell stiffness.
  - Conditions associated with reduced ENaC (ENaC knockdown, spironolactone, amiloride) lead to significant reductions in endothelial stiffness.
  - Future direction: *vascular-specific* ENaC inhibition to lower BP, reduce atherosclerosis *without* hyperkalemic effect
- Gut microbiota and HTN: Olfactory receptors in large arteries in the kidney (and elsewhere in the body) may sense short-chain fatty acid production by gut bacteria and induce a vasodilatory and hypotensive effect.
- Novel potential treatment targets:
  - Plasminogen activator inhibitor-1 (PAI-1) antagonism:
    - PAI-1 is profibrotic and impairs cell migration and extracellular matrix degradation in the vasculature.
    - PAI-1 antagonism has been shown to reduce BP, improve vascular injury, and senescence in hypertensive animal models.
  - ACE2 activation/angiotensin 1-7 (Ang 1-7)peptide:
    - Ang 1-7 is vasodilatory in contrast to AII [whereas AII is converted from angiotensin I by ACE, Ang 1-7 is converted from angiotensin 1 by ACE2].
    - Xanthenone, an ACE2-stimulating agent, has been shown to significantly reduce myocardial, perivascular, and renal interstitial fibrosis in spontaneously hypertensive rats and improve endothelium-dependent vasodilatation.

HTN Treatment Updates

- ACEI, ARB, direct renin inhibitor (DRI) interactions:
  - Aliskiren in the evaluation of proteinuria in diabetes (AVOID) trial: Combination therapy consisting of losartan 100 mg/d and aliskiren (150 mg/d for 3 months and 300 mg/d for 3 months) was minimally beneficial compared with lone losartan therapy in patients with diabetes mellitus type 2 and hypertension (reduction in BP (−2/1 mm Hg), decrease in eGFR decline (−3.8 vs. −2.4 mL/min/1.73 m^2), and 20% reduction in albumin to creatinine ratio) at the expense of higher rate of hyperkalemia, 4.7% versus 17%.
  - Aliskiren in Type 2 Diabetes Using Cardio–Renal Endpoints (ALTITUDE) trial: Patients with diabetic kidney disease receiving combination therapy with

aliskiren and either an ACEI or ARB had reduced proteinuria and SBP by 1 to 2 mm Hg compared with those receiving lone ACEI or ARB therapy at the expense of 25% greater stroke rate and more frequent hyperkalemia.
- Over suppression of RAAS leads to worse outcome.
- Body mass index: Avoiding Cardiovascular Events through Combination Therapy in Patients Living with Systolic HTN (ACCOMPLISH) trial:
  - ACCOMPLISH trial suggests the preferential addition of a CCB over a diuretic to an ACEI in the treatment of HTN in normal-weight patients for improved cardiovascular benefits. In obese high-risk hypertensive patients, however, the choice of adding either a diuretic versus CCB to an ACEI is less important.
  - Proposed mechanism for observed difference: Compared to obese patients, lean individuals are thought to have more prominent RAAS and SNS activities. The use of diuretic in lean patients could further stimulate RAAS and lead to worse cardiovascular outcomes.
- Renal denervation for resistant HTN:
  - Interruption of renal artery afferent signals (i.e., sympathetic stimulation) to brain
  - Simplicity HTN-3 trial: no benefit
  - Concerns regarding procedure:
    - May promote renal artery atherogenesis
    - Interference with denervated kidney ability to tolerate insults such as volume depletion, infection, trauma, drug exposures.
- Chlorthalidone (CTD) versus hydrochlorothiazide (HCTZ):
  - Longer half-life: CTD (~40 hours) versus HCTZ (~4 hours)
  - Chlorthalidone is associated with lower LDL and glucose levels.
  - Meta-analysis: 19% lower cardiovascular event rate for CTD compared with HCTZ.
    - Better nighttime BP control. Other beneficial non-BP related effects may be possible.
    - Further data needed
- Orthostatic hypotension management:
  - Goal: focus on the well-being of patient, not achieving a specific BP level
  - Nondrug: increase fluid and salt intake, avoid getting up quickly or prolonged motionless standing, use of compressive waist-high stockings, raise head of be by 6 to 9 inches, maintain active lifestyle.
  - Drug options: midodrine, fludrocortisone, and pseudoephedrine
    - If supine HTN: consider midodrine as needed basis (prn).
    - If no supine HTN: consider fludrocortisone or midodrine prn. Combination therapy if necessary.
- Sodium glucose transporter-2 (SGLT-2):
  - Expressed in S1 and S2 segments of proximal renal tubule where 90% of glucose reabsorption occurs.
  - Inhibition of SGLT-2 leads to glucosuria, hence glucose control in diabetics, and weight loss due to glucose-derived calories.
  - Inhibition of SGLT-2 also leads to mild BP reduction, presumably via (osmotic) diuretic effect.
- Nondrug, nondiet treatments for HTN: most effective: dynamic, aerobic exercise.

Management of HTN in Stroke

- Ischemic stroke: SBP control < 130 mm Hg has been shown to reduce recurrent strokes (2.25% vs. 2.77% per patient-year) and ICH at the expense of increased risk of orthostasis with syncope: Secondary Prevention of Small Subcortical Strokes (SPS3) trial.

- Hemorrhagic stroke, ICH:
  - What is the optimal BP control goal in acute hemorrhagic stroke?
  - Intensive BP Reduction in Acute Cerebral Hemorrhage Trial (INTERACT 2):
    - 2,974 participants (2/3 were Chinese) with SBP 150 to 220 mm Hg at diagnosis of ICH were randomized to BP control to <140 mm Hg or <180 mm Hg within 1 hour of randomization, with maintenance for the ensuing 7 days or until time of discharge: Trend toward better outcomes noted in early intensive treatment group (attainment of SBP < 140 mm Hg within the first hour).
    - Ongoing study: North American Antihypertensive Treatment of Acute Cerebral Hemorrhage II (ATACH II) trial: study outcome in patients with acute ICH treated to a SBP < 140 mm Hg versus <180 mm Hg. Results expected in 2016.

Management of HTN in CKD and Diabetes Mellitus

- BP goals (KDIGO 2013):
  - Nondiabetic or diabetic with CKD with normal to mild albuminuria: goal BP ≤ 140/90 mm Hg
  - Nondiabetic or diabetic with CKD and moderate to severe albuminuria, or kidney transplant recipients: goal ≤ 130–140/80–90 mm Hg
  - Children with CKD: ≤90th percentile for age, sex, height or ≤50th percentile if any proteinuria.
  - Age > 80 years with CKD: individualize
- Use of ACEI/ARB:
  - Nondiabetics with HTN and albuminuria ≥ 30 mg/d
  - Diabetics and nondiabetics with albuminuria ≥ 300 mg/d
  - HTN and CKD (black patients included)

Access the eBook for self-assessment questions.

Tubular, Interstitial, and Cystic Disorders

Phuong-Chi T. Pham, Monica S. Deshmukh, and Cynthia C. Nast

RENAL TUBULAR DISORDERS AND FANCONI SYNDROME

Fanconi Syndrome

Proximal tubular dysfunction causing excessive renal wasting of low molecular weight (LMW) proteins, glucose, bicarbonate, phosphate, uric acid, carnitine, and others.

Clinical Manifestations of Fanconi Syndrome

- Polyuria, polydipsia, tendency for volume depletion
- LMW proteinuria (non-albumin proteinuria): LMW proteinuria reflects proximal tubular injury and reduced proximal tubular endocytosis and reabsorption of filtered proteins. LMW proteins that may be excreted with proximal tubular injury include amino acids, β2-microglobulin, cystatin C, α1-macroglobulin
- Glucosuria in the absence of hyperglycemia
- Proximal renal tubular acidosis (RTA) due to reduced bicarbonate reabsorption (ammoniagenesis appears to be normal)
- Hypophosphatemia (phosphaturia is typically only seen in early disease; once new steady state has been achieved, phosphate loss in urine matches intake)
- Hypokalemia (likely due to distal potassium loss due to high distal sodium delivery to the epithelial sodium channel (ENaC); high filtered load of K^+ associated with acidemia)
- Hypouricemia due to hyperuricosuria
- Carnitine deficiency: Carnitine is required for the transport of fatty acids from cytosol into mitochondria during the breakdown of lipids for the generation of metabolic energy. Carnitine deficiency has been implicated in poor fatty acid metabolism, reduced antioxidant activities, poor glucose control, and osteoporosis.
- Rickets, osteomalacia, growth failure: likely due to hypophosphatemia, decreased 1,25 vitamin D production in proximal tubule (due to reduced renal 1-α hydroxylase activity), and chronic metabolic acidosis

Conditions Associated with Fanconi Syndrome

- Inherited:
  - Cystinosis: Most common inherited condition associated with Fanconi syndrome; associated with defective tubular reabsorption of **C**ystine, **O**rnithine, **L**ysine, and **A**sparagine, known as COLA. Unlike the other three amino acids,

cystine has low solubility, thus easily crystallizes in tubular lumen to form cystine stones.
  - Others: galactosemia, hereditary fructose intolerance, tyrosinemia type 1, glycogenosis, Wilson disease (inherited disorder involving copper metabolism), oculocerebrorenal syndrome (Lowe syndrome), mitochondrial cytopathies
- Acquired:
  - Heavy metals: lead, cadmium, mercury, platinum
  - Drugs: cisplatin, ifosfamide, imatinib (Gleevac), gentamicin, rifampin, expired tetracycline, tenofovir, didanosine, adefovir, azathioprine (AZA), valproic acid, suramin, streptozocin, ranitidine
  - Other exogenous agents: glue sniffing, diachrome, some herbal medicines
  - Dysproteinemias: multiple myeloma/light chain nephropathy (most common condition associated with Fanconi syndrome in adults), amyloidosis, Sjogren's
  - Others: acute tubular necrosis, nephrotic syndrome

Crystalluria

- Risk factors for drug crystallization: supersaturation of drug level in urine, volume depletion (low urine flow), urine pH, reduced levels of inhibitors of crystallization
- Most drug-crystalluria-induced acute kidney injury (AKI) resolves with drug withdrawal and supportive therapy.
- Drugs associated with crystal nephropathy (Fig. 6.1):
  - Sulfadiazine (used to treat toxoplasmosis):
    - Risks: high dose > 4 to 6 g/d, urine pH < 5.5, volume depletion
    - Crystals are strongly birefringent as "shocks of wheat" or "bow-tie" with an amber color and radial striation.
    - Treatment: volume repletion, urine alkalinization with sodium bicarbonate to pH > 7.15
  - Ciprofloxacin:
    - Risks: alkaline urine (pH > 7.0), elderly patients, volume depletion
    - Typically crystallizes in high urine pH > 7.3, but may occur in acidic pH
    - Crystals may take forms as needles, stars, fan shaped; all with lamellar structures and are strongly birefringent under polarized light.
    - Preventive measures: volume repletion, avoid concurrent use of alkalinizing agents, use with caution in patients > 65 to 70.
  - Acyclovir:
    - Risks: rapid intravenous bolus (500 mg/m^2) for herpes simplex virus–associated encephalitis, volume depletion
    - Crystals are birefringent and needle shaped
    - Preventive measures: use low dose, or slow infusion with normal saline support.
    - Acyclovir is dialyzable.
  - Indinavir (HIV protease inhibitor):
    - Crystallizes at physiologic pH 5.5 to 7.0; soluble at pH of ≤3.5
    - Crystals are pleomorphic and may range from plate-like rectangles, fan shaped, to start burst shaped.
    - Associated with tubular obstruction, chronic tubulointerstitial nephritis (CTIN)
    - Treatment: volume intake of at least 2 to 3 L/d is suggested while on indinavir; dose adjustment in liver disease; avoid concurrent use of

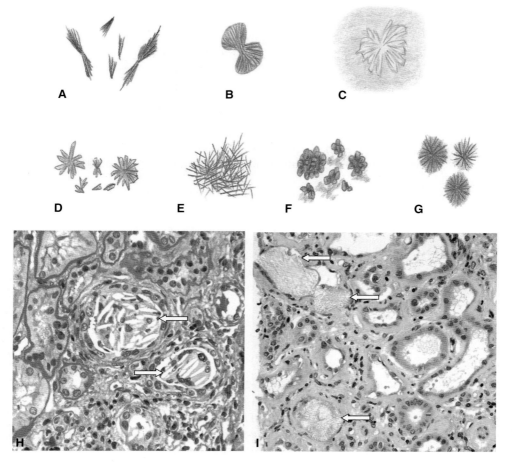

FIGURE 6.1 A–G. Drug-induced crystalluria. **(A)** Amoxicillin **(B)** Sulfonamide **(C)** Sulfadiazene **(D)** Indinavir **(E)** Acyclovir **(F)** Methotrexate **(G)** Ciprofloxacin. **H and I.** Tubular injury due to intraluminal crystals: **(H)** Indinavir crystals are within the lumina of tubules admixed with sloughed epithelium (Periodic acid–Schiff, ×400). **I.** There are clear to yellow crystalline aggregates of oxalate within tubular lumina (*arrows*) with tubular cell flattening, simplification and attenuation, and relative dilatation of tubular lumina (Hematoxylin and eosin, ×250).

trimethoprim–sulfamethoxazole as it can increase indinavir blood levels. Urine acidification difficult to achieve and not recommended.
- Methotrexate:
  - Risks: low urine pH, low volume
  - May cause both tubular obstruction and direct tubular toxicity
  - Treatment: urine alkalinization to pH > 6.0, volume repletion, leucovorin rescue
- Triamterene:
  - Risks: urine pH < 5.5
  - Crystals are spherical shaped, brown in color, appear as maltese crosses under polarized light.
  - Preventive: use low dose, adequate volume intake, avoid concurrent nonsteroidal anti-inflammatory drugs (NSAIDS) use.
  - Treatment: volume repletion, urinary alkalinization

- Orlistat (inhibitor of gastric and pancreatic lipase, induces fat malabsorption):
  - Associated with calcium oxalate deposition within renal tubules and interstitium. Mechanism for calcium oxalate stone formation is thought to be similar to that seen in patients with inflammatory bowel disease.
  - Risks: underlying kidney disease, volume depletion
  - Preventive: avoid use in patients with underlying kidney disease, volume repletion
- Ampicillin (needle shaped)
- Oral sodium phosphate solution used as bowel preparation for colonoscopy:
  - Calcium phosphate precipitations in renal tubular cells as well as tubular lumen
  - Risks: underlying kidney disease, females, and possibly hypertension (HTN) with concurrent use of angiotensin-converting enzyme inhibitor (ACEI) or angiotensin-receptor blocker (ARB)
  - Preventive measures: volume repletion, appropriate dosing, avoid concurrent use with ACEI, ARB, diuretics, and/or NSAIDS; Exercise caution with use in older patients.
- Vitamin C (converts to oxalate, calcium oxalate stones)
- Other drug crystalluria: foscarnet, pseudoephedrine
- Natural sources: star fruit (oxalate), rhubarb leaves (oxalate), cranberry juice (oxalate), ma huang (ephedra), djenkol beans (needle like)

TUBULOINTERSTITIAL NEPHRITIS

Acute Tubulointerstitial Nephritis

Epidemiology of Acute Tubulointerstitial Nephritis

- Prevalence of acute tubulointerstitial nephritis (ATIN) is increasing in recent years.
- Overall prevalence of biopsy-proven ATIN is 2% to 5%.
- Prevalence of biopsy-proven ATIN in patients with acute kidney injury (AKI) is 10% to 15%.

Pathogenesis of ATIN

There are three suggested mechanisms.
- The inciting agent (i.e., infection or drug) acts as a hapten. That is, the inciting agent binds to an otherwise nonimmunogenic native kidney protein and renders it immunogenic.
- Antibodies made against the inciting agent cross-reacts with native kidney antigens.
- Circulating immune complexes formed against the inciting agent deposit into the kidney interstitium and induce an inflammatory immunologic response.

Immunologic response:
- Predominantly cell mediated: kidney biopsy typically reveals predominant T-cell infiltrates in interstitium.
- Less commonly antibody mediated:
  - Most biopsies do not reveal immune complex deposits.
  - In some cases, immune complex deposits may be seen in tubular basement membranes (TBM).

Clinical Manifestations of ATIN

- Classic triad of skin rash, leukocyturia, and fevers:
  - Not common; likely seen in <10% of cases

- Classic triad is uncommonly seen in NSAIDS-induced ATIN.
- More commonly seen with antibiotic-induced ATIN
- AKI:
  - Onset of kidney injury typically occurs within 10 to 20 days of exposure to inciting agent.
  - Kidney injury may occur within 2 to 3 days with re-exposure.
  - De novo kidney injury from a medication previously tolerated may be observed.
- Abnormal urinalysis: leukocytouria, microscopic or gross hematuria, eosinophiluria, white blood cell casts, granular casts, proteinuria. Red blood cell casts reported but *rare*.
  - Eosinophiluria:
    - Poor sensitivity (40% to 91%) and specificity (52% to 95%), but improved specificity if eosinophils is >5% of total leukocyturia.
    - Eosinophiluria may also be seen in urinary tract infections, prostatitis, bladder malignancy, and rapidly progressive glomerulonephritis.
    - Hansel stain for eosinophilia is preferred over Wright stain due to Hansel stain's consistent sensitivity with varying urine pH.
  - Proteinuria:
    - Typically nonnephrotic range (i.e., <1 g/d, or urine protein to creatinine ratio < 1 g/g)
    - LMW proteinuria predominance a.k.a. "tubular proteinuria": albuminuria generally comprises less than 25% of total proteinuria.
    - May be nephrotic if associated with NSAIDS use
- Blood tests: elevated serum creatinine (SCr), leukocytosis with increased eosinophilia, anemia, elevated erythrocyte sedimentation rate, transaminitis. Anti-neutrophil cytoplasmic antibody (ANCA) may be positive without associated glomerular disease.

Histopathology of ATIN

- Light microscopy (LM):
  - Inflammatory infiltrates within the interstitium: Infiltrative lesions can be diffuse, but often are patchy, predominating in the deep cortex and outer medulla. Inflammatory cells are mostly T-cells and monocytes, macrophages, and also plasma cells, eosinophils, and a few neutrophilic granulocytes (Fig. 6.2).
  - Tubulitis may be seen in ATIN. Tubulitis refers to leukocytes and lymphocytes infiltration into tubular epithelium.
  - Granulomas may be seen in ATIN or CTIN associated with sarcoidosis, Sjogren syndrome, granulomatous polyangiitits, infections (e.g., tuberculosis, leprosy, histoplasmosis, xanthogranulomatous pyelonephritis), crystals/foreign bodies (e.g., urate, oxalosis, recreational drug impurities), medications (e.g., sulfas, synthetic penicillins, NSAIDS, thiazides, levofloxacin).
- Immunofluorescent microscopy (IF) and electron microscopy (EM):
  - IF and EM are typically negative because most ATIN have no immune complex deposits.
  - In some instances, antibodies may be formed linearly against antigens or drugs bound to tubular basement membrane (TBM) (e.g., methicillin, NSAIDS, phenytoin, allopurinol).
  - Kidney biopsies from patients with AKI from hantavirus infection may reveal granular immune deposits along the TBM and within glomeruli in 50% of cases.

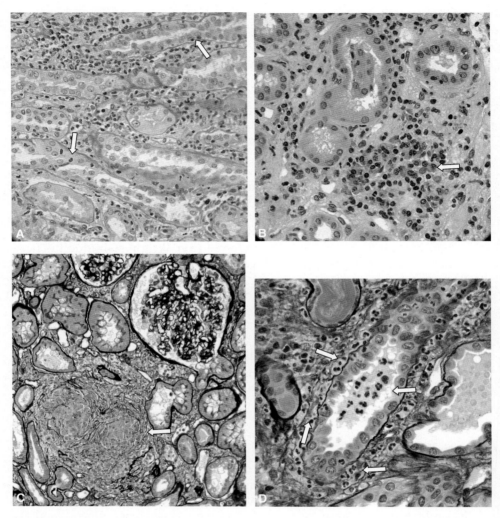

FIGURE 6.2 Acute tubulointerstitial nephritis. **A.** Lymphocytes are in the edematous interstitium and walls of tubules (*arrows*) with acute tubular cell injury (Periodic acid–Schiff, ×250). **B.** Interstitial edema and inflammation with prominent plasma cells (*arrow*) admixed with lymphocytes and plasma cells (Hematoxylin and eosin, ×350). **C.** Granulomatous interstitial nephritis. There is a nonnecrotizing granuloma (*arrow*) in the interstitium composed of epitheliod histiocytes and multinucleated giant cells (Periodic acid methenamine silver, ×200). **D.** Neutrophils are in the interstitium (*arrows*), and tubular walls and lumen in infection (pyelonephritis) (Periodic acid methenamine silver, ×425).

Diagnosis of ATIN

- Gold standard: kidney biopsy
- Urinalysis with abnormalities mentioned earlier
- Gallium scan:
  - Gallium binds to lactoferrin on white blood cells and originally thought to identify conditions with high white blood cell count such as ATIN.
  - Poor sensitivity and specificity and *not* recommended for the diagnosis of ATIN
  - May also be positive in association with glomerular diseases, presumably with concurrent interstitial disease, pyelonephritis, atheroembolic disease, etc.

Causes of ATIN

Eighty-five to ninety-five percent of ATIN are either drug- (adults in the United States) or infection induced (children, developing countries).

- Drug induced:
  - Common drugs associated with ATIN: antibiotics (particularly β-lactams, sulfas), NSAIDS including cyclooxygenase-2 (COX-2) inhibitors, proton pump inhibitors, diuretics, etc.
  - Specific drug-induced ATIN:
    - NSAIDS (and COX-2 inhibitors): These agents may induce kidney injury via various mechanisms:
      - Acute tubular necrosis due to acute afferent arteriolar vasoconstriction and resultant reduction in intraglomerular filtration pressure
      - Interstitial nephritis which may present as acute, chronic, or granulomatous interstitial nephritis
      - Papillary necrosis in patients with underlying ischemic renal disease (e.g., patients with diabetes mellitus and associated arteriosclerosis, sickle cell disease)
      - Three-fourth of NSAIDS-induced ATIN is associated with nephrotic syndrome and glomerular lesions including minimal change disease, membranous glomerulonephropathy, and less commonly, focal segmental glomerulosclerosis (FSGS), membranoproliferative glomerulonephropathy. Risks include older age, chronic use, and use of fenoprofen.
    - Rifampin: Renal injury pattern may reflect pattern of use:
      - Intermittent or interrupted use:
        - Acute tubular necrosis with or without associated interstitial infiltrations, intravascular hemolysis, or thrombocytopenia
        - Patient may present with flu-like symptoms within hours of drug ingestion.
      - Continuous use: interstitial nephritis, light chain proteinuria, or even rapidly progressive glomerulonephritis
    - Allopurinol:
      - Thought to be due to immunologic reactions between the metabolite oxypurinol with purines, ribonucleoproteins, and nucleic acids. Accumulation of oxypurinol increases with reduced kidney function. Dose reduction in chronic kidney disease (CKD) is recommended.
      - Clinical manifestations:
        - Male-to-female ratio estimated to be 2:1
        - Besides ATIN ± granulomas, patients may also develop toxic epidermal necrolysis, exfoliative dermatitis, or diffuse maculopapular rash, hepatic necrosis, and cholangitis.
    - Cimetidine: Histamine stimulates a subset of suppressor T-cells via H_2 receptors. Blockage of H_2 receptors may lead to increased cell-mediated responses.
    - 5-aminosalicylates (sulfasalazine, mesalamine, olsalazine): ATIN typically occurs within the first year of use.
    - Aristolochic acid nephropathy, a.k.a. Chinese herb nephropathy:
      - First reported in Belgium, presumed etiology of Balkan nephropathy
      - Aristolochic acid was mixed in slimming regimens.
      - Affected patients may develop rapidly progressive interstitial nephritis which can progress to end-stage renal disease (ESRD).
      - Associated with uroepithelial malignancy
    - Oxalate nephropathy presenting as ATIN: ascorbic acid (vitamin C), star fruit, orlistat (induces malabsorptive state that promotes gastrointestinal [GI] oxalate absorption), rhubarb leaves

- Drug reaction with eosinophilia and systemic symptoms (DRESS):
  - Clinical manifestations: fevers, facial edema, skin lesions (diffuse macular/papular erythematous lesions with lymphocytic infiltrates, exfoliative dermatitis), lymphadenopathy, multiorgan inflammatory response (e.g., pneumonitis, hepatitis).
  - Laboratory findings: eosinophilia, lymphocytosis, elevated aminotransferase (ALT)
  - Reported responsible agents: phenytoin, phenobarbital, allopurinol, sulfonamides, dapsone, vancomycin, minocycline, raltegravir, vemurafenib, lenalinomide (used for multiple myeloma), β-lactams
  - Treatment: drug withdrawal, supportive care, steroids
- Other recently reported drug-induced ATIN: liraglutide, varenicline, rosuvastatin, ipilimumab (monoclonal antibody that activates the immune system via inhibition of CTLA-4, used in treatment of melanoma), kudzu root (Japanese arrowroot) juice ingestion, linezolid, clindamycin
- Infection-related:
  - May involve various bacteria, viruses, parasites, atypical microorganisms, fungi
  - Granulomatous ATIN may be seen, particularly with fungal, mycobacteria, and parasites.
  - AKI during treatment of infections may result from infection-related ATIN, and not necessarily antibiotic/treatment-related ATIN.
- Glomerular disease-associated tubulointerstitial nephritis (TIN): nonselective proteinuria of proinflammatory proteins and growth factors may induce peritubular inflammatory response, complement activation, and progressive interstitial fibrosis.
- Immune mediated: autoimmune/collagen vascular diseases (e.g., systemic lupus erythematosus (SLE), Sjogren's, essential cryoglobulinemia, primary biliary cirrhosis, tubulointerstitial nephritis and uveitis (TINU)), sarcoidosis
  Tubulointerstitial nephritis and uveitis:
  - Inflammatory disease involving dysregulated T-cells that affect both eyes and kidneys
  - Mechanism of disease not known
  - Commonly seen in young women
  - Clinical manifestations: painful red eyes (uveitis), ATIN, possibly transaminitis
  - Treatment: prednisone 1 mg/kg/d × 3 to 6 months with slow taper. Addition of cytotoxic agent may be necessary (e.g., mycophenolate, calcineurin inhibitor)
- Other causes of ATIN: antineoplastic agents, heavy metals, herbal products, idiopathic

Prognosis of ATIN

- Recovery depends on duration of drug exposure, duration of AKI, and severity of interstitial fibrosis and tubular atrophy.
- Recovery may take several weeks. 50% recover fully, while the other 50% will have elevated serum creatinine.

Management of ATIN

- Supportive, dialysis as needed
- Removal of offending agent

- Role of glucocorticoids:
  - May lead to prompt recovery *if given early*, but not necessarily overall outcome
  - Due to the questionable benefit of glucocorticoids, risks must be minimal.
  - Consider systemic glucocorticoids if severe systemic involvement (e.g., DRESS)

Asymptomatic Bacteriuria: Infectious Diseases Society of America Guidelines 2005

- Asymptomatic bacteriuria is defined differently for different population and manner of urine collection:
  - For asymptomatic women, two consecutive voided urine specimens with isolation of the same bacterial strain in quantitative counts $\geq 10^5$ cfu/mL defines bacteriuria.
  - For asymptomatic men, a single clean-catch voided urine specimen with one bacterial species isolated in a quantitative count $\geq 10^5$ cfu/mL defines bacteriuria.
  - For both asymptomatic women and men, a single catheterized urine specimen with one bacterial species isolated in a quantitative count $\geq 10^2$ cfu/mL defines bacteriuria.
- Pyuria accompanying asymptomatic bacteriuria is not an indication for antimicrobial therapy.
- Screening for and treatment of asymptomatic bacteriuria are *recommended* for the following:
  - Pregnant women should be screened for bacteriuria by urine culture at least once in early pregnancy and be treated if positive results.
    - The duration of antimicrobial therapy should be 3 to 7 days.
    - Periodic screening for recurrent bacteriuria should be done following therapy.
    - No recommendation can be made for or against repeated screening of culture-negative women in later pregnancy.
  - Before transurethral resection of the prostate: Antimicrobial therapy should *not* be continued after the procedure, unless a postprocedural indwelling catheter is needed.
  - Before other urologic procedures with anticipated mucosal bleeding
- Screening for or treatment of asymptomatic bacteriuria is *not* recommended for premenopausal, nonpregnant women, diabetic women, older persons living in the community, elderly institutionalized subjects, persons with spinal cord injury, catheterized patients with indwelling catheters.
- Antimicrobial treatment should be considered for asymptomatic women with catheter-acquired bacteriuria that persists 48 hours after indwelling catheter removal.
- Urinalysis: Positive leukocyte esterase indicates presence of white blood cells; Positive nitrite suggests presence of bacteria that can convert dietary nitrates to nitrite (E. coli, proteus spp., Klebsiella pneumoniae); Nitrite may be absent in presence of bacteria that cannot convert nitrates to nitrite (enterococci, staphylococci, adenovirus)

CHRONIC TUBULOINTERSTITIAL NEPHRITIS

Background

CTIN is characterized by tubulointerstitial scarring and fibrosis, tubular atrophy, with or without significant macrophage and lymphocytic infiltration.

Clinical Manifestations of CTIN

Patients are typically asymptomatic with incidental abnormal laboratory findings:
- Mild proteinuria < 1.5 to 2.0 g/d
- Proteinuria is predominantly LMW proteins.
- "Bland" urinalysis: no (or rare granular) casts, minimal white and/or red blood cells
- Anemia severity out of proportion to degree of kidney injury due to damage of peritubular erythropoietin producing cells
- Other signs of tubular injury may be present: sodium wasting, metabolic acidosis, Fanconi syndrome, nephrogenic insipidus.

Histopathology of CTIN

- Fibrotic hypocellular interstitium (Fig. 6.3)
- Tubular atrophy

Causes of CTIN

- Common causes (drugs, crystals [e.g., calcium phosphate, uric acid, oxalate], infections, autoimmune, obstruction, chronic ischemia, heavy metals)
- Drug-induced CTIN:
  - Analgesic nephropathy:
    - Traditionally referred to the chronic use of the drug mixture containing (phenacetin, paracetamol, or acetaminophen) plus (salicylate) plus a potentially addicting agent (caffeine or codeine). Any of the drugs belonging to the first group can be metabolized to acetaminophen and subsequent toxic metabolites which require glutathione for detoxification. Accumulation of these toxic metabolites may form covalent bonds with kidney tissue and induce tissue injury and vascular endothelial damage. Salicylate is a

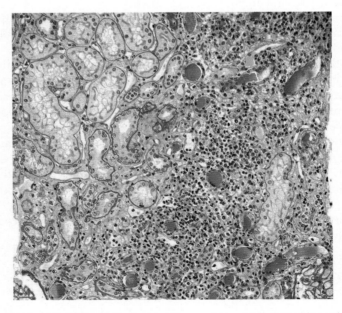

FIGURE 6.3 Chronic tubulointerstitial nephritis. The interstitium contains a lymphocytic infiltrate which is restricted to the area of interstitial fibrosis and tubular atrophy. Note the adjacent preserved tubulointerstitium in the upper left corner, in which there is no inflammation (Periodic acid–Schiff, ×250).

glutathione depletor which can limit the neutralization process of toxic metabolites of acetaminophen.
- Analgesic nephropathy affects predominantly the medulla and papillary tip. Characteristic presentations include CKD, CT revealing papillary necrosis and calcifications, or kidney ultrasound revealing small echogenic kidneys (Fig. 6.4).
- Single analgesic use may also lead to analgesic nephropathy.
  - Acetaminophen:
    - There are data to suggest that chronic, daily, high dose use of acetaminophen may lead to long-term nephrotoxicity in women.
    - Physicians' Health Study (11,000 healthy men): No increased relative risk of CKD with exposure $\geq$ 2,500 pills over a period of 11 years.
    - Nurses' Health Study (1,700 healthy women): >3,000 g of acetaminophen gave an odds ratio of 2.04 for a decrease in glomerular filtration rate (GFR) of >30 mL/min/1.73 m^2 compared to <1,000 g use.
  - Salicylates: Most studies suggest that the long-term use of daily therapeutic dose of aspirin (ASA) alone (i.e., without concurrent use of acetaminophen) do not lead to kidney injury.
  - NSAIDS:
    - High dose of NSAIDS may induce CKD in those with underlying or high risk for kidney injury, but not in healthy individuals.
    - Physicians' Health Study (healthy men): No increased risk of CKD with ingestion of $\geq$2,500 pills.
    - Nurses' Health Study (healthy women): No association with decline in GFR over lifetime use
- Lithium-induced kidney injury:
  - Chronic interstitial nephritis: characterized by cortical and medullary distal and collecting tubular dilatations/cysts, tubular atrophy, and interstitial fibrosis

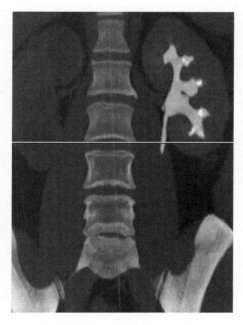

FIGURE 6.4 Papillary necrosis. Coronal postcontrast excretory phase maximum intensity projection (MIP) images showing classic appearance of papillary necrosis.

- Toxic intracellular lithium levels are thought to alter primary cilia function and lead to tubular cyst formation.
- Commonly associated glomerular lesions: global sclerosis, FSGS, minimal change disease
- Lithium may also be associated with nephrogenic diabetes insipidus, distal RTA, hypercalcemia, and hypothyroidism.
- Histopathology (Fig. 6.5): Severe lithium-associated tubulointerstitial nephropathy with diffuse interstitial fibrosis, tubular cysts, dilations, and tubular atrophy (flattened tubular epithelial cells) and relative sparing of glomeruli. Tubular cysts may be evident on CT imaging.
- Management:
  - Discontinue lithium if safe and possible (there are reports of patients committing suicide with lithium discontinuation).
  - Routine CKD management to slow down progression of disease
  - Amiloride may be considered to reduce lithium reabsorption at collecting tubules.
  - Thiazides may be considered in the treatment of nephrogenic diabetes insipidus.
- Famotidine: case report of famotidine-induced autoantibody formation against carbonic anhydrase II in the kidneys
- Infection-related CTIN:
  - Malakoplakia:
    - Rare granulomatous disease of infectious etiology (bacterial, fungal, tuberculosis, etc.)
    - Presents as friable yellow plaques that may involve urinary tract, GI tract, other visceral organs, skin (erythematous nodular lesions, ulcerations, to draining fistulas/abscesses).

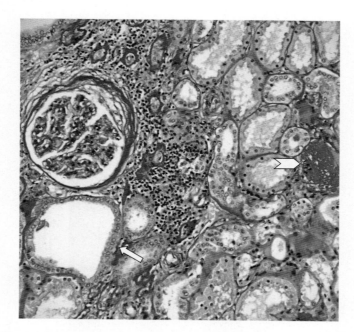

FIGURE 6.5 Lithium-induced chronic tubulointerstitial nephritis. There are focal tubular atrophy and interstitial fibrosis with associated lymphocytic inflammation. A distal tubule shows microcystic dilatation (*arrow*), and there is a globally sclerotic glomerulus (*arrowhead*) (Periodic acid–Schiff, ×200).

- Seen in immunocompromised hosts (e.g., diabetes mellitus, malignancy, malnutrition, alcoholism, immunosuppressive therapy)
- Pathogenesis: thought to be due to poor T-cell function, inadequate killing of bacteria by macrophages, or defective phagolysosomal activity by monocytes. Inadequate levels of intracellular cyclic guanosine monophosphate (cGMP) have been attributed to reduced microtubular function and lysosomal activity, hence ineffective bacterial killing. Accumulation of partially digested bacteria in monocytes or macrophages leads to calcium and iron deposition on residual bacterial glycolipids. The presence of the resulting basophilic inclusion structure, the Michaelis–Gutmann (MG) body, is considered pathognomonic for malakoplakia.
- Diagnosis: urine culture and biopsy
  - Imaging studies may reveal mass-like lesions, mimicking renal cell carcinoma (RCC).
  - Histopathology (Fig. 6.6): Haematoxylin and eosin staining reveals sheets of histiocytes with basophilic inclusions with concentric laminations (MG bodies). These MG bodies may be stained for calcium and iron. EM: MG bodies consist of lysosomes filled with partially digested bacteria. Identification of responsible organism may be possible with bacterial gram staining or immune staining with antibody against *Mycobacterium bovis*.
- Management: surgical, antibiotics (e.g., quinolones, trimethoprim-sulfomethoxazole), bethanecol (choline agonist), ascorbic acid. The latter two agents are thought to increase levels of cGMP.
- Xanthogranulomatous pyelonephritis (Fig. 6.7):
  - Condition associated with chronic obstruction (e.g., staghorn calculi) and urinary tract infections with resulting granulomatous inflammation and diffuse cellular infiltrate of lipid-laden foam cells replacing normal renal parenchyma. CT may reveal low-density masses with associated calcifications resembling malignancy.
  - Clinical manifestations: commonly affect middle-aged women who may present with fevers/chills, chronic flank pain, possibly palpable mass. Urine

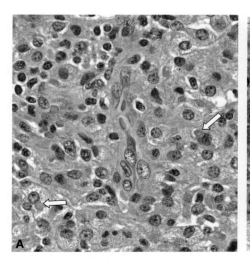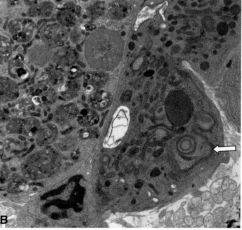

FIGURE 6.6 Malakoplakia. **A.** Interstitial macrophages with abundant granular cytoplasm containing rounded calcifications (Michaelis–Gutmann bodies, *arrows*) (Hematoxylin and eosin, ×600). **B.** Electron micrograph of a macrophage showing forming calcospherule (Michaelis–Gutmann body, *arrow*) (×12,000).

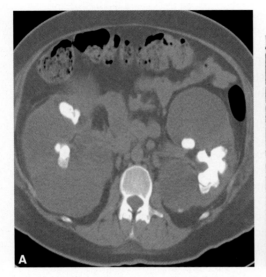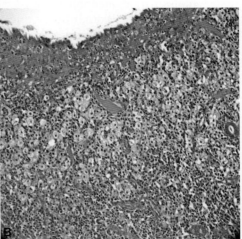

FIGURE 6.7 Xanthogranulomatous pyelonephritis. **A.** Axial and coronal noncontrast CT images showing enlarged kidneys containing staghorn calculi with resulting contraction of the renal pelvices and associated ballooning of the renal calyces and inflammation of the perinephric fat. The appearance of xanthogranulomatous pyelonephritis on CT has been compared to a "bear claw" with the ballooned renal calyces representing the paws. **B.** The renal pelvis and medulla are diffusely infiltrated with foamy (xanthomatous) cells, which are lipid-laden macrophages, and lymphocytes obliterating the normal renal parenchyma (Hematoxylin and eosin, ×200).

cultures may reveal common gram-negative organisms such as *Escherichia coli*, *Klebsiella*, *Proteus* and less commonly staphylococcal species.
- Management: organism specific antibiotics, surgical resection as needed
- Emphysematous pyelonephritis (Fig. 6.8):
  - Life-threatening necrotizing acute pyelonephritis ± obstruction, predominantly seen in diabetic patients that is caused by gas-forming organisms such as *E. coli*, *Klebsiella pneumonia*, *Pseudomonas aeruginosa*, and *Proteus mirabilis*.
  - Gas pockets may be detected on plain abdominal radiograph, ultrasound, or CT.
  - Management: organism-specific antibiotics, relief of obstruction and surgical resection as needed
- HIV immune restoration inflammatory syndrome (IRIS):
  - Seen in patients with prolonged severe immunodeficiency, recently treated for an opportunistic infection, now receiving never-before-seen or intensified antiretroviral therapy with resultant marked viral load reduction, increase in CD4, and multiorgan inflammatory response
  - Kidney involvement may manifest as interstitial nephritis with granulomas.
  - Treatment: prednisone 1 mg/kg/d × 1 month followed by taper
- Heavy metal–associated CTIN:
  - Lead (Pb):
    - Pathogenesis: thought to be due to chronic lead deposition and its associated toxicity in proximal tubules, hyperuricemia, and HTN
    - Clinical manifestations:
      - Chronic: anemia with basophilic stippling, gout, CKD, peripheral motor neuropathies, perivascular cerebellar calcifications, small shrunken kidneys
      - Acute lead intoxication: encephalopathy, abdominal pain, hemolytic anemia, Fanconi syndrome, and peripheral neuropathy

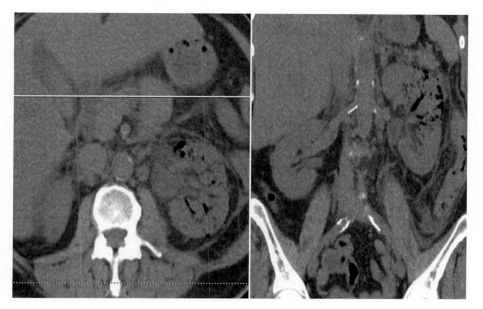

FIGURE 6.8 Emphysematous pyelonephritis. Axial and coronal noncontrast CT images showing crescentic collection of gas within Gerota fascia (indicative of infection within the perinephric spaces) consistent with emphesematous pyelonephritis.

- ■ Management:
  - • Routine CKD management
  - • Consider Pb chelation therapy.
- • Mercury:
  - • Found in alloy and mirror plants, batteries
  - • Mercury dichloride ($HgCl_2$) may also induce acute tubular necrosis in addition to CTIN.
- • Cadmium:
  - • Found in glass/metal alloy plants, electrical equipments
  - • Outbreak of cadium toxicity in Japan due to industrial contamination lead to itai-itai, a.k.a. "ouch ouch" disease because of significant bone pain associated with condition. Kidney involvement includes hypercalciuria, kidney stones, proximal tubular dysfunction, anemia, CTIN.
- • Arsenic:
  - • Found in poison gas, insecticides, weed killers, paints
  - • Proximal RTA and CTIN
- • Other conditions associated with CTIN:
  - • IgG4-related disease:
    - • A condition characterized by dense lymphoplasmacytic infiltrate rich in IgG4-positive plasma cells, storiform fibrosis, with or without associated elevated serum IgG4 concentrations
    - • Mass lesions in various organs including pancreas, enlarged salivary glands, kidneys (TIN), lungs, lymph nodes, meninges, aorta, breast, prostate, thyroid, pericardium, skin, and even bone (destructive lesions resembling granulomatous polyangiitis).

- Patient characteristics:
  - Male predominance (estimated 62% to 83% are males)
  - Older age (i.e., >50 years)
  - Up to 40% with history of allergic diseases (e.g., bronchial asthma or chronic sinusitis)
- Clinical diagnosis:
  - Elevated serum IgG4 (although 30% have normal values)
  - Affected tissue biopsy is characterized by (Fig. 6.9):
    - Dense lymphoplasmacytic infiltrates consisting of lymphocytes, plasma cells, eosinophils, and fibroblasts
    - Ratio of IgG4-bearing plasma cells to IgG-bearing plasma cells > 50% is highly suggestive of IgG4-related disease.
    - Obliterative phlebitis
    - Storiform fibrosis (likened to cartwheel pattern)
- Pathogenesis is thought to involve:
  - Autoimmune process or presence of an infectious agent that trigger an immune response driven predominantly by type 2 helper T (Th2) cells and activation of regulatory T (Treg) cells. The influx of inflammatory cells leads to multiorgan enlargement, cytokine release, eosinophilia, elevated IgG4 and IgE levels, and eventual progression to fibrosis of affected organs.
- Treatment of IgG4-related disease:
  - Glucocorticoids: suggested regimen: prednisolone 0.6 g/kg body weight/d for 2 to 4 weeks, tapered over 3 to 6 months to 5 mg/d and maintain for up to 3 years.

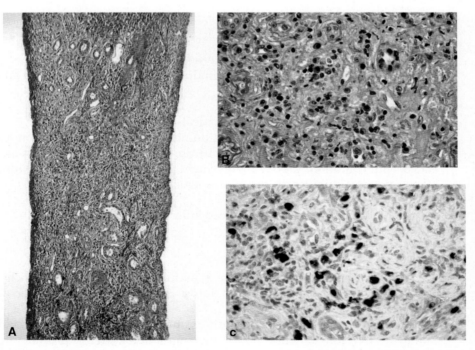

FIGURE 6.9 IgG4-related disease. **A.** There is widespread interstitial fibrosis with varying degrees of tubular atrophy and a heavy inflammatory infiltrate (Masson trichrome, ×100). **B.** There are small aggregates of lymphocytes and plasma cells with surrounding collagen (Hematoxylin and eosin, ×400). **C.** IgG4 immunohistochemical stain showing positive staining in >50% of the plasma cells (×400).

- Others: Azathioprine (AZA), mycophenolate mofetil (MMF), and metho-trexate have been suggested as glucocorticoid-sparing agents.
        - For recurrent or refractory disease, consider rituximab.
    - Relapse may occur.
  - Balkan nephropathy-like CTIN:
    - Arises from chronic exposure to aristolochic acid (environmental or contaminant from herbal preparation)
    - Associated with uroepithelial malignancies
  - Mesoamerican nephropathy:
    - Described in Central America
    - Affects predominantly males, often sugar cane field workers
    - Underlying etiology thought to be due to repeated exposures to severe dehydration and rehydration, hyperosmolality-stimulated aldose reductase activity leading to conversion of glucose to sorbitol and fructose with subsequent metabolism by fructokinase to oxidant mediators. Exacerbating or contributing factors may include concurrent high intake of fructose and/or NSAIDS, contaminated drinking water (e.g., arsenic, pesticides), leptospirosis, and/or genetic susceptibility.
    - Typical manifestations: mild proteinuria, hyperuricemia, hypokalemia
    - Kidney biopsy is characterized by extensive glomerulosclerosis, tubular atrophy, and interstitial fibrosis. Of note, glomerulosclerosis is a prominent feature of this condition which is thought to reflect glomerular ischemic injury.
    - Kidney biopsy is characterized by extensive glomerulosclerosis, tubular atrophy, and interstitial fibrosis.
  - Inflammatory bowel disease is associated with an increased risk of CTIN, independent of exposure to 5-aminosalicylates. Although 5-aminosalicylates may be associated with ATIN.
  - Granulomatous (noncaseating) CTIN: common causes
    - Drugs: sulfas, synthetic penicillins, NSAIDS, thiazides, quinolones
    - Infections: tuberculosis, leprosy, xanthogranulomatous pyelonephritis, histoplasmosis, glandular fever
    - Systemic diseases: granulomatous polyangiitis, sarcoidosis
    - Others: urate, oxalosis
  - Karyomegalic interstitial nephritis:
    - Rare systemic disease noted for bizarre enlarged nuclei found in brain, lung, biliary/intestinal cells, and renal tubular epithelial cells.
    - Patients may present with slowly progressive CTIN and ESRD in late adulthood, transaminitis. Etiology and treatment remain to be defined.
- Diagnosis of CTIN: Kidney biopsy is gold standard.

RENAL CYSTIC DISEASES

Multicystic Kidney Disease

Background

Multicystic kidney disease (MCDK) is a congenital abnormality of the kidney and urinary tract (CAKUT) where irregular cysts replace normal renal parenchyma, leading to a nonfunctional kidney.

Epidemiology

- 0.1%; male-to-female ratio: 1.3 to 1.9:1

Pathogenesis

- Known mutations account for <20% of cases and predominantly include genes involved in glomerular development, ureteric branching, and metanephric mesenchyme
- May be seen with fetal alcohol syndrome

Clinical Manifestations of MCDK

- Age of onset: in utero, may present with oligohydramnios
- Thirty percent of patients have other CAKUT: vesicoureteral reflux in contralateral kidney, neurogenic bladder, duplicating collecting systems, ectopic kidney.
- Ultrasound: typically only involves one kidney. Spontaneous involution with cystic collapse may occur. Higher rate of involution by 10 years is seen with kidney size < 5 cm and more commonly for right than left kidney. Adults may thus present with single functioning kidney, which may be confirmed with a dimercaptosuccinic acid scan (DMSA).
- MCDK is not associated with HTN or malignancy.
- Long-term follow-up for vesicoureteral reflux, albuminuria, and kidney injury is recommended.

Autosomal Dominant Tubulointerstitial Kidney Disease
Background

Autosomal-dominant tubulointerstitial kidney disease (ADTKD) is a form of nephronophthisis (chronic tubulointerstitial disease that progresses to ESRD) that is associated with various mutations (UMOD, MUC1, REN, HNF-1b).

Clinical Manifestations Common to Various ADTKD

- Small kidneys with or without corticomedullary cysts
- Renal insufficiency, bland urine; ESRD by third decade of life with UMOD and sixth decade of life with MUC1 mutations
- Hyperuricemia and gout may be seen in patients with UMOD and REN mutations.
- HTN is uncommon prior to ESRD.
- Genetic testing is indicated for living related kidney donors.

Pathogenesis of ADTKD

- ADTKD—UMOD (a.k.a. uromodulin kidney disease, familial juvenile hyperuricemic nephropathy, medullary cystic kidney disease type 2)
  - Mutation of UMOD which encodes for uromodulin = Tamm Horsfall proteins (THF). Mutated THF proteins are trapped in tubular epithelial cells which lead to tubular cell apoptosis, reactive interstitial fibrosis, and cyst formation.
  - Renal insufficiency, bland urine, ESRD: early third decade of life
  - Early-onset hyperuricemia and gout
- ADTKD—MUC1 (a.k.a. Mucin-1 kidney disease, medullary cystic kidney disease type 1)
  - Mutation of MUC1 which encodes for Mucin-1
  - Age to ESRD: sixth decade of life

- ADTKD—REN (a.k.a. familial juvenile hyperuricemic nephropathy type 2)
  - Mutation of REN which encodes for preprorenin. Mutated preprorenin results in defective translocation to endoplasmic reticulum (ER) and lysozymes for processing into renin. Cytoplasmic accumulation of preprorenin in renin producing cells leads to tubular dilation and fibrosis.
  - Associated with anemia, hyporenin, hypovolemia, early onset hyperuricemia, gout
- ADTKD—HNF-1b (a.k.a. maturity-onset diabetes mellitus of the young type 5, renal cyst and diabetes syndrome)
  - Mutation of HNF-1b which encodes for the hepatocyte nuclear factor-1b
  - Associated with diabetes mellitus

Autosomal Recessive Tubulointerstitial Disease

Background

Rare nephronophthisis with similar histopathology as the autosomal-dominant forms of tubulointerstitial disease. NPHP1-3 are the most common types of NPHP.

Epidemiology

- 1 in 5,000 live births

Pathogenesis

- Multiple single-gene mutations have been implicated in the pathogenesis of NPHP. Responsible genes are those encoding proteins localized to the cilium, basal body, and centrosome in tubular epithelial cells. Causal gene is not known in two-third of NPHP cases.
- Genetic testing is indicated for living related kidney donors.

Clinical Manifestations

- Age of onset: in utero
- Growth retardation
- ESRD by age 30s in general; ESRD by age 3 in NPHP2
- Ultrasound findings are similar to those seen in ADTKD: Kidneys are small to normal size, with increased echogenicity and loss of corticomedullary differentiation. Corticomedullary or medullary cysts may be present. Thin section CT may identify corticomedullary junction cysts.
- Histopathology: classic triad of tubular basement membrane irregularities, tubular atrophy with cyst formation, and interstitial fibrosis with cell infiltration
- Vasopressin-resistant urinary concentration defect with associated polyuria and polydipsia
- Histology with tubular atrophy, interstitial fibrosis, and corticomedullary microcystic dilation of renal tubules.
- Clinical manifestations other than kidney disease in NPHP 1, 2, and 3: retinitis pigmentosa, coloboma, strokes

Management

Blood pressure control if applicable, preferably with renin–angiotensin–aldosterone system (RAAS) inhibitors; consider salt, fluids, with or without fludrocortisone if hypotension/hypovolemia.

Autosomal-Dominant or Spontaneous Germ Line and Somatic Mutation: Tuberous Sclerosis Complex

Background

Autosomal-dominant (or sporadic) tumor-suppressor gene syndrome associated with benign hamartomas of brain, eyes, heart, lung, liver, kidney, skin: angiomyolipomas (AML), oncocytomas, lymphangiomatous cyts; others: renal cysts, glomerulocystic kidney disease (GCKD), RCC (often bilateral and multifocal), FSGS with interstitial fibrosis.

Epidemiology

- 1 in 6,000 live births
- Sporadic mutations occur in approximately 70% of cases.

Pathogenesis

- Mutations in tumor suppressor genes TSC1 or TSC2 encoding for hamartin and tuberin respectively. Both normally form a hamartin–tuberin complex which antagonizes an insulin-signaling pathway and downstream mammalian target of rapamycin (mTOR) that normally regulates cell size and growth rate.
- Compared with TSC1, TSC2-linked disease is typically more severe. TSC2 mutations are five times more common than TSC1 with sporadic mutations. Familial mutations involve TSC1 and TSC2 equally.
- Genetic analysis is positive in 75% to 90%. False-negative genetic testing may occur with de novo somatic mutations.

Clinical Manifestations

- Classic Vogt triad (< 30% of TSC): seizures, mental retardation, facial angiofibromas.
- Most common associated findings: renal AML (60% to 70%) and cysts (20% to 30%). AML may be more severe in women with increased rupture risk during pregnancy and length > 3 cm. Prophylactic surgery or vascular coiling/thrombosis may be considered if >4 cm (Fig. 6.10).
- Lymphangioleiomyomatosis AML may occur almost exclusively in women with or without spontaneous pneumothorax.
- Others: brain: mental retardation, seizures, autism; skin: angiofibromas, hypomelanotic macules; lungs: interstitial disease; RCC (often bilateral and multifocal)

Management

- Annual renal ultrasound screening is recommended.
- mTOR inhibitor everolimus for TSC-related renal AML
- Surgical decompression of large symptomatic cysts refractory to medical therapy
- Nephron-sparing surgical resection of renal carcinoma
- Bilateral nephrectomies are recommended at ESRD (dialysis or transplant).

TSC/PKD1 Contiguous Gene Syndrome

- Deletion mutation involving both *TSC2* and *PKD1* genes resulting in severe polycystic kidney disease
- Occurs in 2% to 3% of patients with TSC; age of onset: first year of life; ESRD by age 20s
- Ultrasound: large kidneys similar to autosomal-dominant polycystic kidney disease (ADPKD)

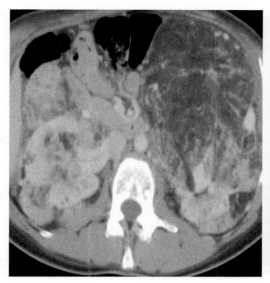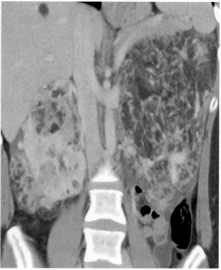

FIGURE 6.10 Renal angiomyolipoma. Axial and coronal postcontrast CT images show very large angiomyolipoma (AML) in both kidneys in a patient with known tuberous sclerosis complex. The left renal AML is very large and at risk for bleeding. Note a small AML in the liver.

Von Hippel–Lindau Disease

Background

Multiorgan predisposition to malignancy due to a germ-line mutation and a subsequent somatic mutation of the VHL gene.

Epidemiology

- 1 in 36,000 live births involving all ethnicities

Pathogenesis

- Autosomal-dominant mutation of VHL gene encoding two VHL proteins. VHL protein is part of the ubiquitin–ligase complex involved in ubiquitination and subsequent degradation of the α subunit of the hypoxia-inducible-factor HIF-1 and HIF-2. Accumulated HIF-α binds to HIF-β, translocate to nucleus, bind to the hypoxia response element to induce transcriptions of vascular endothelial growth factor, erythropoietin, tumor growth factor-β1, platelet-derived growth factor, among others.
- Autosomal mutation occurs in 80% of cases and sporadic in 20%.
- Diagnosis may be made with:
  - One tumor if positive family history, two tumors if no family history, or genetic analysis
  - Renal imaging: normal kidney size with cysts in >50% of cases. Cysts typically present in small number and small size. While not all renal tumors are preceeded by cysts, all renal cysts must be considered preneoplastic.

Clinical Manifestations of VHL Disease

- Onset of disease between 20 and 30s, >90% by age 65

- Retinal or CNS hemangioblastomas, clear cell renal carcinoma, pheochromocytomas (plasma norepinephrine), pancreatic islet tumors, endolymphatic sac tumors, renal and pancreatic cysts, epididymal or broad ligament cystadenomas.
- RCCs in VHL tend to be slower growing than those seen in sporadic cases.

Management

- Annual blood pressure measurements, urinary studies for pheochromocytomas, MRI or CT of kidneys and CNS
- Renal-sparing surgery is appropriate for RCC < 3 cm in size due to the life-long risk for the development of new lesions at different sites. Radioablative therapy is an option for multicentric lesions. Medical therapies with promising results include VEGF tyrosine kinase inhibitors (sunitinib) and mTOR inhibitor rapamycin.

Autosomal Recessive Polycystic Kidney Disease

Pathogenesis

- Mutations of the polycystic kidney and hepatic disease 1 gene (PKHD1) gene encoding fibrocystin/polyductin (FCP), a transmembrane protein found in mitotic spindle, microtubules, and apical primary cilia in biliary and renal tubular epithelia. FCP interacts with polycystin 2 and is thought to play a central role in microtubule formation and function and epithelial proliferation and secretion of renal tubules and biliary ducts.
- Mutations of FCP lead to abnormal dilation of collecting ducts and abnormal remodeling of the biliary system, resulting in renal cystic disease and progressive portal fibrosis respectively. This condition is also known as "congenital hepatic fibrosis."
- Genetic testing is available.

Epidemiology

- Occurs in 1 of 20,000 live births; carrier rate: 1 in 70

Clinical Manifestations

- Majority of patients present in utero or at birth.
- In utero presentation includes enlarged echogenic kidneys with poor kidney function, thus oligohydramnios. The latter may lead to abnormal fetal development with Potter phenotype consisting of pulmonary hypoplasia, characteristic facies, and spine and limb deformities.
- Perinatal mortality is estimated to be 25%.
- ESRD is reached in >60% by age 10.
- Findings of echogenic or cystic kidneys and congenital hepatic fibrosis in childhood is specific for autosomal-recessive polycystic kidney disease (ARPKD).
- Ultrasound: radially arrayed dilated collecting ducts spanning from cortex to medulla. ARPKD cysts are not discrete sacs as seen in ADPKD, TSC, and VHL disease; CT: striated nephrogram due to stasis of contrast media in dilated tubules
- Hepatobiliary complications: hepatosplenomegaly, portal HTN, ascending cholangitis, cholangiocarcinoma
- Patients may present with combined severe kidney and liver disease, or mild disease of one organ and severe disease of the other, mild disease of both organs, or isolated hepatic fibrosis and nonobstructive dilation of intrahepatic bile ducts (Caroli disease).

Management

- Blood pressure control with RAAS inhibitors
- Maintain high index of suspicion for ascending cholangitis.
- Kidney transplantation is preferred in ESRD. Combined kidney liver transplantation should be considered in case of extensive portal HTN. Parental organ donation is generally possible if normal imaging studies of kidneys and liver due to recessive nature of disease.

Autosomal-Dominant Polycystic Kidney Disease

Epidemiology

- Incidence estimated to be 1 in 500 to 1,000 live births.
- ADPKD affects 12.5 million people worldwide, both genders, and all ethnic groups equally.
- ADPKD accounts for up to 10% of patients with ESRD and fourth leading cause for renal replacement therapy worldwide.

Pathogenesis

- Implicating factors involved in cystogenesis and growth include reduction in intracellular calcium, increased intracellular cAMP, increased epithelial chloride fluid secretion via cystifc fibrosis transmembrane conductance regulator channels, and increased epithelial cellular proliferation.
- Renal cysts are thought to develop from a "two-hit" mechanism:
  - First "hit": full or partial loss of functional polycystin (or even overexpression of polycystin in rodents) AND
  - Second "hit": Somatic inactivation of normal allele
- PKD1 and PKD2 encode for polycystin (PC) 1 and 2, respectively. PC1 and PC2 form a polycystin complex on primary cilium on the apical surface of renal tubular and biliary epithelial cells. The PC complex functions as a mechanosensor that regulates flow-mediated calcium entry into cells, which in turn triggers calcium release from the ER into the cytoplasm (this is known as "calcium-induced calcium release"). PC2 is also present in the ER, where it interacts with inositol triphosphate and ryanodine receptors to signal calcium release into the cytoplasm from intracellular stores.
- Mutations of PC1, PC2 lead to altered intracellular calcium homeostasis. The reduced intracellular calcium level enhances accumulation of cAMP, an important mediator of cystic growth. cAMP accumulation occurs via increased adenylyl cyclase activity and possibly decreased phosphodiesterase I activity.
  - cAMP stimulates chloride-driven fluid secretion into cysts.
  - While cAMP inhibits cell proliferation under normal conditions, it stimulates cell proliferation in calcium deprived states. The proliferative effect of cAMP may be enhanced by epithelial growth factor (EGF)-like factors present in cyst fluid.
  - Note that ADH can increase cAMP levels via activation of adenylate cyclase.
- PC1 on the cell surface also interacts with tuberin. A disrupted tuberin–PC1 interaction is thought to cause a loss of downstream inhibition of the mTOR. Activation of mTOR leads to increased protein synthesis and cell proliferation.
- Family history may be absent in 10% to 15% of patients with ADPKD due to de novo mutations, mosaicism, mild disease from PKD2, nontruncating PKD1 mutations, or misdiagnosis.
- Despite large-sized kidneys, ADPKD cysts only involve <1% to 2% of all nephrons.

Epidemiology
- Relative frequencies of PKD1 and PKD2 are 65% to 70% and 25% to 30%, respectively.
- Disease may manifest in <1% of cases.

Clinical Manifestations
- PKD1 have more cysts and larger kidneys compared with PKD2. Cystic growth rates are similar between PKD1 and PKD2. The lower number of cysts, a.k.a. "lower cyst dose," in PKD2 is thought to result in later development of ESRD in PKD2 compared with PKD1.
- Clinical findings from the consortium for radiologic imaging studies of PCKD (**CRISP**):
  - The value of MRI in the study of PCKD:
    - Cyst volume increase may be detected within 6 months
    - Renal blood flow may be used as a marker of disease severity. The decline in kidney function and disease progression of ADPKD appears to be closely linked with the decline in renal blood flow.
  - PKD1 is a more severe disease compared to PKD2 because in PKD1 more cysts develop earlier, not grow faster.
  - Cystic growth and increase in total kidney volume (TKV) is a continuous and steady process that is patient specific. At 3-year follow-up, the mean annual growth rate was 5% to 6%.
  - PKD1 typically reaches ESRD by age 40s and PKD2 by age 60s.
- Ultrasound diagnostic criteria for PKD1, PKD2, and unknown genotype:
  - At-risk individuals age 15 to 39 years: three or more cysts unilateral or bilateral
  - 40 to 59 years: two or more cysts in each kidney
  - >60 years: more than four cysts in each kidney
  - NOTE: Diagnosis in children is controversial. In the United States, presymptomatic screening for at-risk children is currently not recommended.
- MRI-based criteria for disease exclusion in at-risk individuals and below age 40: "the finding of fewer than 5 renal cysts by MRI is sufficient for disease exclusion." - KDIGO 2015.
- However, for kidney donors at risk for PCKD (positive family history) and age < 40 years or have in utero presentation or unilateral disease, direct mutation analysis for PKD1 and PKD2 is warranted.
- Preimplantation genetic diagnosis is available for ADPKD.
- Risks for progression:
  - Patients with TKV > 600 mL per meter of patient height or kidney length > 17 cm likely progress to stage 3 CKD within 8 years.

$$\text{TKV/height} = \text{sum of [kidney length} \times \text{width} \times \text{depth (cm)} \times \pi/6]$$
$$\text{of both kidneys/height (m),}$$

  - Urine albumin excretion
  - HTN (particularly if onset prior to age 35)
  - Male gender
  - Low birth weight
  - Higher plasma copeptin level is associated with higher TKV and urinary albumin excretion and reduced GFR and effective renal blood flow.
  - Others: sickle cell trait, dyslipidemia

- Stones:
  - Cyst burden (high TKV) is associated with hematuria and nephrolithiasis.
  - Uric acid stones are most common and less commonly, calcium oxalate.
  - Increased stone risk is thought to be due to urinary stasis from cyst compression, reduced urinary citrate excretion, low urinary pH presumably due to defective ammonium excretion, hypercalciuria, and hyperuicosuria.
- HTN:
  - Occurs even prior to reduction in GFR in 60% of patients, thought to be due to RAAS activation from cyst expansion into renal parenchyma
  - Absence of nocturnal BP dipping (40% of patients)
- Left ventricular hypertrophy (even in normotensive patients, up to 25%)
- Pain (back, abdomen, head, chest, legs)
- Cyst infections:
  - Most common: *E. coli*; treat with fluoroquinolones or trimethoprim–sulfamethoxazole for better cystic penetration for 4 to 8 weeks, up to 3 months; vancomycin or erythromycin if streptococcal or staphylococcal infection, metronidazole or clindamycin if anaerobic organisms; drainage or surgical intervention may be necessary.
  - 18-fluorodexoyglucose-positron emission tomography may be considered to identify infected cyst.
- RCC: recent retrospective study revealed 5% malignant neoplasms with elective nephrectomy in patients with ADPKD. The incidence of clinically significant RCC in those with ESRD is not increased compared with that of other kidney diseases. Detection of RCC may be improved with MRI with and without gadolinium.
- Polycystic liver disease occurs in >85% of patients by age 25 to 34 and 94% by age 35 to 46 (CRISP study). Liver function is often preserved, but can be complicated with transaminitis, cyst infections, and hepatic venous outflow obstruction (Budd Chiari). Progressive disease may be seen with pregnancies, oral contraceptives, and hormonal replacement therapy.
- Cerebral aneurysms (most often in the anterior circulation of circle of Willis):
  - Asymptomatic cerebral aneurysms may be detected in 5% of patients without a family history and up to 20% in those with a family history.
  - High risk of rupture for aneurysms > 10 mm in diameter.
  - Mutations in the 5′-flanking region of the *PKD1* gene are more likely to have cerebral aneurysms compared to those at the 3′-end.
  - Screening indications: family history of aneurysm, previous known aneurysms, high-risk occupations (e.g., pilots), kidney transplantation, pregnancy, elective surgery. Screening recommendations apply to those with good life expectancy.
    - Small unruptured aneurysms require regular follow-up, 6 to 24 months.
    - Patients with family history and negative screening should be rescreened in 5 to 10 years.
    - Screening study of choice is time-of-flight MRI without gadolinium.
- Other associations: cardiac valve abnormalities (mitral valve prolapse, aortic. mitral, tricuspid regurgitation), pericardial effusions, asymptomatic bronchiectasis, inguinal/umbilical hernia (may be problematic with peritoneal dialysis), diverticulosis (increased risk of perforation in kidney transplant recipients)

Management

- Dietary:
  - Salt restriction 2 to 3 g/d (increased urinary sodium correlates with increased TKV over time)

- Minimize caffeine intake (caffeine is a methylxanthine that increases intracellular cAMP levels in cultured renal epithelial cells which could potentially accelerate cystic growth).
- Adequate free water intake to minimize ADH secretion (goal urine osmolality ~250 mOsm/kg with caution not to cause hyponatremia. Note, however, although this practice is commonly practiced, its benefit has not been proven)
- Control HTN:
  - RAAS inhibitors are first-line BP-lowering agents in combination with lifestyle modification and sodium-restricted diet. Selection of second-line agent is controversial and should be based on patients' comorbidities.
  - HALT-PKD (60-month follow up for TKV, 96-month for eGFR decline):
    - ACEI alone can adequately control HTN in most patients. The addition of ARB did not provide any additional benefits.
    - Lowering BP below goal (target 95-110/60-75 mm Hg) in young patients with good kidney function reduced the annual TKV growth rate (5.6% vs. 6.6%), renal vascular resistance, urine albumin excretion, and left ventricular mass. The rate of decline in eGFR, however, was not significantly different.
  - ACEI or ARB is associated with reducing left ventricular mass index and proteinuria.
  - Use of diuretics is associated with higher increase in TKV compared to RAAS inhibitors.
  - There are concerns that CCB may accelerate cystic growth.
- ESRD/Renal replacement therapy:
  - 5-year survival of ADPKD patients undergoing hemodialysis is superior to those with other kidney diseases.
  - Compared with arteriovenous grafts and fistulas, the use of catheters for HD in ADPKD is associated with an increased risk for renal and liver cyst infections.
  - Peritoneal dialysis is not contraindicated. However, there is a higher risk of abdominal wall hernia. Overall survival rate and peritonitis rates are similar to those seen in nondiabetic PD patients.
  - ADPKD patients have been reported to have higher hemoglobin levels and lower requirement for erythropoiesis stimulating agents.
  - Kidney transplantation:
    - Deceased ADPKD kidneys with good function and relatively small size may still be considered for recipients who consent.
    - Noted post-transplant complications: GI complications (e.g., perforation from diverticulosis), erythrocytosis, urinary tract infections, thromboembolic complications
- Direct medical therapies of ADPKD:
  - ADH (vasopressin) V2 receptor antagonists (tolvaptan): Tolvaptan has been shown to slow down TKV rate of growth and eGFR decline rate. Renal toxicity and other adverse effects (transaminitis) are of great concerns currently. (Tolvaptan in patients with ADPKD: TEMPO study)
  - Increased signaling of the mTOR complex 1 is thought to enhance cystic growth in ADPKD. Two clinical studies involving sirolimus, however, have not shown benefits in TKV or kidney function at 18-month follow-up. Notably, urine albumin to creatinine ratio was higher in the sirolimus group. (Sirolimus for ADPKD [SUISSE] study)

- Everolimus (mTOR inhibitor): slowed TKV increase but no slowing of eGFR decline detected over a 2-year study period
- Somatostatin analogs:
    - Beneficial effects have been shown in small randomized controlled trials.
    - A Long-Acting Somatostatin on Disease Progression in Nephropathy due to ADPKD (ALADIN): somatostatin analog octreotide-LAR resulted in a trend for smaller TKV increase and better secondary outcome of kidney function; small study. Ongoing larger trial in the Netherlands.
    - Not yet recommended due to lack of larger trials
- HMG-CoA reductase inhibitor (statin): The use of pravastatin in children treated with ACEI revealed slower rates of TKV growth and reduced rate of GFR decline.
- Management of ADPKD associated complications:
    - Pain:
        - Sequential approach based on the World Health Organization's pain relief ladder is recommended.
        - Others: celiac plexus blockade, radiofrequency ablation, spinal cord stimulation, laparoscopic or percutaneous transluminal catheter-based denervation
    - Gross hematuria:
        - Observation, hospitalization if severe, fluid support as needed
        - Prolonged hematuria (i.e., >7 days) dictates further evaluation for neoplasm.
    - Polycystic liver disease:
        - For severe polycystic liver disease, aspiration, sclerotherapy, fenestration, partial or segmental liver resection, or liver transplantation may be considered.
        - Somatostatin analogs use is restricted to clinical trials or compassionate use.
        - Cyst infections are best treated with percutaneous drainage and prolonged therapy with fluoroquinolones.
- Pregnancy:
    - Increased risk for progression of liver cysts
    - Increased risk for pregnancy-induced HTN and preeclampsia
    - Multiple pregnancies (>3) are associated with a greater risk for GFR decline.

Medullary Sponge Kidney

Epidemiology/Pathogenesis

- Incidence is likely underestimated because many patients are asymptomatic, but medullary sponge kidney (MSK) is thought to affect 1 in 5,000 people.
- Sporadic or familial clustering as autosomal-dominant inheritance with variable penetrance
- Thought to involve developmental defect in medullary pyramids and may occur with other developmental defects or tumors

Clinical Manifestations

- Generally asymptomatic, incidental finding
- May be complicated by hematuria, infections (urinary tract infections), nephrolithiasis (pure calcium phosphate (apatite) or mixture with calcium oxalate)
- Decreased concentrating defect and urinary acidification (incomplete distal RTA with hypercalciuria, hypocitraturia, alkaline urine), the latter leads to bone mineralization defect and stone formation; pre-calyceal duct ectasias
- MSK usually does not lead to ESRD.

Histopathology

Bilateral multiple spherical or oval cysts (1 to 8 mm) detected in papillae that may contain apatite concretions and may communicate with the collecting system.

Diagnosis

- Abdominal radiographs revealing radiopaque concretions (calcium stones) (Fig. 6.11)
- Excretory urography revealing spherical cysts or diffuse linear striations due to contrast retention by dilated medullary and papillary collecting ducts. These findings may also be described as "bouquet of flowers" or "paintbrush" sign.
- Nonenhanced CT may reveal echogenic hyperdense foci in the medulla from stones/nephrocalcinosis.

Management

- Nephrolithiasis:
  - 24-hour urine stone risk analysis: e.g., hypercalciuria, hypocitraturia
  - High fluid intake; potassium citrate 10 to 20 mEq 2 to 3 doses daily to achieve high normal citraturia but with urine pH < 7.5 to avoid calcium phosphate precipitation; thiazides if recurrent stones
- Urinary tract infections:
  - Antibiotics per sensitivity
  - Aggressive and prolonged therapy is generally recommended, particularly if coagulase-negative *Staphylococcus* is present.

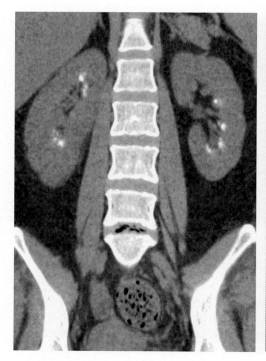 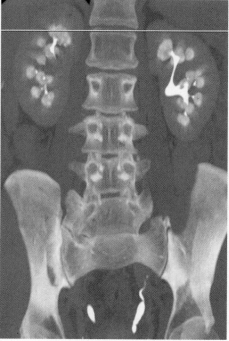

FIGURE 6.11 Medullary sponge kidney with classic "paintbrush" appearance. Coronal noncontract CT images showing amorphous and course pyramidal calcifications in both kidneys. Postcontrast excretory phase maximum intensity projection (MIP) images show a "paintbrush" like appearance to the renal calyces.

Simple Cysts

- Thought to originate from distal convoluted tubule or collecting ducts
- Increasing prevalence with increasing age
- Male-to-female predominance: 2 to 3:1
- Associated with smoking, HTN, reduced renal mass, increased body mass index, reduced kidney function
- Similar to ADPKD, circulating levels of copeptin levels (validated surrogate for vasopressin) is associated with kidney length and function.
- Generally asymptomatic, but may be associated with HTN, erythrocytosis
- Infected cysts may develop thickened walls, calcifications.
- Large cysts associated with severe HTN may be considered for drainage.
- Kidney transplantation: Growth rate of simple cysts does not increase with kidney donation whether they are in the donor or recipient. Simple cysts do not adversely affect renal outcomes.

Acquired Cystic Kidney Diseases

Conditions Associated with Acquired Cystic Kidney Diseases

- Chronic hypokalemia: cysts typically localized to renal medulla; resolution possible after correction of hypokalemia (e.g., adrenalectomy for functioning tumors)
- CKD-associated acquired cystic kidney diseases (ACKD) (see Chronic Kidney Disease Complications in Chronic Kidney Disease chapter):
  - Development of >3 to 5 macroscopic cysts in individuals without a hereditary cystic disease is required for the diagnosis of ACKD. ACKD typically involves >25% of renal parenchyma.
  - Increased risks with CKD vintage, 80% to 100% have ACKD by 10 years on dialysis.
  - May regress with successful kidney transplant
  - ACKD may transform into adenomas and RCC
    - Unlike sporadic clear cell RCC, ACKD-associated RCC are typically multifocal and bilateral with lower proliferative activity and metastatic disease.
    - ACKD-associated RCC are histologically distinct with eosinophilic cytoplasm with calcium oxalate crystal deposits in cribriform, tubulocystic, and papillary architecture.
  - Annual ultrasound screening (or at least 3 years after onset of dialysis with frequency increased to every 1 to 2 years if ACKD is present) is indicated in ESRD patients with good life expectancy. Interpretation is generally based on Bosniak classification.
- Bosniak classification of cysts (initially defined for CT, now often used for ultrasound):
  - I: Benign simple cyst; hairline thin wall; no septation, calcification, or solid components; no enhancement with contrast CT
  - II: Benign cyst with a few hairline thin septations ± "perceived" enhancement may be present; fine calcification in cyst wall or septation(s). Uniformly high-attenuation lesions < 3 cm, well marginated; no enhancement with contrast CT
  - IIf (f is for follow-up): Cysts with multiple hairline thin septa or minimal smooth thickening of wall/septa; "perceived" enhancement of septa/wall; calcification of wall/septa that may be thick and nodular; no measurable contrast enhancement.

- III: "Indeterminate" cystic masses with thickened irregular or smooth wall/septa; measurable enhancement. Contrast enhancement implies vascularized mass, thus possible malignancy. Although possibly benign, surgery is generally indicated.
  - IV: Malignant cystic masses that also contain enhancing soft tissue components
- General management per Bosniak classification:
  - Class I and II are benign. Six- to twelve-month follow-up may be warranted in ESRD patients.
  - Class IIf requires follow-up within 3 to 6 months.
  - Class III and IV are considered malignant until proven otherwise. Surgical evaluation is required.
- Management: bed rest, analgesics; if no resolution, consider renal embolization or laparoscopic nephrectomy.

Multilocular Cystic Nephroma, a.k.a. Papillary Cystadenoma, Benign Cystic Nephromas

- Well-circumscribed, multiseptated, generally benign, cystic lesions typically classified as Bosniak III on CT that require surgery to exclude malignancy (Fig. 6.12).
- Thought to arise from hamartomatous origin, embryonic metanephric blastema, or variant of Wilms tumor.
- Follows a bimodal age and sex pattern: boys 3 months to 4 years; women 40 to 60 years of age.
- Complications: flank pain, hematuria, calculi, urinary tract infections. Carcinomatous degenerations may occur.

Glomerulocystic Kidney Disease

- Glomerulocystic kidney disease (GCKD) may be present as a familial dominant or sporadic condition or infantile manifestation of ADPKD. GCKD is characterized by cystic dilation involving Bowman space and proximal tubules.

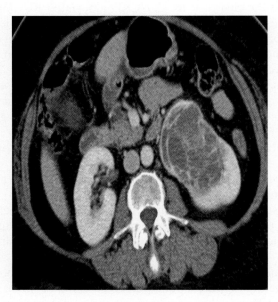

FIGURE 6.12 Multilocular cystic nephroma. Axial postcontrast CT image showing a well-circumscribed multilocular cystic mass with septal enhancement. This lesion is indistinguishable from renal cell carcinoma on imaging.

- Ultrasound may be notable for increased echogenicity of renal cortex with minute cysts. Associated renal medullary dysplasia and biliary dysgenesis may be found in infants with familial or sporadic GCKD.
- GCKD can present as an isolated condition or as part of a disease syndrome involving a heritable malformation syndrome or dysplastic kidneys. Familial hypoplastic GCKD presents with relatively small kidneys with medullocalyceal abnormalities and variable associations with gynecologic abnormalities and maturity-onset diabetes of the young type 5 (MODY5).

NOTES REGARDING RENAL CYSTIC DISEASES

- Kidney size:
  - Large: ADPKD, TSC-PKD1 contiguous gene deletion syndrome
  - Normal to small: MSK
  - Small: nephronophthisis (autosomal-dominant or -recessive tubulointerstitial disease)
  - Unilateral atrophic kidney: multicystic kidney disease
- Classic ultrasound of CT findings:
  - Radially arrayed dilated collecting ducts spanning from cortex to medulla: ARPKD
  - "Paintbrush," "bouquet of flowers": MSK
- Associations:
  - Renal malignancy: von Hippel–Lindau disease (often bilateral involvement), tuberous sclerosis complex (TSC)
  - Seizures, mental retardation: TSC
  - Cerebral aneurysms: ADPKD
  - AML (may present with retroperitoneal bleed), angiofibromas: TSC
  - Kidney stones (uric acid): ADPKD
  - Multiple small medullary stones/nephrocalcinosis: MSK

SUMMARY OF RENAL CYSTIC DISEASES

- Multicystic kidney disease
  - Congenital abnormality of kidney and urinary tract where irregular cysts replace normal renal parenchyma; spontaneous involution of cysts may lead to unilateral atrophic nonfunctioning kidney; association with vesicoureteral reflux
- Nephronophthisis: Tubulointerstitial kidney diseases (small kidneys)
  - Autosomal dominant:
    - Mutations of uromodulin (Tamm Horsfall protein), mucin 1, prorenin, or HNF-1b; early hyperuricemia and gout are associated with UROMOD and REN mutations.
  - Autosomal recessive:
    - NPHP1-3, multiple other syndromes associated with small kidneys and often abnormal eye findings (e.g., retinitis pigmentosa)
- Autosomal-dominant or spontaneous germ line and somatic mutation: TSC
  - Tuberous sclerosis: hamartomas, AML
  - TSC/PKD1 continuous gene deletion syndrome: enlarged polycystic kidney disease similar to ADPKD

- Von Hippel–Lindau disease: associated with multiorgan malignancies including RCC, pheochromocytoma, pancreatic islet cell tumor/cysts, hemangioblastomas
- Polycystic kidney disease
  - Autosomal recessive
    - Kidneys are enlarged in utero and infancy but may reduce in size with age due to fibrosis; association with hepatobiliary fibrosis, ascending cholangitis, ultrasound notable for radially arrayed dilated collecting ducts spanning from cortex to medulla.
  - Autosomal dominant
    - Enlarged kidneys; PKD1 reaches ESRD by fourth decade versus sixth decade by PKD2; association with polycystic liver disease
- Medullary sponge kidney disease
  - Bilateral multiple spherical cysts (1 to 8 mm) or diffuse linear striations arise from distal convoluted tubules or collecting ducts in that papillae +/− calcium apatite concretions. Classic CT finding of "paintbrush" or "bouquet of flowers" sign
- Acquired cysts
  - Simple cysts: increased with age; may be associated with reduced renal mass, increased body mass index, reduced kidney function
  - Acquired cystic kidney disease (associated with CKD)
- Others:
  - Bengin (multilocular) cystic nephroma (may appear malignant, i.e., Bosniak class III), glomerulocystic kidney disease (familial, sporadic, or infantile manifestation of ADPKD)

Access the eBook for self-assessment questions.

Glomerular/Vascular Diseases

Phuong-Chi T. Pham, Cynthia C. Nast, Jeffrey M. Miller, and Phuong-Thu T. Pham

GENERAL PRINCIPLES IN THE MANAGEMENT OF GLOMERULAR DISEASES

Kidney Biopsy Indications

- Proteinuria > 1 g/d
- Unexplained acute kidney injury (AKI)
- Extrarenal manifestations suggestive of systemic diseases (e.g., small vessel vasculitis, pulmonary renal syndromes)
- Unexplained dysfunction of transplant kidney
- Isolated microscopic hematuria: case specific, for example, evaluation for living donation, patient reassurance

Repeat Kidney Biopsy Indications (KDIGO 2012)

- Uncharacteristic deterioration of kidney function for kidney disease in question
- Changes in clinical or laboratory parameters suggestive of change in injury pattern within the same diagnosis (e.g., conversion of membranous to diffuse proliferative lupus nephritis [LN])
- Unclear reason for rapid decline in kidney function
- Determination of "point of no return" of kidney disease (stop, continue, or intensify therapy)

Tissue Adequacy

- Diagnosis possible with just one glomerulus: membranous nephropathy
- Glomerular diseases that typically require a higher number of glomeruli: focal segmental glomerulosclerosis (FSGS), necrotizing glomerulonephritis with antineutrophil cytoplasmic antibodies (ANCA)
- Generally, a lesion that only affects 5% of glomeruli, at least 20 glomeruli are needed (e.g., FSGS).

General Management Considerations for Glomerular Diseases

- Hypertension:
  - Lifestyle modifications: salt restriction, weight optimization, exercise, smoking cessation
  - Maintain BP goal < 140/90 mm Hg.

- There are (limited) data to support lower target BP < 125/75 mm Hg if protein-uria > 1 g/d.
- Clinical data support angiotensin-converting enzyme inhibitor (ACEI) or angiotensin-receptor blocker (ARB) as first-line therapy if safely tolerated.
- Proteinuria:
  - ACEI or ARB may reduce proteinuria by 40% to 50%.
  - Combination may result in additive antiproteinuric effect, but side effects may also be additive and unacceptable.
- Hyperlipidemia:
  - Statin use should be per standard guidelines for those with increased cardio-vascular risks.
  - Statins (HMG CoA reductase inhibitors) have not been proven to reduce cardio-vascular events in nephrotic syndrome. However statin use is recommended for hyperlipidemia associated with membranous glomerulonephropathy (MGN).
  - The renoprotective effect of statins in slowing GFR decline is not established.
- Nephrotic edema:
  - Intravenous loop diuretics should be considered if anasarca is present; bowel wall edema limits oral medication absorption.
  - Resistant edema: add thiazide, metolazone, amiloride, or spironolactone to loop diuretics; consider albumin infusion, although this is of unproven benefit.
  - Dietary sodium restriction 2.0 g daily
- Hypercoagulability:
  - Increased risk in patients with nephrotic syndrome with serum albumin < 2.5 g/dL
  - Anticoagulation with heparin or warfarin (target international normalized ra-tio [INR] 2-3) if known arterial or venous thrombosis or pulmonary embolism
  - Consider anticoagulation if serum albumin < 2.0 to 2.5 g/dL *and* one or more of the following: proteinuria > 10 g/d, body mass index > 35 kg/m^2, family his-tory of thromboembolism with documented genetic predisposition; New York Heart Association class III or IV congestive heart failure, recent abdominal or orthopedic surgery, or prolonged immobilization.
  - During heparin anticoagulation, a higher-than-average dose may be required because part of action of heparin depends on antithrombin III, which may be lost in urine of nephrotic patients.
- Risk of infection:
  - Spontaneous bacterial peritonitis may occur in nephrotic patients with ascites: empirical antibiotics should include benzylpenicillin (pneumococcal infection).
  - In cases with repeat infections, consider intravenous immunoglobulin 10 to 15 g to keep serum IgG > 600 mg/dL (limited evidence).
  - Pneumococcal vaccination with both heptavalent conjugate vaccine (7vPCV) and 23-valent polysaccharide vaccine (23vPPV) and annual influenza vaccination

NEPHRITIC GLOMERULAR DISORDERS AND VASCULITIS/VASCULOPATHY

Immunoglobulin A Nephropathy

Background

- Most common glomerulonephropathy (GN) worldwide
- Highest incidence among Eastern Asians, common in Native Americans, and very low incidence in African Americans

- Among biopsy-proven immunoglobulin A nephropathy (IgAN), 15% to 25% reach end-stage renal disease (ESRD) within 10 years and 20% to 40% by 20 years.
- Despite being slowly progressive, IgAN comprises 10% to 20% of ESRD due to high prevalence.

Pathogenesis (Multistep Model)

- Elevated circulating levels of galactose-deficient at hinge region of IgA1 *(Gd-IgA1) are produced*, presumably due to genetic factors; mistrafficking of B cells from mucosal to systemic compartments may also be responsible (likely influenced by genotype).

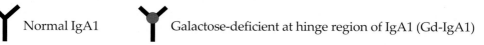

Normal IgA1   Galactose-deficient at hinge region of IgA1 (Gd-IgA1)

- *Antibodies directed against the underglycosylated hinge region of Gd-IgA1 are produced,* likely driven by molecular mimicry.

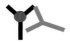

- Antibodies directed against Gd-IgA1 are produced. Antibodies may be of IgA or IgG class.
- *The immune complexes (IC) are deposited in the kidneys* (the IC are either preformed in circulation or formed in situ against previously deposited Gd-IgA1).
- Deposited IC *activate complement cascade (C3) and induce mesangial cell proliferation,* matrix deposition, and activation, all leading to irreversible kidney damage.

Common Associations/Etiologies

- IgAN may occur as a primary or secondary glomerulonephritis.
- Primary isolated IgAN:
  - May occur at any age, but typically in older patients
  - Kidney involvement only
  - IgA rheumatoid factor may be positive in 30% of affected patients.
- Primary systemic Henoch–Schonlein purpura (HSP):
  - Typically occurs in first decade of life, but may occur at any age
  - Systemic manifestations: palpable purpura affecting extensor surfaces (>90%), abdominal pain +/− (bloody) diarrhea (50%), arthritis, positive IgA rheumatoid factor (50% to 60%), IgA ANCA titers
- Secondary causes generally involve organs that produce or clear IgA, conditions that stimulate IgA production, or autoimmune diseases:
  - Skin: dermatitis herpetiformis, psoriasis, psoriatic arthritis
  - Liver: alcoholism, primary biliary cirrhosis, cirrhosis; hepatitis B, chronic schistosomiasis. Cirrhotic liver has reduced capacity to metabolize/clear IgA.
  - Gastrointestinal tract: inflammatory bowel disease, celiac disease, ulcerative colitis, Crohn's
  - Pulmonary: sarcoidosis, idiopathic hemosiderosis, cystic fibrosis, bronchiiiolitis obliterans, ANCA disease involving upper respiratory tract
  - Neoplasia: lung, larynx, pancreas, mycosis fungoides

- Infection: HIV, leprosy
- Systemic or immunologic disorders: systemic lupus erythematosus, rheumatoid arthritis, cryoglobulinemia, ankylosing spondylitis, Sjogren's, Behcet's, Reiter's, familial immune-mediated thrombocytopenia, autoantibody IgA-mediated Goodpasture's

Clinical Manifestations

IgAN may present with various patterns of clinical presentation:
- Episodic macroscopic "gross" hematuria:
  - More common in children
  - Association with upper respiratory tract infection or gastroenteritis (gross hematuria occurs concurrently or within 3 days of onset of infection and typically resolves by 3 days) with or without accompanying flank or loin pain
  - Prolonged remission of clinical signs is common.
- Asymptomatic (incidental finding) hematuria and proteinuria:
  - More common in adults
  - Hypertension and impaired kidney function may be present at diagnosis.
  - Remission is uncommon.
- Gross hematuria with concurrent AKI
- Nephrotic syndrome
- Slowly progressive chronic kidney injury
- Rapidly progressive (crescentic) glomerulonephritis

Histopathology

- Light microscopy (LM): mesangial expansion and hypercellularity, may be segmental and global glomerulosclerosis, endocapillary hypercellularity, crescents (Fig. 7.1)
- Immunofluorescent microscopy (IF): mesangial deposits of IgA, dominant or co-dominant with IgG or IgM $\pm$ C3. Staining of anything other than IgA is equal to or less intense than IgA.
- "MEST" Oxford Classification for IgAN:
  - **M**esangial proliferation (>50% glomeruli = M1)
  - **E**ndocapillary proliferation: most active lesion which suggests best indication for therapy (>1 occluded glomerular capillary = E1)
  - **S**egmental sclerosis (>1 segment of sclerosis = S1)
  - **T**ubular atrophy and interstitial fibrosis (T0 = 0% to 25%, T1 = 26% to 50%, T2 > 50%)
  - "M1," "S1," "T1," and T2 are associated with worse prognosis and are additive

Prognostic Indicators

- NOTE: *Well-established* presenting factors indicating worse prognosis for IgAN: *proteinuria* $\geq$ 1 g/d, *hypertension* (DBP $\geq$ 95 mm Hg) or normotensive on antihypertensive therapy, *SCr* $\geq$ 1.5 mg/dL, kidney biopsy with greater degree of tubular atrophy and interstitial fibrosis
- Novel markers using available techniques/samples: clinical risk score based on (presenting GFR, hemoglobin, albumin, and systolic blood pressure) genetic risk score, glomerular density measurement (number of nonsclerotic glomeruli per biopsied cortical area)
- Emerging tests: Gd-IgA1 levels, antiglycan autoantibodies, markers of oxidative stress or fibroblast, urine and serum proteomics, gene expression analyses

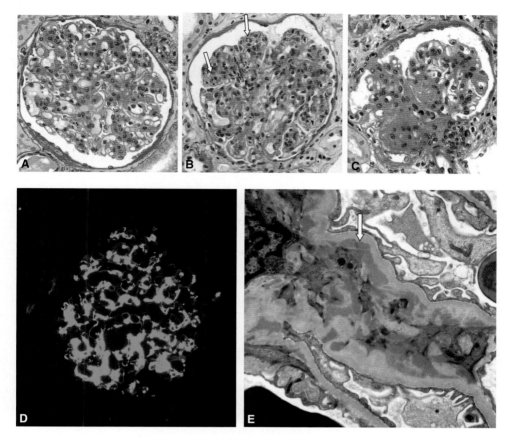

FIGURE 7.1 IgA Nephropathy. **A.** Global mesangial hypercellularity (M1 lesion) (Periodic acid–Schiff, ×400). **B.** Endocapillary hypercellularity with luminal occlusion (*arrows*) (E1 lesion) (Periodic acid–Schiff, ×400). **C.** Mesangial hypercellularity and segmental glomerulosclerosis (M1 and S1 lesions) (Periodic acid–Schiff, ×400). **D.** Global mesangial IgA (×275). **E.** Mesangial electron dense deposits, prominent in the paramesangial region (*arrow*) with a single subepithelial deposit (×14,000).

Management (KDIGO 2012)

- All patients:
  - BP control < 130/80 mm Hg; consider <125/75 mm Hg if presenting proteinuria > 1 g/d
  - ACEI or ARB is "recommended" if proteinuria > 1 g/d, otherwise ACEI/ARB is "suggested."
  - Aldosterone blockers may also be considered for antiproteinuric and antifibrotic effects.
  - Low-sodium diet
  - Consider tonsillectomy if recurrent tonsillitis
  - Use of fish oil is suggested in patients with proteinuria > 1 g/d despite 3 to 6 m of optimized ACEI/ARB and blood pressure control. Note that the benefit of fish oil is marginal on proteinuria. However, the use of ACEI has been shown to enhance the effect of fish oil.
- Mild disease: normal GFR, proteinuria < 500 mg/d; benign histology (noncrescentic), normotensive: observation

- Moderate or severe disease: proteinuria > 1 g/d or ≥ 0.5 to 1 g/d with clinical or histologic features suggesting risk of progression (mesangial hypercellularity, endocapillary proliferation, segmental sclerosis):
  - Glucocorticoids $\times$ 6 months (if GFR > 50 mL/min/1.73 m^2): two suggested regimens
    - Intravenous bolus of 1 g methylprednisolone $\times$ 3 days at months 1, 3, and 5, followed by oral prednisone at 0.5 mg/kg on alternate days $\times$ 6 months
    - Oral prednisone at 0.8 to 1.0 mg/kg/d $\times$ 2 months then reduced by 0.2 mg/kg/d per month for the next 4 months.
  - Consider cytotoxics (*poor data on preferred agent: KDIGO suggests cyclophosphamide (CYC) based on one low-quality study; mycophenolate mofetil (MMF) not suggested due to conflicting data and possible risk for delayed pneumonia*)
- End-stage or advanced disease: GFR < 30 mL/min/1.73 m^2, biopsy with severe global glomerulosclerosis and tubular atrophy, interstitial fibrosis: immunosuppressive therapy is not recommended.
- Crescentic IgAN: rapidly progressive glomerulonephritis, >30% to 50% cellular or fibrocellular crescents on biopsy: pulse followed by high dose oral glucocorticoids; consider adding CYC.
- AKI associated with macroscopic hematuria in IgAN: repeat kidney biopsy if there is no improvement after 5 days from onset to rule out crescentic IgAN.

RENAL AND SYSTEMIC VASCULITIDES

Classification of Vasculitis

- Large-sized vessels: aorta, renal artery
  - Granulomatous arteritis: giant cell or Takayasu arteritis (Table 7.1)
  - Patients > 50 years of age: giant cell arteritis
  - Patients < 50 years of age: Takayasu arteritis

Table 7.1	Large-sized vasculitis: giant cell versus Takayatsu arteritis	
	Giant Cell Arteritis	**Takaysu Arteritis**
Age of onset	Typically >50	10–20 y old; very rare after age 50
Female-to-male ratio	4:1	9:1
Pathogenesis	Unknown	Unknown
Clinical manifestations	Headaches, temporal artery tenderness, blindness, deafness, jaw claudication, tongue dysfunction, reduced pulses, extremity claudication; > 50% have polymyalgia rheumatica (stiffness and aching of neck, hips, shoulders); renal involvement rare compared with Takaysu; hypertension possible	Reduced pulses, vascular bruits, claudication, renal ischemia due to renal artery stenosis or aortic coarctation; hypertension possible
Pathology	Renal arteries may be involved, but significant disease is rare.	Ischemic renal disease relatively common; Glomerular lesion possible: nodular mesangial matrix expansion, mesangiolysis
Treatment	Same for both conditions: glucocorticoids (prednisolone 1 mg/kg/d for 1 mo, followed by slow taper over several months. Persistent disease requires prolonged glucocorticoid $\pm$ cytotoxic agents (cyclophosphamide); patients with giant cell arteritis should also be on low-dose aspirin to reduce thrombotic risks. Surgical bypass or angioplasty may be required when disease is quiescent.	

- Medium-sized vessels: renal artery, medium-sized vessels within the kidneys (interlobar artery, arcuate artery)
  - Necrotizing arteritis: polyarteritis nodosa (PAN) or Kawasaki disease (Table 7.2). NOTE: microaneurysms in PAN may resemble small grapes or "beads on a chain" within the kidneys on angiogram.
  - *Without* mucocutaneous lymph node (MCLN) syndrome: PAN
  - *With* MCLN syndrome: Kawasaki disease

Table 7.2	Medium-sized vasculitis: polyarteritis nodosa versus Kawasaki arteritis	
	Polyarteritis Nodosa (PAN)	**Kawasaki**
Age of onset	Age 40–60	Young children, peaks at age 1, typically <5 y old
Epidemiology	1:1 female:male; no race predilection	More common in Asians and Polynesians than Caucasians and Blacks; occasional endemic or epidemic pattern, sporadic
Pathogenesis	Unknown; immune-complex trigger (e.g., hepatitis B) suggested but not confirmed; *absence of ANCA*	Not clear; possible precipitating factors: infectious agent or environmental toxin; both cell- and antibody-mediated mechanisms possible
Clinical manifestations	Fevers, malaise, weight loss, arthralgias, myalgias, skin ulcers, purpura, livedo reticularis, infarction, ulceration, mononeuritis multiplex, abdominal pain, bloody stools, flank pain, hematuria, hypertension, life-threatening retroperitoneal bleed due to arterial aneurysm rupture rare, testicular pain, stroke, confusion, cardiomyopathy, pericarditis. *No mucocutaneous lymph node involvement*	*Mucocutaneous lymph node syndrome*: fevers, mucosal inflammation, swollen red (strawberry) tongue, polymorphous erythematous rash, indurative edema of extremities, erythema of palms/soles, desquamation from tips of digits, conjunctival injection, lymphadenopathy, coronary arteritis (possible myocardial infarction). Renal arteritis is uncommon.
Pathology	Renal artery, interlobar, arcuate, interlobular arteries (involvement of capillaries, arterioles, venous beds *exclude* PAN)	Small and medium arteritis with necrotizing inflammation, frequently involving coronaries and renal arteries (interlobar, arcuate, interlobular arteries)
	Nodular inflammatory lesions and aneurysms in arteries	Pseudoaneurysm formation and thrombosis may occur.
	Acute arterial lesion: segmental transmural fibrinoid necrosis ± leukocyte infiltration; chronic changes: arterial wall erosions from necrotizing inflammation into surrounding perivascular tissues leading to appearance of enlarged lumen, hence "pseudoaneurysm" and propensity for thrombosis and rupture.	
	NOTE: LM changes of involved vessels are indistinguishable from ANCA-associated GN.	
Treatment	If no hepatitis B: glucocorticoids ± cytotoxic agent (e.g., cyclophosphamide)	Aspirin and IV Ig
	Glucocorticoids alone may be adequate if benign (younger age, no cardiac, gut, or renal involvement). If hepatitis B+: high-dose glucocorticoids tapered over 2 wk followed by antiviral therapy ± plasma exchange	Disease is typically self-limited. Recurrence is rare if promptly treated. NOTE: glucocorticoids may *increase* risk of coronary artery aneurysms.

- Small-sized vessels: Smaller vessels within the kidneys (interlobar artery, arcuate artery, interlobar artery, arterioles)
  - Immune complex deposits in vessel walls:
    - Cryoglobulins: cryoglobulin deposits often affecting both skin and glomeruli
    - IgA-dominant deposits (HSP): vasculitis involving skin, gut, and glomeruli, with associated arthritis/arthralgias
    - Systemic lupus erythematosus (SLE) or rheumatoid arthritis
    - Others: postinfectious, hypocomplementemic urticarial (anti-C1q) vasculitis
  - Circulating ANCA with paucity of vascular or glomerular immunoglobulin staining:
    - Granulomas and no asthma: granulomatous polyangiitis (Wegener's)
    - Eosinophilia, asthma, and granuloma: eosinophilic granulomatosus with polyangiitis (Churg–Strauss)
    - No asthma or granulomas: microscopic polyangiitis

ANCA Vasculitis

What Is ANCA?

- ANCA are antineutrophil cytoplasmic auto**antibodies** directed against various *antigens*:
  - ANCA directed *against* proteinase 3 (anti-PR3) → cytoplasmic pattern (c-ANCA)
  - ANCA directed *against* myeloperoxidase (anti-MPO) → nuclear pattern (p-ANCA)
  - ANCA directed *against other* antigens/proteinases (e.g., human neutrophil elastase [HNE], lysozyme). ANCAs directed against other antigens/proteinases often give perinuclear (p)-ANCA pattern. The pathogenic roles of these atypical ANCAs are unclear.
    - Cystic fibrosis: ANCA directed against bactericidal/permeability-increasing protein
    - Cocaine adulterated with levamisole: all with MPO-ANCA and 50% with positive PR3-ANCA in a series reported from Massachussetts General Hospital involving 30 patients. Others suggest ANCA directed against HNE. Affected patients may present with purpuric to necrotic skin lesions that may involve earlobes and nose. Renal manifestations may include ANCA-associated GN or renal infarction.
- Cytoplasmic (c-ANCA) or perinuclear (p-ANCA) pattern reflects an artifact that occurs with alcohol fixation of neutrophils. All antigens above (including MPO) are cytoplasmic in vivo.
- While c-ANCA is anti-PR3, and p-ANCA is typically anti-MPO, c-ANCA and p-ANCA can bind to other proteinases (other than the respective PR3 and MPO) that are not necessarily pathogenic. Testing for ANCA should therefore include both indirect immunofluorescent microscopic assay (IFA) and enzyme immunoassay (EIA). The former is to check for c- or p-ANCA pattern, and the latter is to check for the specificity of ANCA against specific enzymes, that is proteinase 3, myeloperoxidase, or other enzymes.
- NOTE:
  - Classic PAN does *not* have ANCA; hence, ANCA testing may be used to differentiate between ANCA vasculitides and PAN.
  - 30% of patients with antiglomerular basement membrane (anti-GBM) positive sera and 25% of patients with idiopathic immune-complex crescentic GN have concurrent ANCA.

- 5% of patients with ANCA-positive sera also have anti-GBM positive sera.
- Patients with concurrent anti-GBM and ANCA antibodies:
  - Thought to be either fortuitous coexistence of both anti-GBM and ANCA or anti-GBM develops following glomerular basement membrane (GBM) injury from ANCA-associated GN.
  - Disease course is similar to anti-GBM GN in early disease, but relapse pattern is similar to ANCA disease. Lone anti-GBM GN typically does not relapse.
- Evidence for ANCA involvement in pathogenesis of small-vessel vasculitis:
  - ANCA titers correlate with disease activity within the same individual.
  - Drug-induced ANCA production (propylthiouracil, methimazole, hydralazine, pencillamine) is associated with pauciimmune crescentic GN and small-vessel vasculitis.
  - Report of neonate with GN and pulmonary hemorrhage from transplacental passage of MPO-ANCA IgG.
- Proposed chain of events involved in ANCA-induced vasculitis:
  - Priming of neutrophils by cytokines (e.g., from a viral infection) leads to:
    - Increased neutrophil expression/trafficking of cytoplasmic ANCA *antigens* (e.g., PR3 or MPO) onto cell surfaces, where they are accessible to ANCA. The **ANCA:** *antigen* interaction in cytokine-primed neutrophils leads to the following:
      - Neutrophil release of IgG from granules, toxic oxygen metabolites, inflammatory mediators into surroundings *and*
      - Adherence of activated neutrophils to endothelial cells, both leading to *endothelial cell injury and/or death, hence vasculitis*
- Of note, the onset of ANCA small-vessel vasculitis is frequently associated with an influenza-like syndrome, an indicator of high levels of circulating cytokines, thought to serve as priming factors for neutrophils.

Clinical Manifestations

- See Table 7.3 for well-characterized ANCA syndrome specific clinical manifestations.
- In general ANCA-associated GN may present with relatively low degree of proteinuria and hematuria, acute nephritis with necrosis and new crescents, rapidly progressive nephritis with crescentic GN, or slowly progressive nephritis.
- Nonspecific signs and symptoms of necrotizing vasculitis: cutaneous purpura, papular/ulcerated lesions, peripheral neuropathy (mononeuritis multiplex), nonspecific muscular/joint pain, evidence of gastrointestinal bleed, tendency for venous thrombosis
- Histopathology: ANCA-associated (pauciimmune) crescentic glomerulonephritis often has crescents in different stages simultaneously (acute, subacute, and chronic) due to the relapsing nature of the disease

Natural History/Prognosis

- Five-year renal and patient survival are approximately 65% to 75%.
- Poor prognostic risks: older age, higher presenting SCr/dialysis need, pulmonary hemorrhage
- NOTE: Risks for higher relapse rates include respiratory tract involvement and PR3-ANCA serology.

Table 7.3	ANCA syndromes			
	Microscopic polyangiitis (MPA) c-ANCA (PR3): 40% p-ANCA (MPO): 50% negative ANCA: 10-30%	Granulomatosis with polyangiitis (GPA) c-ANCA (PR3): 80-90% p-ANCA (MPO): 10-20% negative ANCA: 5-10%	Eosinophilic granulomatosis with polyangiitis (EGPA) c-ANCA (PR3): 10% p-ANCA (MPO): 60% negative ANCA: 30%	Pauci-immune glomerulonephritis c-ANCA (PR3): 20% p-ANCA (MPO): 70% negative ANCA: 10%
Age	Fifth to seventh decade; Slight male predominance; More common in White than Black			
Lungs	Necrotizing vasculitis *without* granulomatous inflammation	Necrotizing granulomatous lesions; upper respiratory involvement more common than MPA: may include sinusisitis, rhinitis, otitis media, ocular inflammation; bone destruction leading to saddle-nose deformity	Asthma; eosinophil-rich and granulomatous inflammation	
Kidneys	Often rapidly progressive disease but can be indolent acute or chronic nephritis		Less frequent kidney involvement. Kidney disease is less severe than MPA or GPA	ANCA positive glomerulonephritis *but* without classic manifestations or symptomology for MPA, GPA, or EGPA
Gastro-intestinal	50% of patients with MPA, GPA, or EGPA may have abdominal pain, bloody stool with mesenteric ischemia/intestinal infarction/performation, pancreatitis, hepatitis			
Skin	Nodular cutaneous lesions rare	Skin nodules due to dermal or subcutaneous arteritis and necrotizing granulomatous infiltration		
Neurologic	Peripheral neuropathy, usually mononeuritis multiplex pattern; Up to 70% in EGPA, 50% GPA, 30% MPA			
	Central nervous system involvement less common, may present as vasculitis within meninges			
Other organ involvement	20% cardiac involvement (e.g., heart blocks, ventricular hypokinesis).	20% cardiac involvement	Eosinophilia: systemic/infiltration 50% cardiac involvement	

- Others:
  - MPO-ANCA patients tend to present with worse renal impairment and more chronic changes. However, if MPO-ANCA is diagnosed early, it may be associated with better renal outcome compare with PR3-ANCA.
  - Patients with eosinophilic granulomatous polyangiitis (Churg–Strauss) typically present with less-severe kidney involvement.

Management (KDIGO 2012)

- Initial treatment:
  - CYC (0.75 g/m^2 IV q 3 to 4 weeks or 1.5 to 2.0 mg/kg/d orally; reduce dose if age > 60 years or GFR < 20 mL/min/1.73 m^2) and corticosteroids (methylprednisolone 500 mg IV pulse daily × 3 days, followed by 1 mg/kg/d × 4 weeks, not exceeding 60 mg daily, taper over 3 to 4 months)
  - Rituximab (375 mg/m^2 weekly × 4) and corticosteroids may be used as alternative initial treatment in patients without severe disease or in whom CYC is contraindicated.
  - There is no evidence that either agent above is superior to the other: Remission–induction Regimens for ANCA-Associated Vasculitis "RAVE" trial. Rituximab therapy was not inferior to daily CYC treatment for induction of remission in severe ANCA-associated vasculitis. Note however, RAVE trial excluded patients with severe pulmonary hemorrhage requiring mechanical ventilation or severe renal impairment with SCr > 4.0 mg/dL due to current episode of renal disease activity.
  - All trials report similar adverse effect profiles for rituximab and other immunosuppressive therapies used in the treatment of ANCA vasculitis.
  - Plasmapheresis:
    - Recommended if:
      - Patients require dialysis at presentation or present with rapidly increasing SCr.
      - Concurrent diffuse pulmonary hemorrhage
    - Suggested if concurrent ANCA vasculitis and anti-GBM GN
    - Plasmapheresis regimen:
      - 60 mL/kg body weight; replacement fluid is 5% albumin. Fresh-frozen plasma may be used at end of apheresis session to replace coagulant factors.
      - Vasculitis: seven treatments over 14 days if diffuse pulmonary hemorrhage, daily until bleeding stops, then every other day, up to total of 7 to 10 treatments.
      - Vasculitis in association with anti-GBM antibodies: daily for 14 days or until anti-GBM antibodies are undetectable
      - *Must* monitor daily prothrombin time and fibrinogen and replace with fresh frozen plasma (FFP) and cryoprecipitates respectively as needed to correct any coagulopathy associated with removal of coagulant factors with apheresis.
- Maintenance therapy:
  - Discontinue CYC/further immunosuppressive therapy if patients remain dialysis-dependent and free of extrarenal manifestations after 3 months.
  - Otherwise, maintenance therapy is recommended.
  - Maintenance therapy for at least 18 months is suggested.
  - Choice of maintenance therapy:
    - Azathioprine (AZA) 1 to 2 mg/kg/d orally is recommended.
    - MMF may be suggested, up to 1 g twice daily, if intolerant of AZA.
    - Methotrexate (initially 0.3 mg/kg/wk, maximum of 25 mg/wk) for maintenance therapy in patients intolerant of both AZA and MMF, but not if GFR < 60 mL/min/1.73 m^2.
    - Trimethoprim–sulfamethoxazole as adjunct to maintenance therapy in patients with upper respiratory tract disease is suggested. (Prevents "priming" of neutrophils.)

- Relapse:
  - Same therapy as initial therapy is recommended if patients present with severe relapse (e.g., life- or organ-threatening).
  - Otherwise, reinstitution of immunosuppressive therapy or increasing intensity with agents other than CYC, including reinstitution or increasing dose of glucocorticoids, with or without AZA or MMF is suggested.
- Resistant disease:
  - Addition of rituximab is recommended.
  - Suggested alternatives: IV immunoglobulin or plasmapheresis
- Disease monitoring: changing immunosuppression (i.e., intensifying or reinitiation therapy) with changing (i.e., increasing) ANCA titer alone is not recommended.
- Avoid over-immunosuppression, provide *Pneumocystis jiroveci* (*Pneumocystis carinii*) prophylaxis and be vigilant with infectious complications in ALL patients receiving immunosuppressive therapy.

Kidney Transplantation

- Delaying transplantation until complete remission for 6 to 12 months is recommended. (opinion-based)
- Delaying transplantation in patients in complete remission but with positive ANCA is *not* recommended. Also see Kidney Transplantation chapter.

ANTIGLOMERULAR BASEMENT MEMBRANE DISEASE

Epidemiology

- Incidence: 0.5 to 0.9/million/year (predominantly Caucasians); rare in other ethnicities
- Slight male predominance
- Peak 20 to 30, and smaller peak at 60 to 70 years old

Clinical Manifestations

- Disease may develop over weeks to months.
- May occur with mild respiratory symptoms or incidental microscopic hematuria with disease progressing over months to years

Pathogenesis

- Autoimmunity with antibody formation against the noncollagenous (NC1) domain of type IV collagen chain, $\alpha 3(IV)NC1$, a.k.a. the "Goodpasture antigen" or
- Antibodies to any other GBM constituents, $\alpha 3$-$\alpha 5(IV)$ chains
- These type IV collagen chains are also present in alveolus, cochlea, parts of eye (corneal basement membrane and Bruch membrane), choroid plexus of brain, and some endocrine organs, thus symptoms related to injury of these organs are also possible.

Histopathology

- LM: glomerular crescents without mesangial hypercellularity. Crescents are in the same stage (all active, all subacute, or all chronic) due to "one-shot" anti-GBM antibody production (in contrast to presence of crescents different stages with ANCA GN) (Fig. 7.2)
- IF: glomerular capillary wall IgG in a linear pattern

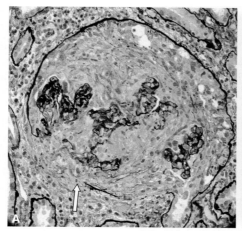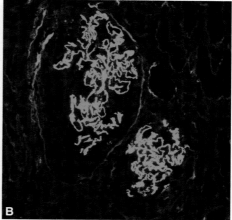

FIGURE 7.2 Antiglomerular basement membrane antibody nephritis. **A.** Cellular crescent causing destruction of Bowman capule segmentally (*arrow*) (Jones silver, ×400). **B.** Linear capillary wall staining for IgG (×200).

Differential Diagnoses

- Specific binding to GBM
  - Anti-GBM disease with kidney involvement only
  - Alport syndrome after renal transplantation
- Nonspecific binding to GBM: diabetes mellitus (DM), light-chain disease, fibrillary GN, SLE

Predisposing factors:

- HLA-DR2: HLA-DRB1*1501
- HLA-DR4: DRB1*1501 or DR4
- DR1 and DR7 confer strong and dominant protection.

Precipitating factors:

- Underlying exposure to hydrocarbons, cigarette smoking, pulmonary infection, and fluid overload leads to an initial alveolar injury which allows the preformed anti-GBM antibodies to access and attack the alveolar membranes, thus leading pulmonary hemorrhage. Pulmonary hemorrhage may be seen on chest radiographs as "fluffy, fleeting infiltrates," due to rapid onset and rapid clearing.
- Prior kidney injury/inflammation may predispose the kidney to the development of anti-GBM disease. Again, the existing injury to the GBM allows anti-GBM antibodies access to the GBM to cause anti-GBM disease.

Prognostic Indicators

- Higher-presenting SCr and higher percentage of crescents portend worse prognosis.
- Need for dialysis, particularly if in association with 100% crescents

Management (KDIGO 2012)

- Methylprednisolone 500 to 1,000 mg/d intravenously for 3 days, followed by prednisone, 1 mg/kg/d based on ideal body weight (maximum 80 mg/d) with slow taper to off by 6 months, *plus*

- CYC: 3 mg/kg/d orally. For patients older than 55, reduce dose to 2.5 mg/kg/d × 2 to 3 months, *plus*
- Plasmapheresis: one 4 L exchange daily with 5% albumin. Add 150 to 300 mL fresh-frozen plasma at the end of each session if patients have pulmonary hemorrhage, or have had recent surgery, including kidney biopsy. Plasmapheresis should be performed for 14 days or until anti-GBM antibodies become undetectable.
- NOTE:
  - Maintenance immunosuppressive therapy for anti-GBM glomerulonephritis is *not* recommended. This disease is not characterized by frequently relapsing course. Antibodies tend to disappear spontaneously after 12 to 18 months. Recurrence, if occurs, presents at a mean time of 4.3 years, range 1 to 10 years. Recurrence may manifest as kidney involvement or pulmonary hemorrhage. Treatment is similar to initial regimen outlined earlier.
  - *Exception* to immunosuppressive therapy initiation: patients who are dialysis-dependent at presentation and have 100% crescents in an adequate biopsy sample, and do not have pulmonary hemorrhage
  - *Routine daily coagulation laboratory tests should be performed with additional FFP replacement as needed* to correct any plasmapheresis-induced coagulopathy due to removal of coagulant factors.
  - Corticosteroids should be started prior to tissue diagnosis if high suspicion due to rapidly progressive disease. Following diagnosis confirmation, add CYC and plasmapheresis.

Kidney Transplantation

- Defer transplantation until anti-GBM antibodies are undetectable for at least 6 months.
- Recurrent of disease is very unusual when transplant is performed six months or longer after antibody disappearance.
- New-onset anti-GBM disease following kidney transplantation should raise the possibility of Alport syndrome in the native kidneys.

LUPUS NEPHRITIS

Epidemiology

- It is estimated that 60% of patients with SLE will develop clinically significant LN in the course of the disease.
- Age:
  - The majority of patients who develop LN are younger than 55 years old.
  - Severe nephritis is more common in children than elderly patients.
- Gender difference (female-to-male ratio) is noted for female predominance and varies with age:
  - 2:1 in prepubertal children
  - 4:1 in adolescents
  - 8 to 12:1 in adults
  - 2:1 in adults age greater than 60
  - Renal outcome portends worse prognosis in males than females.
- Race-related demographics:
  - SLE is more common in African Americans and Hispanics than whites.
  - Severe LN is more common in African Americans and Asians than in other ethnic groups.

Pathogenesis

- *Production of autoantibodies* by mature B cells (plasma cells) against nuclear antigens (e.g., double stranded DNA (dsDNA), ribonucleoproteins, complement factors (e.g., C1q). This process may be driven by:
  - Antigenic mimicry: antibodies against bacterial or viral peptides cross-react to self-antigens.
  - Impaired clearance of apoptotic bodies
  - Polyclonal hyperactivity of the B-cell system or defects of T-cell autoregulation leading to high antibody production
  - Anti-double stranded DNA (anti-dsDNA) antibody response driven by histone-specific T-helper cells
- *IC deposition*: deposition of circulating IC in GBM or direct binding of nucleosomal antigens to GBM followed by in situ autoantibody-binding activates both complement-dependent and independent inflammatory cascades.
- *IC clearance*:
  - ICs are normally cleared by the C1 complement complex. Binding of C1 complex to IC leads to downstream complement activation and opsonization of the IC for phagocytosis.
  - C1q is a component of the C1 complex. Upon binding of C1 complex to IC, C1 complex undergoes conformational change, exposing antigenic sites of C1q, which then leads to autoantibody formation against C1q. High autoantibody titers against C1q have been suggested to correlate with active lupus.
- *Inflammatory effects* following impaired apoptotic bodies clearance and/or IC formations and roles of other inflammatory cells:
  - Neutrophils:
    - NETosis: a process whereby upon exposure to microorganisms, neutrophils release nuclear components, granule proteins, and chromatin to form an extracellular matrix (ECM), referred to as "neutrophil extracellular traps" (NETs) to "trap," destroy, and clear the invading microorganisms. NETs comprise of DNA and histones along with various peptides and proteinases such as high-mobility group protein box-1, cathelicidin, myeloperoxidase, neutrophil elastase, matrix metalloproteinase 9, and proteoglycan recognition protein short. NETs may serve as a source of autoantigens in SLE.
    - There are data to suggest that NETs are complement activators and can play a role in increasing C1q deposition.
  - Basophils:
    - Cross-linking of IgE to its receptors (FcκRI) on basophil surface leads to the secretion of histamine and proinflammatory cytokines by basophils.
    - There are data to suggest that increased titers of both dsDNA-IgE and dsDNA-IgG predict SLE disease activity better than dsDNA-IgG titers alone.
    - Activated basophils secrete cytokines (IL-4 and IL-6) and express the MHC-II and B cell-activating factor BAFF (also known as B-Lys), which can enhance plasma cell survival and autoantibody production amplification loop.
    - Other functions of activated basophils: promotion and regulation of TH2 adaptive immune responses, antigen presentation to T cells, plasma cell differentiation and support, monocyte polarization and recruitment, and inflammatory site organization.
  - Macrophages/monocytes:
    - NETs containing LL37 stimulate NLRP3 inflammasome in monocytes and result in IL-1β and IL-18 release, NETosis, and amplification of the proinflammatory state.

- Polymorphism in the IL-18 gene promoter with associated increased IL-18 production may promote SLE susceptibility.
- Autoreactive B-cells and T-cells due to defective regulatory mechanisms.
- Advances in SLE targeted therapy:
  - Belimumab: human monoclonal antibody that selectively neutralizes B-cell activating factor (BAFF)
    - FDA approved for treatment of ANA/anti-dsDNA positive adults with high disease activity despite standard therapy
    - Short-term clinical trials suggest reduced SLE activity, flare rates, and corticosteroid need
  - Sifalimumab: human monoclonal antibody that inhibits several IFN-α subtypes[1]
  - Rontalizumab: humanized mouse monoclonal anti-IFN-α-antibody.
  - Omalizumab: recombinant humanized monoclonal antibody that blocks the binding of IgE to the FcεRI receptor.

Diagnosis

- Routine laboratory findings:
  - Microscopic hematuria ± red blood cell casts, proteinuria ± nephrotic syndrome
  - Serologies: positive antinuclear antibody (sensitive, not specific), anti-Smith (specific), anti-dsDNA, hypocomplementemia (particularly low C3). Anti-Smith is specific for the diagnosis of SLE. Anti-dsDNA and hypocomplementemia correlate with kidney disease activity.
- Histopathology (Fig. 7.3): International Society of Nephrology/Renal Pathology Society classification of LN:
  - Class I: Minimal mesangial LN: normal glomeruli by LM; mesangial immune deposits by IF alone or by both IF and EM.
  - Class II: Mesangial proliferative LN: mesangial hypercellularity and matrix expansion on LM; mesangial immune deposits by both IF and EM.
  - Class III: focal LN (<50% of glomeruli are involved)
    - Class III(A): Active lesions (leukocytes, karyhorrexis, cellular or fibrocellular crescents, large subendothelial deposits forming "wire loops" or "hyaline thrombi")
    - Class III(A/C): Active and chronic lesions
    - Class III(C): Chronic lesions (segmental or global glomerulosclerosis, fibrotic crescents)
  - Class IV: Diffuse LN (≥50% glomeruli)
    - Diffuse segmental (IV-S) or global (IV-G)
    - Class IV(A): Active lesions
    - Class IV(A/C): Active and chronic lesions
    - Class IV(C): Chronic lesions
  - Class V: Membranous LN (>50% subepithelial deposits with or without mesangial hypercellularity)
  - Class VI: Advanced sclerosing LN (≥90% globally sclerosed glomeruli without residual activity)

Management (KDIGO 2012)

- Class I LN:
  - Benign, no long-term adverse effect on kidney function

---

[1]Ongoing clinical trials.

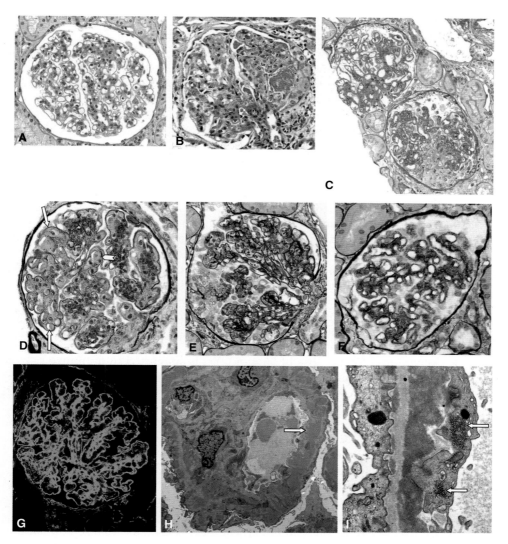

FIGURE 7.3 Lupus nephritis. **A.** Mesangial proliferative (Class II) (Periodic acid–Schiff, ×400). **B.** Segmental proliferation with leukocytes and a necrotizing/crescentic lesion (Masson trichrome, ×400). **C.** Active focal lupus nephritis (Class III). There is segmental involvement of <50% glomeruli with proliferative features. In chronic focal lupus nephritis, there is focal scarring/sclerosis (Periodic acid–Schiff, ×200). **D and E.** Active diffuse lupus nephritis (Class IV). In (**D**) there are large subendothelial deposits forming wire loop lesions (*arrows*) and hyaline thrombi (*arrowhead*). In (**E**) there is more leukocytic infiltration with a segmental cellular crescent. **F.** Membranous lupus nephritis (Class V). Capillary walls are thickened with subepithelial deposits and spikes, with mild segmental mesangial hypercellularity (**D–F** Jones silver, ×200). **G.** Global mesangial and capillary wall staining for IgG in mixed diffuse and membranous lupus nephritis (Class IV + V) (×400). **H.** EM showing large subendothelial (wire loop) (*arrow*), mesangial and segmental subepithelial electron dense deposits (×6,000). **I.** Tubuloreticular inclusions (*arrows*) in endothelial cell cytoplasm beneath subendothelial deposits. Small subepithelial deposits are also present (×29,000).

- Disease-specific therapy not necessary. Routine chronic kidney disease (CKD) progression risk reduction management.
- Class II LN:
  - <1 g/d proteinuria: routine CKD progression risk reduction management and management of extrarenal manifestations of SLE as needed.
  - >3 g/d proteinuria: Treatment with corticosteroids or calcineurin inhibitors (CNIs) as described for MCD/FSGS is suggested.

- Class III and class IV LN initial induction therapy:
  - Initial therapy with corticosteroids plus either CYC or MMF.
  - Corticosteroids: oral prednisone 1 mg/kg, taper over 6 to 12 months per clinical response. Initial IV methylprednisolone (e.g., 5 to 10 mg/kg × 3 days may be considered at induction for aggressive disease—NOTE: dosing and duration have not been tested in any randomized controlled trials [RCTs]).
  - CYC
    - Intravenous cyclophosphamide (IV CYC):
      - "NIH regimen": (0.5 to 1.0 g/m^2) given monthly for 6 months
      - Euro-Lupus regimen: (500 mg) given every 2 weeks for 3 months (equivalent efficacy as NIH regimen in Caucasians).
        - Euro-Lupus study was limited to less severe patients (severe disease was defined as >50% segmental glomerular necrosis or crescents and rapidly progressive kidney failure).
        - Whether efficacy of Euro-Lupus is similar to that of NIH regimen in class III/IV or in non-Caucasians is not known.
    - Oral cyclophosphamide (PO CYC): 1.0 to 1.5 mg/kg/d (maximum dose 150 mg/d) for 2 to 4 months.
      - Similar efficacy to IV CYC in prospective observational studies.
      - Some but not all investigators suggested more adverse effects with PO CYC compared with IV CYC.
    - Safety notes for use of CYC:
      - Maximum lifetime dose of 36 g of CYC is suggested to minimize risk of hematologic malignancies.
      - Dose reduction with renal insufficiency (20% and 30% reduction for CrCl 25 to 50 and 10 to 25 mL/min, respectively
      - Adjust CYC dose to keep nadir leukocyte count ≥ 3,000/μL (typically occurs in 10 to 14 days for IV CYC and 1 week for PO CYC)
      - Use sodium-2-mercaptoethane (mesna) to minimize bladder toxicity
      - Fertility protection while on CYC treatment:
        - Women: leuprolide, ovarian tissue cryopreservation
        - Men: testosterone (efficacy poorly established), sperm banking
- MMF: 750 to 1,500 mg twice daily for 6 months
  - MMF was shown to have similar efficacy as PO CYC in Chinese population; severe LN were excluded.
  - Aspreva Lupus Management Study (ALMS), RCT involving patients with class III, IV, and V LN: MMF had an equivalent response rate for induction compared with IV CYC at 6 months, with similar incidence of adverse events including serious infections and deaths.
    - Post hoc analysis of ALMS indicated inferior outcomes with CYC compared to MMF in black, Hispanic, and mixed-race patients (patients considered to have more resistant LN).
- CYC versus MMF for induction therapy:
  - If disease worsens as evidenced by increasing SCr or proteinuria during the first 3 months of therapy with either CYC or MMF, switch therapy (e.g., from CYC to MMF or vice versa) or use alternative therapy (see options below). Consider rebiopsy.
    - Definitions of response:
      - Complete response: return of SCr to baseline, plus a decline in urine protein to creatinine ratio (uPCR) < 500 mg/g

- Partial response: stabilization ($\pm 25\%$) or improvement of SCr *plus* $\geq 50\%$ decrease in uPCR where final uPCR is <3,000 mg/g
- Response rates appear equivalent, but current data suggest a trend for more relapses, prolonged proteinuria > 1 g/d, and persistent SCr > 2 mg/dL in MMF compared to CYC induction therapy.
- CYC RCTs included patients with more severe LN compared to MMF trial. CYC may thus be preferred over MMF in patients with severe LN.
  - Other alternative therapies:
    - AZA: AZA + corticosteroids had similar induction response rate compared with that for IV CYC + corticosteroids at 2 years. AZA had fewer adverse effects, but had higher late relapse rate, risk of doubling of SCr, and more chronic changes on late follow-up biopsies.
    - Cyclosporine (CSA): 4 to 5 mg/kg/d
      - Comparable remissions to IV CYC
      - Nephrotoxicity limits use in patients with elevated SCr.
    - Tacrolimus (TAC): comparable remission rates between combination TAC (4 mg/d) + MMF (1 g/d) + glucocorticoids and IV CYC (0.75 g/m^2) for 6 months (Chinese RCT).
    - Adding rituximab to standard MMF + corticosteroids for induction therapy provided no added benefit and is not recommended.
- Class III and IV LN maintenance therapy:
  - Either AZA (1.5 to 2.5 mg/kg/d) or MMF (1 to 2 g/d in divided doses) *and* low-dose oral corticosteroids ($\leq$10 mg/d prednisone equivalent) is recommended.
    - With the exception of the ALMS trial where MMF is a better maintenance agent compared to AZA in composite treatment failure endpoint (death, ESRD, kidney failure, sustained doubling of SCr, or requirement for rescue therapy), AZA and MMF generally have comparable maintenance efficacy.
    - Maintenance therapy with AZA or MMF has been suggested to be superior to CYC based on risk of death and development of CKD.
  - Use of CNIs is suggested for patients who cannot tolerate MMF or AZA.
  - Duration of maintenance is not known, but suggested to be at least 1 year. Average duration of immunosuppressive therapy from 7 RCTs was 3.5 years.
  - If disease relapses during tapering period, go back to previous level of immunosuppression that controlled disease.
- Monitoring of LN:
  - Serial proteinuria and SCr
  - Hematuria may persist for months even with improved proteinuria and SCr.
  - Complement levels (up to 80% sensitivity) and anti-double-stranded DNA antibodies (up to 70% to 80%)

Lupus and Pregnancy

- Measurable SLE disease activity is present in 40% to 50% of pregnancies, with LN occurring in up to 75% of these cases.
- Active SLE during pregnancy is associated with:
  - Increased risk of preeclampsia to 30% compared to 5% in the general population
  - Increased risk of fetal death and preterm birth
- Active LN during pregnancy is associated with:
  - Increased maternal adverse outcomes including increased risk of gestational HTN, preeclampsia, and maternal death. There is evidence to suggest that

LN classes III and IV may be associated with greater risk for hypertension/preeclampsia compared to other LN classes.
- Likely increased risks of preterm birth, intrauterine growth restriction, stillbirth, and neonatal death. (Inconsistent findings in the literature.)
- Risk factors for adverse outcomes in pregnancy:
  - Active disease at conception
  - Antiphospholipid antibodies
  - HTN, proteinuria, reduced GFR in the first trimester
  - Chronicity of disease
- Management of antiphospholipid syndrome (APS)/nephrotic syndrome during pregnancy:
  - Adverse outcomes of APS and positive antiphospholipid antibodies: late fetal loss (after 10 weeks of gestation), increased relative risk of preeclampsia
  - Women with APS and arterial thrombotic events are also at high risks for stroke and maternal morbidity and mortality.
  - Routine screening for antiphospholipid antibodies is recommended.
- Anticoagulation:
  - For women with known APS receiving chronic anticoagulation: convert warfarin to unfractionated heparin (UFH) or low-molecular-weight heparin (LMWH) during pregnancy.
  - For women with no known history of thrombotic events, but with obstetric criteria for APS of having either ≥3 pregnancy losses or late pregnancy loss, prophylactic anticoagulation consisting of a low dose aspirin with either UFH or LMWH should be initiated
  - For women with antiphospholipid antibodies but not meeting clinical criteria for APS, clinical surveillance with either antepartum aspirin or prophylactic UFH or LMWH is suggested.
  - For patients with nephrotic syndrome, prophylactic anticoagulation should be considered.
- Differentiating between lupus flare and preeclampsia in a woman with AKI:
  - Lupus flare: AKI may occur any time including prior to 20 weeks of gestation and postpartum, presence of hypocomplementemia, red blood cell casts, and leukopenia
  - Preeclampsia: AKI only occurs after 20 weeks of gestation with absence of findings seen with lupus flare above.
- Management of SLE/LN in pregnancy per KDIGO 2012:
  - Delay pregnancy until complete remission
  - Use of CYC, MMF, ACEI, and ARB is not recommended due to potential teratogenicity.
  - Methotrexate is teratogenic and is contraindicated in pregnancy. Methotrexate should be discontinued ≥3 months prior to conception.
  - Hydroxychloroquine maintenance therapy should be continued during pregnancy. Discontinuation of hydroxychloroquine may lead to lupus flares including LN.
  - LN patients who become pregnant while being treated with MMF be switched to AZA.
  - Patients with LN relapse during pregnancy should be treated with corticosteroids, and if necessary, AZA.
  - Patients receiving corticosteroids or AZA during pregnancy should not be tapered until at least 3 months postpartum.
  - Administration of low-dose aspirin during pregnancy is suggested to reduce risk of fetal loss.

POSTINFECTIOUS, POSTSTREPTOCOCCAL GN

Epidemiology

- Decreased incidence in industrialized countries
- Traditionally disease in children, now seen in debilitated elderly, patients with chronic alcoholism, DM, or IV drug abuse, and in poor communities due to lack of early medical care, antibiotics, and/or fluorinated water. Fluorinated water reduces expression of virulence factors in *Streptococcus pyogenes*.

Pathogenesis

- Likely C3-mediated. Previously thought to be Ab-mediated against bacterial antigens: glyceraldehyde-3-phosphate dehydrogenase (GAPDH), streptococcal pyrogenic exotoxin B (SPEB) and its more immunogenic precursor zymogen.
- Incubation is ~2 weeks after throat infection versus several weeks post skin infections.

Clinical Manifestations

- Hypertension, edema, hematuria "coca cola urine," azotemia common in adults, less commonly, nephrotic syndrome

Laboratory Findings

- Positive *Streptoccocus* culture in up to 70% during epidemics; 20% to 25% of sporadic cases
- Antistreptolysin O (ASO) titers are increased in >2/3 of cases with poststreptococcal GN (PSGN) post throat infection
- Anti-DNAse B titers are increased in 73% of post impetigo cases (greater than two times normal)
- Others: streptozyme panel (ASO, anti-DNAse B, antihyaluronidase, antistreptokinase) is more sensitive and is positive in >80%
- C3 is decreased in >90%; C4 typically normal; serum IgG and IgM elevated in 80%
- Cryoglobulins and rheumatoid factor are increased in up to 1/3 of cases.
- Anti-DNA and ANCA may be positive in rare cases and are of unknown clinical significance.

Histopathology

- LM: Leukocytes, often neutrophils, in and occluding glomerular capillaries (large "bloodless" glomeruli). Crescents may be present (Fig. 7.4)
- IF: Irregular granular capillary and mesangial strong staining for C3 usually with small amounts of IgG and/or IgM. Has been described as "starry sky," "garland" and "mesangial" patterns likely related to timing of biopsy
- EM: Large single subepithelial "hump" or "gumdrop" shaped deposits often at the mesangial waist or notch area where the capillary meets the mesangium

Natural History/Prognosis

- Typically resolves within a few weeks
- Prognosis is excellent in children
- Elderly: azotemia (60% to 70%), congestive heart failure (40%), early mortality (25%)
- Mild proteinuria < 500 mg/d may persists for several months.
- Microscopic hematuria may persists up to a year.

> **NOTE** Hypocomplementemia should resolve within a month, otherwise, consider misdiagnosis of SLE or MPGN.

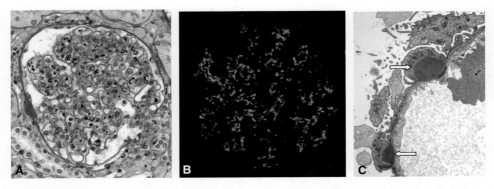

FIGURE 7.4 Postinfectious (infection-related) glomerulonephritis. **A.** Endocapillary hypercellularity with many leukocytes, including neutrophils, occluding glomerular capillary lumens (Periodic acid–Schiff, ×400). **B.** Irregular granular C3 in glomerulus (×400). **C.** Individual "hump"-shaped subepithelial deposits (*arrows*) (×19,000).

Management

- Penicillin (PCN) or erythromycin for 7 to 10 days if PCN allergic even if no persistent infection to decrease antigenic load
- Preventive antimicrobial therapy considerations:
  - At risk populations during epidemics
  - Siblings of affected individuals with *Streptococcal* infection within 2 to 3 weeks
- Other supportive therapies: dialysis support, treatment of hypertension

MEMBRANOPROLIFERATIVE GLOMERULONEPHRITIS, A.K.A. MESANGIOCAPILLARY GLOMERULONEPHRITIS

Epidemiology

- MPGN is a glomerular injury pattern common to a heterogeneous group of diseases.
- Most commonly presents in childhood but can occur at any age
- Accounts for 7% to 10% of all cases of biopsy-confirmed GN
- Third or fourth leading cause of ESRD among primary GN

Histopathology

- LM:
  - Mesangial hypercellularity, endocapillary proliferation, and capillary wall remodeling (with formation of double contours), all leading to lobular accentuation of glomerular tufts (chunky segments/pieces) (Fig. 7.5).
  - Glomerular changes are due to deposition of complement factors with or without immunoglobulins in the glomerular mesangium and along capillary walls.
- EM: Subendothelial deposits with mesangial migration and interposition with duplication of basement membrane forming capillary double contours, variable mesangial deposits, subepithelial and intramembranous deposits in type III MPGN. Traditional classification of MPGN was based on EM findings:
  - MPGN I: subendothelial deposits
    - Idiopathic
    - Secondary causes: subacute/chronic infections, hepatitis C > B, cryoglobulinemia, lymphoproliferative malignancies, carcinomas, C2 or C3 deficiency, autoimmune disease, C3 glomerulopathy
  - MPGN III: MPGN type I features with additional subepithelial and/or intramembranous deposits.

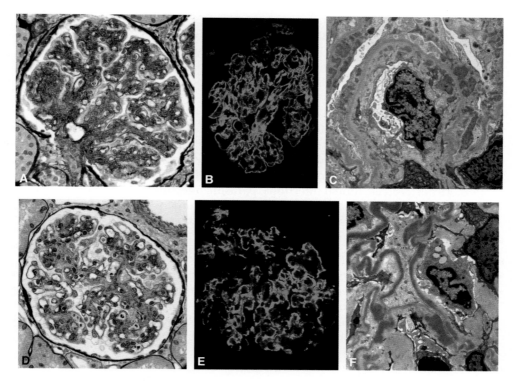

FIGURE 7.5 Membranoproliferative glomerulonephritis. **A.** Lobular hypercellular glomerulus (Jones silver, ×400). **B.** IgG in a peripheral granular and mesangial pattern in immune complex–mediated MPGN (×250). **C.** Subendothelial deposits with new basement membrane deposition forming a double contour in immune complex–mediated MPGN. There also are scattered subepithelial deposits (×10,000). **D.** Dense deposit disease showing silver negative material in widened mesangial regions and capillary walls (Jones silver, ×400). **E.** Coarse linear and segmental coarse granular C3 deposition in dense deposit disease (×400). **F.** Electron dense transformation of capillary basement membranes and segmental mesangial matrix in dense deposit disease (×10,000).

- MPGN II: dense deposits in GBM, a.k.a. "dense-deposit disease," **"DDD"**
  - Idiopathic
  - Secondary causes: complement dysregulation due to deficiency or mutations of complement regulatory proteins, autoantibody formation against regulatory proteins, C3 nephritic factor autoantibodies (C3NeF), familial and acquired partial lipodystrophy
- MPGN I and MPGN III may be either immune complex–mediated or complement-mediated GN.
- IF: Findings from IF studies may define the underlying pathogenesis of the MPGN.

> **NOTE** Current classification of MPGN is based on its underlying pathogenesis as immune complex-mediated, complement-mediated, or neither.

Immune Complex–Mediated MPGN:
- Involves classical pathway
- IF typically shows *both* Ig and complement deposits.
- Proposed sequence of events:
  - Chronic increase in immunoglobulin production due to infections, autoimmune disease, or monoclonal gammopathies leads to:
  - Binding of the immunoglobulins to GBM and activation of the complement cascade and induction of inflammatory changes (cellular or proliferative), followed by a:

- Reparative phase where new mesangial matrix is formed (mesangial expansion) along with new GBM formation (duplication of GBM "tram tracks or double contours"). New GBM formation may entrap capillary wall deposits ± inflammatory cells, mesangial, and endothelial cells, leading to thickened appearance of capillary walls and formation of double contours along capillary walls.
- Conditions leading to increased Ig production:
  - Infections: chronic viral infections (e.g., hepatitis C >> B ± cryoglobulins); bacterial infections (endocarditis, shunt/indwelling catheter nephritis, abscesses; common organisms: *Staphylococcus, Mycobacterium tuberculosis*, streptococci, *Propioibacterium acnes, Mycoplasma pneumoniae, Brucella, Coxiella burnetii, Nocardia, Meningococcus*; fungal infections, parasitic infections
  - Autoimmune diseases: systemic lupus erythematosus, Sjögren syndrome, rheumatoid arthritis, mixed connective tissue diseases
  - Paraproteinemias: monoclonal gammopathies ± cryoglobulins

Complement-Mediated MPGN:
- Involves complement dysregulation in the alternative pathway
- Dysregulated complement activation leads to abnormal C3 convertase activity and resultant inflammatory changes, endothelial/GBM/podocyte injury, and subsequent reparative phase similar to that seen with immune complex–mediated injury. With the exception of DDD, EM *cannot* distinguish between immune complex–mediated and complement-mediated MPGN.
- Dysregulation of complement activation may occur via different mechanisms:
  - Antibody formation against:
    - C3 convertase (antibodies against C3 convertase are also known as C3 nephritic factor (C3NF)—C3NF binds to and stabilizes C3 convertase, thereby prolonging its half-life and allowing continuing activation of the alternative pathway.
    - Complement regulators (Factor H, I, or B)
  - Mutations of complement regulators: factor H, factor I, membrane cofactor protein MCP/CD46, complement factor H-related protein CFHR5, CFHR 3-1
  - Allele variants: C3, MCP
  - Dysregulation of alternative pathway may be subdivided into **DDD** and C3 glomerulonephritis (**C3GN**) based on EM findings. Both disease entities, however, are thought to be part of a continuum of the same condition. Differences in histopathology are likely due to the degree or site, or both, of the dysregulation of the alternative pathway. Certain allele variations of complement regulating proteins may be associated with DDD, while others (e.g., CFHR5) with C3GN.
    - **DDD**: Characterized by osmiophilic, sausage-shaped, wavy, dense deposits that replace GBM and also occur in mesangium (old classification: MPGN II). MPGN II is associated with partial lipodystrophy and ocular drusen.
    - **C3GN** is characterized by mesangial, subendothelial, and sometimes subepithelial and intramembranous deposits (old classification: MPGN I or MPGN III).

MPGN without IC or complement:
- May be seen with thrombotic microangiopathies (TMA)
- Pathologic characteristics: absence of immunoglobulins or complements on IF; absence of electron-dense deposits in mesangium or capillary walls on EM
- Associated conditions: thrombotic thrombocytopenic purpura or hemolytic-uremic syndrome, atypical hemolytic-uremic syndrome, antiphospholipid antibody

syndrome, drug-induced TMA, malignant hypertension, radiation nephritis, bone marrow transplant-associated nephropathy, connective tissue disorders

Clinical Manifestations

- Asymptomatic hematuria and proteinuria
- Acute nephritic syndrome
- Nephrotic syndrome
- CKD
- Rapidly progressive glomerulonephopathy

Diagnosis

Complement levels:
- IC-mediated MPGN: typically low C3 *and* low C4
- Complement-mediated MPGN: typically low (but may be normal) C3 and normal C4
- Serologies per kidney biopsy:
  - Immunofluorescence with both immunoglobulin and complement deposits:
    - Blood cultures, polymerase chain reaction and serologic tests for viral (e.g., hepatitis B, C, cytomegalovirus (CMV), bacterial, occult infections, malaria, and fungal infections (per local prevalence and/or symptoms)
    - Cryoglobulins, (consider rheumatoid factor: 70% cross-reactivity with cryoglobulins)
    - Serum protein electrophoresis and immunofixation, serum free light chains
    - Screening for autoimmune disorders, particularly SLE
  - Immunofluorescence with complement deposits alone (with or without dense deposits on EM):
    - Evaluation of alternative pathway: serum complement levels, serum membrane-attack complex levels, alternative pathway functional assay, hemolytic complement assay
    - Retinal scan to evaluate for ocular drusen
    - Consider genetic analysis for mutations and allele variants of complement factors and assays for presence of autoantibodies to complement-regulating proteins, including C3 nephritic factor.
    - Evaluation of monoclonal gammopathy (particularly in older individuals)
  - Immunofluorescence without immunoglobulin or complement deposits: C3, complement factor H, ADAMST13, blood smear for schistocytes, LDH, indirect bilirubin, platelet count and volume

Management

Routine:
- Use ACEI or ARB for proteinuria as safely tolerated.
- Anticoagulation and antiplatelet therapy such as combination of aspirin plus dypiridamole are of unclear long-term benefit.

Specific therapy:
- Idiopathic MPGN: *all* MPGN patients must be evaluated for secondary causes.
- KDIQO suggests that patients with presumed idiopathic MPGN accompanied by nephrotic syndrome *and* decline in kidney function may be treated with either PO CYC or MMF *and* alternating or daily steroids, with initial therapy limited to 6 months.

- Secondary MPGN: Treat underlying disease (i.e., infections, monoclonal gammopathy, autoimmune disease) if applicable.
  - Rituximab may be beneficial if monoclonal gammopathy but without overt hematologic malignancy.
  - Consider plasmapheresis if association with symptomatic cryoglobulinemia.
- Glucocorticoids as monotherapy in adults: currently undefined
- Rapidly progressive disease or crescentic glomerulonephritis: Limited data but may consider CNI, high-dose pulse steroids as monotherapy or in combination with AZA, CYC, or MMF.
- MPGN due to complement dysregulation due to factor H abnormality or C3 nephritic factor autoantibody formation:
  - Glucocorticoids + cytotoxic agents
  - Consider plasmapheresis in severe cases.
- MPGN due to congenital mutations leading to complement dysregulation:
  - Consider therapy that inhibits membrane attack complex (MAC) formation (e.g., eculizumab), particularly if high serum levels of MAC.
  - Eculizumab is an anti-C5 monoclonal antibody that inhibits C5 activation.
    - Eculizumab has been shown effective in the treatment of atypical HUS due to complement dysregulation in the alternative pathway.
    - Eculizumab may be effective in some patients with DDD.

Kidney Transplantation

- High recurrence rates: MPGN I (15% to 50%), DDD (80% to 100%)
- DDD: universal recurrence (80% to 100%)

NEPHROTIC/HEAVY-PROTEINURIC GLOMERULAR DISORDERS

Minimal Change Disease

Background

Most common cause of nephrotic syndrome in children (70% to 90% of nephrotic syndrome in children < 10 years of age); 50% in older children; 10% to 15% of primary nephrotic syndrome in adults

Pathology

- LM: normal glomeruli (Fig. 7.6)
  - Tubules may have acute injury and luminal proteinaceous material due to heavy proteinuria.
  - Other glomerulonephropathies that may present with minor changes on LM include: IgM nephropathy, C1q nephropathy, minimal mesangial LN.
- IF: no immunoglobulin or complement deposition
- EM: podocyte foot process effacement (>75%)

Clinical Manifestation

- NOTE: classic presentation of MCD is sudden onset of edema (i.e., days to weeks) as opposed to slowly progressive edema seen with MGN and most forms of FSGS, except tip variant.
- Nephrotic syndrome

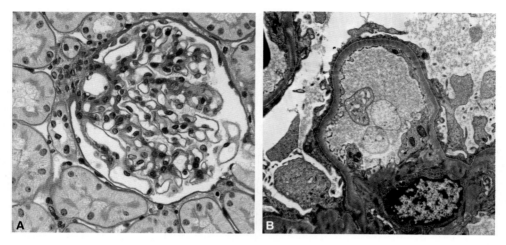

FIGURE 7.6 Minimal change disease. **A.** Normal glomerulus (Periodic acid–Schiff, ×400). **B.** Extensive podocyte foot process effacement over normal capillary basement membrane (×14,000).

- Microscopic hematuria is seen in 20% to 25% in children, but more commonly in adults.
- AKI at presentation: common and often improve with diuresis, treatment of anasarca. Renal vein thrombosis should also be considered.

Pathogenesis

- T-cell dysfunction (likely immature and relatively undifferentiated T cells (CD34+) rather than mature T cells (CD34−) have been implicated in the pathogenesis of MCD):
  - MCD improves with measles (known to modulate cell-mediated immunity).
  - MCD seen more commonly in patients with Hodgkin disease
  - Atopic individuals are at higher risk for MCD.
- B-cell dysfunction:
  - Rituximab (chimeric monoclonal antibody that depletes the B-20 cells) may improve steroid sensitive disease, suggesting a possible role for a glomerular permeability factor produced by B or T cells through pathways regulated or stimulated by B cells.
  - Glomerular permeability factor possible, likely T_H2-derived cytokines, e.g., interleukin IL-13. IL-13 induces CD80 expression, which can induce podocyte fusion and proteinuria. Notably, IL-13 is associated with allergic states, conditions associated with MCD.
- Alterations in GBM, loss of negative charges induced by circulating factor
- Defect/alterations of key proteins in slit diaphragm, e.g., mutation of NPHS2 (nephrin) gene
- Drug-induced direct injury to podocytes

Clinical Conditions Associated with MCD

- Malignancies: lymphomas, Hodgkins, non-Hodgkins leukemia, rarely solid organ tumors
- Allergy, atopy, insect/bee stings, pollens, house dust
- Immunizations

- Drugs: NSAIDS and selective COX-2 inhibitors (long-term use), pamidronate, alendronate (both bisphosphonates are also associated with FSGS), lithium, D-penicillamine, tiopronin, γ-interferon, sulfasalazine and 5-aminosalicylic acid derivatives, antimicrobials (rifampin, PCN derivatives)

Management of MCD (KDIGO 2012)

Initial episode:
- Prednisone or prednisolone at 1 mg/kg/d (maximum 80 mg/d) or alternate day dose of 2 mg/kg (maximum 120 mg) for ≥4 to 16 weeks as dictated by remission. NOTE: Daily and alternating steroid dosing are equivalent in terms of complications and achieving remission.
- Once remission occurs, slowly taper to off for up to 6 months.
- For glucocorticoid relative contraindications or intolerance (e.g., uncontrolled diabetes, psychiatric conditions, severe osteoporosis), consider PO CYC or CNIs
- For patients with infrequent relapses, restart glucocorticoids as mentioned earlier.

Frequent relapsing (i.e., ≥2 within 6 months or ≥4 within 12 months) or steroid dependent (two relapses on steroid taper or within 1 month of ending therapy) MCD:
- Oral CYC 2 to 2.5 mg/kg/d for 8 weeks is suggested.
- CNI: cyclosporine 3 to 5 mg/kg/d or TAC 0.05 to 0.1 mg/kg/d in divided doses for 1 to 2 years for those who relapse despite CYC or those who wish to preserve fertility
- MMF 500 to 1,000 mg twice daily for 1 to 2 years for those who are intolerant to corticosteroids, CYC, and CNIs

Supportive therapy:
- For severe AKI, renal-replacement therapy may be necessary in combination with immunosuppressive therapy above.
- Statins not be used to treat hyperlipidemia as risk of coronary artery disease is *not* increased with MCD. Benefit of statin's anti-inflammatory property has not been proven.
- ACEI or ARBs use is *not* suggested in normotensive individuals with MCD for the *sole purpose* of lowering proteinuria.

> **NOTE**
> - In case of steroid resistant or frequent relapsing MCD, consider erroneous diagnosis due to poor tissue sampling. Rebiopsy to evaluate for FSGS should be considered.
> - There are limited data that patients with steroid dependent/frequent relapse MCD may benefit from rituximab.

FOCAL SEGMENTAL GLOMERULOSCLEROSIS

Background

- FSGS is the most common cause of nephrotic syndrome in African American adults and most common cause of GN-related ESRD in Black and White patients in the United States.
- FSGS refers to a morphologic pattern of glomerular injury that may arise from a *primary* podocytopathy or *secondary* adaptive process involving nephron mass reduction, reflux nephropathy, viral or drug toxicity, genetic mutations, or other glomerular disease.
- Histopathologic findings: segmental increase of mesangial matrix with obliteration of capillaries, sclerosis, hyalinosis, foam cells, podocyte hypertrophy with or without hyperplasia, and adhesions between glomerular tuft and Bowman capsule.
- NOTE: The *deep* inner juxtamedullary glomeruli are preferentially affected in early primary FSGS. Renal biopsies containing <15 glomeruli or only cortical glomeruli cannot exclude FSGS.

Classification of FSGS

- FSGS arising from primary alteration of glomerular epithelial cell:
  - Occurs with podocytopathies (e.g., genetic disorders), drugs, viral infections and primary FSGS. See Etiologies of FSGS below.
  - Sudden onset edema and proteinuria
  - Nephrotic syndrome (proteinuria > 3.5 g/d and serum albumin < 3.5 g/dL)
  - Widespread foot process effacement of nonsclerotic glomeruli on EM
- FSGS arising from reduced nephron mass or glomerular adaptations to injurious insults. See Etiologies of FSGS below.
  - Development of edema and proteinuria are usually slowly progressive.
  - Does not typically present with nephrotic syndrome
  - EM generally reveals <80% segmental foot process effacement of nonsclerotic glomeruli.
- FSGS arising from focal proliferative GN or hereditary nephropathies such as Alport syndrome.

Genetic Predisposition to FSGS

- APOL1: located on chromosome 22, in linkage disequilibrium with MYH9, codes for apolipoprotein L-1
- Missense mutations of APOL1 are thought to predispose patients of African descents (rather than MYH9 in earlier reports) to an excess risk of FSGS, HIVAN and chronic hypertensive nephrosclerosis. Greatest risk: mutation of 2 alleles.
- The same APOL1 mutations are protective against *Trypanosoma brucei*, a parasite spread by tsetse flies in Africa.

Etiologies of FSGS

- Primary FSGS:
  - Presence of the soluble form of urokinase receptor (suPAR) was previously thought to be a candidate in the pathogenesis of primary FSGS. This has been largely disproved.
  - Cardiotropin-like cytokine circulating factor has also been implicated in primary FSGS.
  - Pathogenic circulating factor for primary FSGS remains unknown.
- All other etiologies of FSGS:
  - Familial/genetic: mutations including nephrin (NPHS1), podocin (NPHS2), α-actinin 4, transient receptor potential cation 6 (TRPC6), WT1, informin-2, SCARB2 (LIMP2), formin (INF2), CD2-associated protein, mitochondrial cytopathies
  - Virus: human immunodeficiency virus type-1, parvovirus B19, simian virus 40, CMV, Epstein–Barr virus
  - Drugs: heroin, interferons α, β, and γ), lithium, pamidronate, alendronate, sirolimus, anabolic steroids, CNIs
  - Adaptive structural–functional responses
    - Reduced renal mass: low birth weight, oligomeganephronia, premature birth, unilateral kidney agenesis, reflux uropathy, chronic allograft nephropathy, advanced renal disease with reductions in functioning nephrons
    - Initially normal renal mass: hypertension, DM, atheroemboli/acute vaso-occlusive process, obesity, increased lean body mass, anabolic steroids (body builders), cyanotic congenital heart disease, sickle cell anemia
  - Malignancy (lymphoma)

- Association with any underlying glomerular diseases: IgAN, LN, pauci-immune focal necrotizing and crescentic GN, hereditary nephritis (Alport syndrome), membranous glomerulopathy, TMA

Histopathology of FSGS Variants

- **Not-otherwise-specified (NOS)** FSGS:
  - Generic form of FSGS, not meeting any variant below (Fig. 7.7)
  - Associations: most common subtype, can occur with primary or secondary including genetic forms; other forms can evolve into NOS over time
  - Clinical features: variable
- **Perihilar** FSGS:
  - Lesions at glomerular **vascular pole** thought to reflect increased filtration pressures at the afferent arterioles associated with compensatory demand, glomerular hypertrophy, foot process effacement typically not severe and segmental
  - Associations: adaptive FSGS (see Etiologies of FSGS)

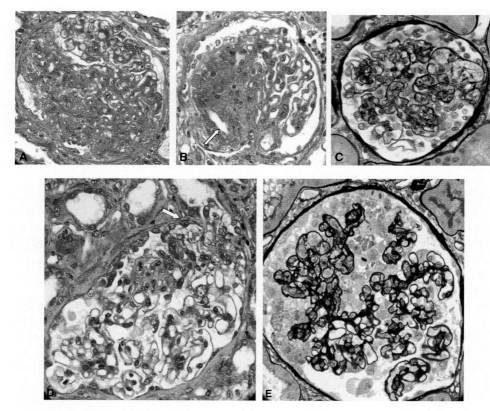

FIGURE 7.7 Focal and segmental glomerulosclerosis. **A.** Not otherwise-specified variant. Segmental capillary obliteration, podocyte hypertrophy, adhesions to Bowman capsule and insudative lesions not at the tip or perihilar region (Masson trichrome, ×400). **B.** Perihilar variant. Segment of sclerosis is adjacent to the arteriolar pole (*arrow*) and characterized by capillary obliteration, insudative lesions (orange) and overlying halo formation (podocyte detachment with deposition of new light-blue basement membrane material) (Masson trichrome, ×400). **C.** Cellular variant. Segmentally, capillaries contain foam cells and leukocytes in association with podocyte hypertrophy (Jones silver, ×400). **D.** Tip lesion variant. Podocyte hypertrophy and capillary obliteration are adjacent to the tubular pole (*arrow*). Note the sclerotic segment protruding into the proximal tubular lumen (Mason trichrome, ×400). **E.** Collapsing variant. Capillary wall collapse and luminal obliteration with podocyte hypertrophy, hyperplasia, and cytoplasmic vacuoles and protein droplets (Jones silver, ×400).

- Clinical features: typically subnephrotic proteinuria and normal serum albumin levels
- **Cellular** FSGS:
  - Least common variant
  - Expansile segmental lesion with **endocapillary hypercellularity**, often including foam cells and infiltrating leukocytes; variable glomerular epithelial cell hyperplasia
  - Severe foot-process effacement typical on EM
  - Associations: usually primary, but may be seen with secondary causes
  - May represent early stage in the evolution of FSGS or tip lesion without proper glomerular orientation
  - Clinical features: typically nephrotic syndrome
- **Tip** lesion FSGS:
  - Segmental lesion involving **tubular pole**, with either adhesion to tubular outlet or confluence of hypertrophic podocytes and tubular epithelial cells, may herniate into proximal tubule, often foam cells.
  - Compared with other variants, tip lesion has the least tubular atrophy and interstitial fibrosis; severe foot-process effacement is typical.
  - Tip lesion is more common in white race.
  - Associations: usually primary; thought to be mediated by physical stresses on paratubular segment due to convergence of protein-rich filtrate on tubular pole
  - Clinical features: usually abrupt onset of nephrotic syndrome; best prognosis, highest rate of response to glucocorticoids compared to all other FSGS variants
- **Collapsing** FSGS:
  - **Implosive glomerular-tuft collapse** with hypertrophy and hyperplasia of overlying epithelial cells; **hyperplastic glomerular epithelial cells** may fill urinary space, resembling crescents; severe tubular injury; tubular microcysts common; severe foot-process effacement
  - Associations: primary or secondary
  - Clinical features: most aggressive variant of primary FSGS, black racial predominance and severe nephrotic syndrome; worse prognosis, poor response to glucocorticoids.

Management of FSGS (KDIGO 2012)

- Routine therapy for all FSGS variants: RAAS inhibition and dietary sodium restriction
- Primary FSGS with subnephrotic proteinuria:
  - If no response or worsening of disease to routine therapy above, add glucocorticoids daily or alternate $\times$ at least 4 weeks, continue high dose up to a maximum of 16 week trial (prednisone 1 mg/kg (maximum 80 mg) daily or 2 mg/kg (maximum 120 mg) alternate day
  - If still no improvement or intolerance to glucocorticoids, (e.g., uncontrolled diabetes, psychiatric conditions, severe osteoporosis), consider CNI.
  - Once remission is achieved (complete remission: proteinuria < 0.3 g/d, normal SCr and serum albumin > 3.5 g/dL; partial remission: proteinuria 0.3 to 3.5 g/d, stable SCr or change in SCr by <25%), taper steroids slowly over 6 months.
  - Steroid-resistant FSGS (persistence of nephrotic syndrome after 4 months of prednisone at 1 mg/kg/d): CNI *plus* prednisone
    - Cyclosporine is thought to exert an antiproteinuric effect on the podocyte actin cytoskeleton independent of its immunosuppressive effect.

- Cyclosporine 3 to 5 mg/kg/d in divided doses (target levels 125 to 175 ng/mL) for at least 4 to 6 months (or TAC 0.1 to 0.2 mg/kg/d in two divided doses (target levels 5 to 10 ng/mL).
- If complete or partial remission, continue CNI for at least 12 months, followed by slow taper (reduce dose by 25% every 2 months).
- If no remission by 6 months, discontinue therapy.
- For steroid resistant FSGS and cyclosporine intolerance, combination of MMF and high-dose dexamethasone (0.15 mg/kg/d for 4 to 6 months, then taper off over 4 to 8 weeks) is suggested. Other options: ACTH gel (ACTHAR), rituximab, pirfenidone (anti-fibrotic agent), fresolimumab (anti-TGFβ antibody)
- Steroid dependent FSGS: two relapses during or within 2 weeks of completing steroid therapy: treatment is similar to relapsing MCD in adults. Relapse is defined as proteinuria > 3.5 g/d after complete remission has been obtained.
- Primary FSGS with nephrotic range proteinuria:
  - Glucocorticoids daily or alternate day × 16 week trial
  - If no improvement or intolerance to glucocorticoids, consider CNI.
- Adaptive FSGS: no immunosuppressive therapy; encourage weight loss if obese.
- Secondary FSGS: treat underlying disease or removal of etiologic agents

Kidney Transplantation

- Recurrence occurs in 20% to 50% of primary FSGS.
- Risks for recurrence:
  - Children younger than 15 years old
  - Rapid course of ESRD (<3 years in native kidneys)
  - Heavy proteinuria prior to transplantation
  - Loss of previous allografts to recurrence
- Plasmapheresis used in the early course of disease recurrence have been met with variable success.

MEMBRANOUS GLOMERULONEPHROPATHY

Epidemiology

- Less than 5% in children and 15% to 50% in adults with nephrotic syndrome
- Male-to-female ratio is 2:1
- US Renal Data System: 0.5% of end-stage kidney disease population
- HLA-associated inherited risks reported
- Familial forms reported but rare

Histopathology

- LM:
  - Variably thick capillary walls; *no* hypercellularity or inflammatory changes (Fig. 7.8)
  - Methenamine (Jones) silver staining: projections of GBM between deposits giving a characteristic spike like pattern (stage 2). Resorption of subepithelial and intramembranous immune deposits leads GBM thickening with lucencies or double contours (stages 3 to 4)
  - Glomerular leukocyte infiltration may occur in association with malignancy; polymorphonuclear leukocytes (PMN) infiltrates with renal vein thrombosis

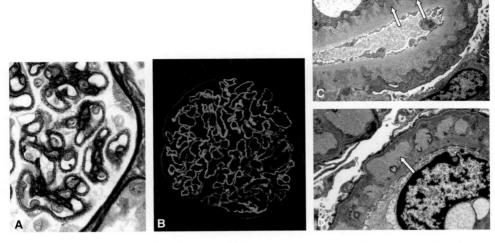

FIGURE 7.8 Membranous glomerulonephropathy. **A.** Global subepithelial deposits with intervening spikes of basement membrane material (Ehrenreich and Churg stage 2) (Jones silver, ×600). **B.** Immunofluorescence for IgG showing granular capillary wall staining (×400). **C.** Subepithelial electron dense deposits (*arrows*) with intervening spikes of basement membrane material (×14,000). **D.** Predominantly cleared intramembranous deposits (*arrow*) with new subepithelial layer of basement membrane material in stage 4 (×14,000).

- Concurrent FSGS is present in up to 30% and may portend worse prognosis, example, rapid progression and poor response to therapy.
- Tubulointerstitial injury and fibrosis are common; may indicate advanced disease.
- EM:
  - Diffuse subepithelial granular electron dense deposits that parallel IgG staining
  - In idiopathic MGN, deposits are not seen in mesangial or subendothelial sites, whereas in secondary MGN, there may be mesangial hypercellularity and deposits in mesangial ± endothelial sites.
  - Foot process effacement
- IF: IgG and complement components deposits
  - Generally, staining for IgG4 dominates in idiopathic MGN (iMGN), whereas IgG1, 2, and/or 3 dominate in secondary MGN.
  - C3 is present in ~50% of patients and likely reflects active, ongoing immune deposit formation and complement activation. C1 and C4 are usually absent, indicating involvement of alternative pathway in association with podocyte injury. Minimal C3 staining suggests inactive or very early disease.
  - Strong capillary staining for C1q, C3, IgG, IgM, and IgA, a.k.a. "full house," is associated with membranous lupus.

Pathogenesis
- Antibody–antigen (Ab–Ag) formation at podocytes leads to complement activation, formation of C5b-9.
  - Ab–Ag complexes are capped and shed to form subepithelial deposits. C5b-9 complexes (a.k.a. MACs) are incorporated into multivesicular bodies and transported by podocyte into urinary space.
  - Increased intracellular sublytic levels of C5b-9 activate podocytes, leading to release of oxidants and proteases that would lead to injury of underlying GBM.

- What are the responsible *antigens* that lead to the development of MGN?
  - Antigens associated with "idiopathic" MGN (iMGN):
    - Phospholipase A_2 receptor 1 antigen expressed on podocyte surface: antibodies made against PLA2R1 are anti-PLA2R1 antibody, IgG4 subtype (80% of iMGN).
      - Anti-PLA2R1 correlates with disease activity
      - Anti-PLA2R1 predicts outcome: lower titer is associated with better rate of spontaneous remissions and time to remission in those requiring therapy.
    - Thrombospondin type-1 domain-containing 7A antigen (THSD7A) (10% of iMGN)

> **NOTE** iMGN is a diagnosis of *exclusion*. Secondary evaluation must still be performed even when biopsy findings suggest iMGN. iMGN is more common in adults, but secondary MGN is more common in children (e.g., in association with hepatitis B).

  - Antigens associated with secondary MGN:
    - Autoimmune (dysregulated autoantibody formation against self-antigen): SLE, diabetes, rheumatoid arthritis, mixed connective tissue disease, dermatomyositis, ankylosing spondylitis, Crohn disease, graft versus host disease, temporal arteritis, Sjögren's, bullous pemphigoid, autoimmune thyroid disease
    - Infectious antigens (think of chronic active infections): hepatitis B (presence of HBsAg, HBcAg and usually HBeAg) >> C, syphilis, tuberculosis, HIV, enterococcal endocarditis, leprosy, filariasis, malaria, schistosomiasis, hydatid disease
    - Drugs/toxins: captopril, gold penicillamine, nonsteroidal anti-inflammatory drugs, COX-2 inhibitors, hydrocarbons, mercury, formaldehyde, lithium, clopidogrel
    - Malignancies (tumor antigen): solid organs (lungs, GI, breast, kidney, etc.).
    - Neutral endopeptidase (NEP—antigen expressed on podocytes)—Mothers without NEP may make antibodies (Abs) against fetal NEP and transfer the Abs to the fetus. These infants are born with nephrotic syndrome.

Clinical Manifestations

- Gradual onset (as opposed to acute onset in MCD and often FSGS tip variant)
- Nephrotic syndrome common (60% to 80%), benign urinary sediment
- Microscopic hematuria (25% to 50%)
- Complements are typically normal, but can be low in ~50% of HBV-associated MGN
- *Increased risk* for thromboembolic disease (e.g., deep vein thrombosis, renal vein thrombosis, pulmonary embolism) (40%)
- Blood pressures normal to mildly elevated
- Dyslipidemia, increased cardiovascular risk
- Up to five times increased incidence of associated malignancy especially in those > 65 years old
- Resolution may occur within 1 week (NSAIDS) to years (gold, penicillamine), following withdrawal of responsible drugs.
- Natural history of iMGN: one-third rule: one-third achieves spontaneous remission, 1/3 remains the same, one-third slowly progresses to renal failure.
- Risks for worse renal outcome: older age, male gender, hypertension, severe hypoalbuminemia, reduced GFR, severe proteinuria (e.g., >8 g/d lasting >6 m), increased

urinary IgG, β_2-microglobulin, or C5b-9 excretion, biopsy with marked tubulointerstitial disease, glomerular focal sclerosis, or extensive GBM damage (overly thickened membrane, presence of lucencies due to resorbed immunoglobulin complexes)

- Risk stratification for iMGN disease progression (see Management section for immunosuppressive options):
  - Low risk (<5% chance of progression):
    - Normal kidney function and proteinuria < 4 g/d
    - Conservative management: if disease deteriorates, initiate immunosuppressive therapy
  - Medium risk:
    - Normal kidney function and persistent proteinuria ≥ 4 and <8 g/d
    - Conservative management for 6 m: if no improvement or deterioration of disease, initiate immunosuppressive therapy.
  - High risk:
    - Abnormal kidney function and/or persistent proteinuria > 8 g/d
    - Conservative management ≤ 6 m, if no improvement, initiate immunosuppressive therapy

Management (KDIGO 2012)

- Conservative management for all patients regardless of risks of progression:
  - ACEI or ARB as tolerated
  - Statin (if LDL > 100 mg/dL)
  - BP control < 130/80 mm Hg, consider ≤125/75 mm Hg if presenting proteinuria > 1 g/d
  - Evaluate for secondary causes particularly malignancy for older patients > 60 years old (i.e., chest CT, kidney ultrasound, urine cytology, mammography, upper endoscopy, colonoscopy, prostate ultrasound and biopsy, colposcopy as clinically appropriate and indicated)
  - Prophylactic anticoagulation therapy with oral warfarin (with heparin bridging) **may be considered** for iMGN patients with nephrotic syndrome, serum albumin < 2.0 to 2.5 g/dL *and* ≥1 of the following: proteinuria > 10 g/d, body mass index > 35 kg/m^2, prior history of thromboembolism, family history of thromboembolism with documented genetic predisposition, NYHA class III or IV congestive heart failure, recent abdominal or orthopedic surgery, or prolonged immobilization. It is reasonable to maintain anticoagulation over duration of nephrotic syndrome when serum albumin < 3.0 g/dL.
- Immunosuppressive therapy for iMGN should be considered in patients with nephrotic syndrome *and* at least *one* of the following:
  - Urinary protein excretion persistently exceeds 4 g/d *and* remains >50% of baseline value during an observation period of at least 6 m.
  - Presence of severe, disabling, or life-threatening symptoms related to nephrotic syndrome
  - SCr increases by ≥30% within 6 to 12 m from time of diagnosis, but baseline eGFR still ≥30 mL/min/1.73 m^2.
  - *Do not* use immunosuppressive therapy if SCr is persistently >3.5 mg/dL or eGFR < 30 mL/min/1.73 m^2 *and* reduction of kidney size on ultrasound *or* concomitant severe or potentially life-threatening infections.
- Other considerations:
  - A conservative management trial may be justified in patients with proteinuria < 4 g/d, improved proteinuria with conservative management, and preserved kidney function.

- Initiation of immunosuppressive therapy is indicated for patients with declining kidney function, disabling symptoms, or "full-blown" nephrotic syndrome persisting for ≥6 m.
- Risks versus benefits for those with advanced disease do not justify the use of immunosuppressive therapy (e.g., advanced interstitial fibrosis and tubular atrophy at biopsy, SCr > 3.5 mg/dL, or evidence of shrunken kidneys).

Immunosuppressive Therapy Options for iMGN

Ponticelli Protocol

- Months 1, 3, 5: methylprednisolone 1 g/d × 3 days, followed by oral methylprednisolone 0.5 mg/kg/d × 27 days (Table 7.4)
- Months 2, 4, 6: oral chlorambucil (0.15 to 0.2 mg/kg/d) or PO CYC (2.0 mg/kg/d) × 30 days

Table 7.4	Therapeutic options for idiopathic membranous glomerulonephropathy	
Treatment	**Efficacy**	**Comments**
Steroids alone	Not effective	Not recommended
Steroids + alkylating agents: cyclophosphamide or chlorambucil	Increase probability of complete or partial remission; improve long-term kidney survival	Cyclophosphamide is preferred over chlorambucil due to better safety profile. See text for Ponticelli regimen. Efficacy confirmed by randomized controlled trials. Caution: leukopenia, oncogenic risks (>36 g cumulative dose), gonadotoxicity. For iMGN resistant to initial steroids + alkylating agent therapy, switching to CNI therapy, and vice versa, is recommended.
Calcineurin inhibitors (CNI): cyclosporine or tacrolimus	Increase probability of complete or partial remission	Monitor CNI levels regularly and with unexplained rise in SCr. Discontinue if no partial or complete remission after 6 mo of therapy. Contraindicated for SCr > 2 mg/dL. Relapse is frequent after drug withdrawal. Caution: nephrotoxicity, hypertension risks. *Cyclosporine* 3.5–5 mg/kg/d orally in two equally divided doses 12 h apart *plus prednisone* 0.15 mg/kg/d × 6 m. Start at lower range and increase as safely tolerated. *Tacrolimus* 0.05–0.075 mg/kg/d orally in two divided doses 12 h apart, *without prednisone* for 6 to 12 m. Start at lower range and increase slowly as safely tolerated.
Mycophenolate mofetil (MMF)	May be effective if given with steroids—*not* when given alone	Limited data. MMF vs. cyclosporine for iMGN: similar complication rates. MMF may not be as effective as cyclosporine in terms of remission and relapse.
Adrenocorticotropic hormone (ACTH)	May be effective	Limited data. Awaiting randomized controlled trials. High cost
Rituximab	May be effective	Optimal dose and treatment duration unclear. No head-to-head comparison with other treatments. High cost

- Comments:
  - CYC is recommended over chlorambucil due to better safety profile.
  - Monitor SCr, urinary protein excretion, serum albumin, and white blood cell (WBC) count every 2 weeks × 2 months, then every month × 6 months.
  - Hold chlorambucil or CYC if WBC count < 3,500/mm^3 until recovery to >4,000/mm^3. Opinion: Restart at ~25% reduced dose.

Definitions of Complete and Partial Remission of iMGN

- Complete remission (CR): Urinary protein excretion < 0.3 g/d (or urine protein to creatinine ratio (uPCR) < 0.3 g/g creatinine), confirmed by two values at least 1 week apart, accompanied by a normal serum albumin concentration and normal SCr.
- Partial remission (PR): Urinary protein excretion < 3.5 g/d (or uPCR < 3.5 g/g creatinine), and a ≥50% reduction from peak values; confirmed by two values at least 1 week apart, accompanied by an improvement of normalization of serum albumin concentration and stable SCr.

PARAPROTEIN-RELATED DISORDERS

Multiple Myeloma and the Kidney

Epidemiology

- Kidney involvement is common:
  - 40% of patients present with SCr > 1.5 mg/dL.
  - Survival is associated with kidney function following treatment of multiple myeloma.

Renal Manifestations (Combination of Lesions May Be Present in Same Patient)

- Tubular involvement:
  - Light-chain (Bence Jones) cast nephropathy a.k.a. "myeloma kidney":
    - Most common renal presentation (40% to 60%) in association with elevated SCr
    - Pathogenesis: acute or chronic kidney injury due to filtration of toxic light chains leading to tubular injury and intratubular cast formation and obstruction.
    - Histopathology: (Fig. 7.9) LM: Light chain casts which are angulated, fractured or coarsely granular staining orange on Masson trichrome and PAS negative in distal tubules. Casts are often surrounded or engulfed by multinucleated giant cells. IF: casts stain strongly for the abnormal light chain, with minimal staining for other immune reactants.
    - Associated with "proteinuria mismatch." Proteinuria from cast nephropathy arises from the large amount of filtered free light chains (FLC) "Bence Jones protein," which, unlike albumin, are not well detected by the routine urinalysis dipstick. That is, while a urine dipstick may indicate "trace" or "1+" proteinuria, the actual quantification of proteinuria from a 24-hour urine collection or uPCR would be equivalent to "≥3+" proteinuria. Proteinuria mismatch may also be unmasked by the addition of sulfosalicylic acid (SSA) to the urine sample because SSA precipitates all proteins including all albumin as well as light chains.
    - Fanconi syndrome: proximal tubular injury due to the reabsorption and accumulation of crystallized nondegradable toxic variable domain fragments

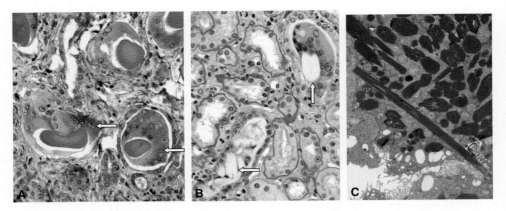

FIGURE 7.9 Light-chain lesions. **A and B.** Light-chain (Bence Jones) cast nephropathy. **A.** Orange light-chain casts with adjacent and engulfing multinucleated giant cells (*arrows*) (Masson trichrome, ×400). **B.** Periodic acid–Schiff negative light-chain casts (*arrows*), the upper right cast surrounded by a giant cell (Periodic acid–Schiff, ×400). **C.** Crystalline tubulopathy. Light chain depositing as electron dense crystals in tubular cells (×7,500).

of the filtered light chains. Patients may present with various proximal tubular transport defects including proximal renal tubular acidosis, phosphate wasting, uricosuria (hence hypouricemia), euglycemic glucosuria, and aminoaciduria.

- Histopathology: (Fig. 7.9) LM: Crystalline inclusions (stain as light blue on H&E) with tubular damage may be seen in proximal tubular cells. EM: proximal tubular cells are filled with electron-dense light-chain crystals with needle, rod, rhomboid, or rectangular shapes
  - Distal tubular dysfunction
- Interstitial involvement:
  - Plasma cell infiltration
  - Interstitial nephritis
- Glomerular involvement:
  - Primary amyloidosis (20% to 30%), (AL, ALH, or rarely AH)
    - Two-third of cases are from λ-light chains
    - Light chains are partially metabolized in macrophages then secreted. The metabolized fragments may precipitate into granular deposits and β-pleated fibrils as "amyloid," which is Congo-red positive.
    - Amyloid depositions within the kidney leading to extensive mesangial and GBM injury can manifest as significant albuminuria and nephrotic range proteinuria. Since routine urinalysis with a dipstick can detect albuminuria well, "proteinuria mismatch" is not characteristic of renal amyloidosis in contrast to that seen in myeloma kidney/cast nephropathy.
    - In the case of predominant interstitial and vascular involvement, progressive kidney injury occurs but with minimal proteinuria.
  - Monoconal Immunoglobulin Deposition Disease (MIDD) involves the deposition of monoclonal light chain (80%), and less commonly heavy chain (10%), or both (10%) in the mesangium and tubular and GBMs.
    - Monoclonal κ-light chain is most common with MIDD (two-third of cases)
    - Same pathogenesis as amyloidosis, but light chain fragments in this case do not form β-pleated fibrils and are Congo red negative.
    - As GBM is affected and significant albuminuria can occur, MIDD does not present with proteinuria mismatch.

- Others: MPGN, monoclonal cryoglobulinemia, proliferative GN with mono-clonal Ig deposits (PGNMID), intraglomerular IgM deposits with resultant thrombi formation (Waldenstroms macroglobulinemia), immunotactoid GN, fibrillary GN, and rarely MCD.
  - NOTE:
    - MPGN associated with monoclonal gammopathy often presents with both IgG and C3 deposits, or less commonly, IgM and C3 deposits. Rarely, some monoclonal Ig proteins and/or their fragments can inhibit comple-ment alternative pathway regulatory proteins (CfH or C3Bb) and induce a "complement-only" form of GN. Older patients with C3GN should there-fore also be evaluated for a monoclonal gammopathy.
    - PGNMID and immunotactoid GN may present with hypocomplemente-mia in 1/3 of cases.
    - Immunotactoid GN is much more commonly associated with monoclonal gammopathy/lymphoproliferative disease than fibrillary GN.
    - Fiber size difference: Amyloid fibrils are smallest with diameter 10 nm, fibrillary fibrils are 15 to 25 nm, immunotactoid microtubules are 30 to 50 nm and cryoglobulin microtubules are 20 to 30 nm.
    - See Table 7.5 and Figure 7.10: Electron microscopy: amyloidosis, fibrillary immunotactoid and cyroglobulin fibrils/microtubules
- Other complications associated with paraproteinemia:
  - Hypercalcemia: nephrocalcinosis, interstitial nephritis, reduced renal perfu-sion due to hypercalcemia induced vasoconstriction, intratubular calcium salt precipitations.
  - Hyperuricemia: acute uric acid nephropathy, interstitial nephritis
  - Light-chain deposition in muscle leading to rhabdomyolysis
  - Hyperviscosity syndrome:
    - Associated with excessive formation of abnormal polymers of IgA or IgG3 or κ-light chains
    - Clinical manifestations: blurred vision, neurologic symptoms, confusion, oral/nasal bleeding, heart failure, kidney injury/acute tubular necrosis
    - Treatment: plasmapheresis if obvious symptoms regardless of serum viscos-ity index. Serum viscosity index may not correlate well with symptoms.
  - Volume depletion:
    - Hypercalcemia-induced nephrogenic diabetes insipidus
    - Reduced oral intake
    - Cardiomyopathy (e.g., amyloid involvement)
  - Treatment related:
    - Drugs (NSAIDS), antibiotics
    - Use of intravenous contrast dye with computed tomography
    - Bisphosphonates (zolendronate: acute tubular necrosis; pamidronate, zolen-dronate: FSGS)

Diagnosis

- Nonspecific clues suggesting the possibility of paraproteinemia, multiple myeloma:
  - Urine studies:
    - Routine urinalysis is typically "bland."
    - Urine-free light chains > 1,500 mg/L, proteinuria mismatch, and low per-centage of albuminuria compared to total proteinuria indicate myeloma cast nephropathy.

Table 7.5	Amyloidosis, fibrillary glomerulonephropathy, and immunotactoid glomerulonephropathy		
	Amyloidosis	**Fibrillary GN**	**Immunotactoid GN**
Clinical manifestations	Depends on type of amyloid; Typical: waxy skin, easy bruising, enlarged muscles, liver, tongue, heart failure, abnormal cardiac conduction, proteinuria, peripheral, autonomic neuropathy, coagulopathy	Mean age 50 y; hematuria, proteinuria, nephrotic syndrome, hypertension, elevated serum creatinine	Older population compared to fibrillary GN; one-third of patients have *hypocomplementemia*
Clinical associations	Primary (AL) predominantly due to monoclonal Ig light chain fragments and secondary (AA) due to chronic inflammatory diseases; periodic fever syndromes (e.g., familial Mediterranean fevers)	Idiopathic; may be associated with malignancy, low association with monoclonal gammopathy (15%); autoimmune diseases; hepatitis C	Idiopathic; *frequent* association with chronic lymphocytic leukemia and B cell lymphomas, 60%–70% with monoclonal gammopathy; cryoglobulinemia and lupus; hepatitis C
Monoclonality	Yes—AL	Oligotypic (IgGl + IgG4) much more common than monotypic deposits	Predominantly monoclonal
Light microscopy	Nodular or diffuse pink deposits of amorphous materials in mesangial matrix and basement membranes of capillary loops, arteriolar walls; nodular lesions resemble diabetic Kimmelstiel–Wilson nodules	Focal mesangial or diffuse proliferative, or membranoproliferative or membranous glomerulonephritis	Same as fibrillary GN
Immunofluorescent microscopy		Mesangial or glomerular capillary wall deposits for IgG, C3, *both* κ and λ light chains; Clq depositions possible	Monoclonal Ig deposition with a restricted light chain, *either* κ *or* λ
Electron microscopy	10 nm fibrils	Randomly arranged fibrils 16–24 nm; more randomly arranged than immunotactoid	30–50 nm microtubules
Congo-red stain	Positive; may be negative in very early disease, heavy-chain amyloidosis	Negative	Negative
Management	Serum-free light chains: treat underlying disease. Dialysis support; kidney transplant in dialysis-related amyloidosis; liver transplant in certain hereditary amyloidosis NOTE: Fat pad biopsy is recommended over biopsies of liver or kidneys due to lowest bleeding complications.	Annual screening for associated diseases: complete blood count with differential, serum immunofixation and free light chains, hepatitis C; treat underlying disease; use of ACEI or ARB; use of immunosuppressive therapy per findings on LM; dialysis support; renal transplant is an option, although controversial in those with monoclonal gammopathy. Recurrence in graft is common, but rate of progression in idiopathic cases may be slower than that observed in native kidneys.	

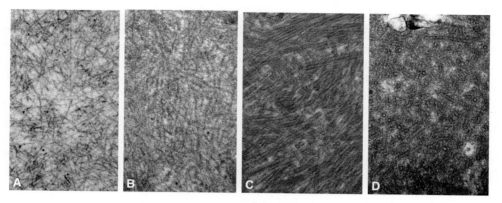

FIGURE 7.10 Fibrillary deposits. **A.** Amyloid. Haphazardly arranged 10-nm fibrils. **B.** Fibrillary glomerulonephritis. Randomly arranged 15- to 25-nm fibrils. **C.** Immunotactoid glomerulonephritis. Parallel arrays of 35- to 50-nm microtubules, often monoclonal. **D.** Cyroglobulin. Randomly arranged to clusters of 20- to 30-nm curved microtubules (All, ×72,000).

- Glucosuria in the absence of hyperglycemia; phosphaturia; renal tubular acidosis
- Chemistries:
  - Low to positive serum anion gap
  - Hypercalcemia
  - Hyperphosphatemia out of proportion to degree of kidney failure if high levels of serum FLC as they may give falsely high phosphate levels
  - High serum total protein to albumin ratio
  - Low complements in PGNMID and immunotactoid GN
- Testing options for monoclonal gammopathy:
  - Serum (or urine) protein electrophoresis (SPEP or UPEP): SPEP separates serum proteins into five general regions in the order of albumin, α_1, α_2, β, and γ based on their charge and size. The various immunoglobulin classes (IgG, IgA, IgM, IgD, and IgE) are usually of γ mobility, but they may also be found in the β-γ and β regions, and occasionally extend into the α_2-globulin area.
  - An "M"-spike indicates the presence of a "M"onoclonal protein. Each M-protein consists of two heavy polypeptide chains of the same class: γ (IgG: IgG1-IgG4), α (IgA: IgA1, IgA2), μ (IgM), δ (IgD), ε (IgE). The paired heavy chains are associated with two light chains of the same type (κ or λ), not both.
  - "Polyclonal gamma globulin" on SPEP does not indicate a monoclonal gammopathy, but a polyclonal immunoglobulin production in response to various conditions including liver disease, connective tissue, nonspecific inflammatory disorders.
  - SPEP is a useful screening procedure but it may miss a small M-protein spike or falsely identify a polyclonal increase in Ig or non-Ig as an M-protein spike. Identification of the actual makeup of the M-protein requires immunofixation. In serum (or urine) protein immunofixation electrophoresis (IFE), antibodies directed against the heavy and light chains (anti-γ, anti-mu, anti-α [IgG, M, A] and anti-κ and anti-λ) are added following the initial electrophoresis procedure to identify overproduction of any corresponding chain.
  - Direct assay for serum-free light chain (Bence Jones) is more sensitive in establishing the diagnosis of monoclonal gammopathy than either SPEP or IFE.

However, it must be noted that the quantity of both κ and λ light chains may be increased with poor kidney function due to reduced renal excretion. The abnormal ratio of κ to λ light chains (i.e., outside the range of 0.26 to 1.65 for normal kidney function and 0.37 to 3.1 for poor kidney function) better serves to indicate a monoclonal gammopathy in patients with advanced CKD than the actual quantity of κ and λ light chains.

- NOTE: Serum-free light chain assay is particularly important in the diagnosis of nonsecretory myeloma, AL amyloidosis (patients with amyloidosis may not have active myeloma), and light-chain-only myeloma.
- Evaluation of suspected monoclonal gammopathy (International Myeloma Working Group):
  - Serum protein electrophoresis with immunofixation
  - 24-hour urine protein electrophoresis
  - Serum FLC

Histopathology

- Amyloidosis
  - LM: Amyloid stains as silver and PAS negative material in mesangial regions and/or capillary walls. It is Congo red positive and displays apple green birefringence when viewed with polarized light (Fig. 7.11).
  - IF: Smudgy amorphous staining for the appropriate light and/or heavy chain. If it is a non-AL amyloid (AA amyloid, transthyretin, Lect2, fibrinogen Aα), there is no light chain or immunoglobulin staining.
  - EM: 10 nm haphazardly arranged fibrils.
- Monoclonal immunoglobulin deposition disease (MIDD)
  - LM: Glomeruli may appear nodular identical to diabetic glomerulosclerosis, mesangial proliferative, crescentic or normal (Fig. 7.12).
  - IF: Diffuse strong linear staining of all renal basement membrane and extracellular material for the abnormal light and/or heavy chain.
  - EM: Coarse granular electron dense material along/within glomerular and tubular basement membranes.

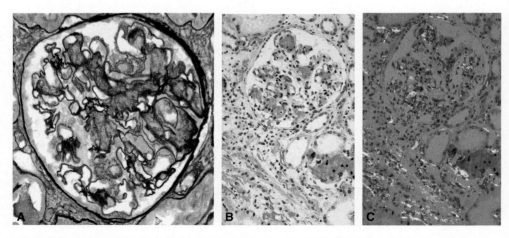

FIGURE 7.11 Amyloidosis. **A.** Silver negative material in mesangial regions and capillary walls (Jones silver, ×400). **B.** Positive Congo red stain in glomerular and interstitial amyloid (×200). **C.** Polarized Congo red stain showing apple green birefringence in the amyloid (×200).

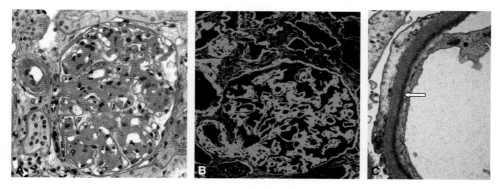

FIGURE 7.12 Monoclonal immunoglobulin deposition disease. **A.** Thickened and somewhat nodular mesangial regions; this may mimic nodular diabetic glomerulosclerosis (Periodic acid–Schiff, ×400). **B.** Strong linear κ light-chain staining of all basement membrane and extracellular material (×300). **C.** Dark granular electron dense material along the glomerular capillary basement membrane; it also involves tubular basement membranes (*arrow*) (×19,000).

Management

- Volume repletion with normal saline is key.
- Management of hypercalcemia:
  - Administration of normal saline as safely tolerated
  - Corticosteroids ± bisphosphonates (pamidronate > zolendronate (due to dosing problem with severe kidney failure in the latter; calcitonin if refractory to bisphosphonates or rapid calcium reduction is needed).
  - Hemodialysis if severe hypercalcemia (serum calcium > 18 mg/dL)
- Avoid contrast studies, NSAIDS, nephrotoxic medications
- Chemotherapy for underlying multiple myeloma, common regimens:
  - Bortezomib (Velcade, proteasome inhibitor) + CYC + dexamethasone
  - Bortezomib + melphalan + prednisone
  - Lenalidomide (Revlimid) + dexamethasone
  - Melphalan + prednisone + thalidomide
  - Thalidomide + dexamethasone
  - Bortezomid + lenalidomide + dexamethasone

> **NOTE** Reduction of serum FLC with chemotherapy predicts renal response in multiple myeloma. Plasma exchange has not been shown to improve kidney function in MM.

- Treatment of AL amyloidosis:
  - Nonmyeloablative chemotherapy and autologous stem cell transplantation (ASCT)
    - Preferred therapy, but high risk of serious complications
    - Criteria of eligibility for ASCT: NT-probrain natriuretic peptide < 5,000 ng/mL, troponin T < 0.06 ng/mL, age < 70 years, <3 organs involved, SCr < 1.7 mg/dL
  - Triple therapy if cannot tolerate ASCT:
    - CYC + thalidomide (or lenalidomide or bortezomib) + dexamethasone
    - Melphalan + lenalidomide + prednisone
  - Double therapy if cannot tolerate triple therapy: oral melphalan and dexamethasone
- Dialysis support as necessary
- Plasmapheresis in the presence of hyperviscosity

Other Fibrillary Disorders

- Fibronectin GN: autosomal-dominant disorder associated with massive deposition of fibronectin.
- Collagenofibrotic (collagen III) GN: GN associated with massive accumulation of atypical type III collagen fibrils in mesangium and subendothelial space
- Nail–patella syndrome and hereditary multiple exostoses syndrome (or hereditary multiple osteochondromas syndrome) with nephrotic syndrome and associated glomerular fibrillar collagen deposition

ALPORT SYNDROME AND THIN BASEMENT MEMBRANE

Epidemiology

- Alport syndrome involves inherited nephritis, sensorineural hearing loss, and ocular abnormalities.
- Prevalence ~1/50,000 live births

Pathogenesis

- Background: There are six genetically distinct collagen type IV chains (α1, α2, α3, α4, α5, α6) that form three triple helical protomers [α1, α1, α2], [α3, α4, α5], and [α5, α5, α6], where
  - [α1, α1, α2] protomer is present in all basement membranes.
  - [α3, α4, α5] protomer is present in **kidney**, lung, testis, cochlea, and eye.
  - [α5, α5, α6] protomer is present in **skin**, smooth muscle, esophagus, and **kidney.**
  - COL4A1 and COL4A2 at 13q34, encodes α1, α2 respectively.
  - COL4A3 and COL4A4 at 2q35-37, encodes α3, α4 respectively.
  - COL4A5 and COL4A6 on *chromosome X*, encodes α5, α6 respectively.

> **NOTE**   Mutations of α5 and α6 chains are X-linked.

- Disease state:
  - Mutations affecting any of the α3, α4, or α5(IV) chains impair the deposition of the entire triple helical complex into the GBM collagen network, leading to alterations in the GBM composition that predispose the kidney to glomerulosclerosis
  - In most patients with α5(IV) mutations, the α3, α4, and α5(IV) chains are all absent from the GBM despite continuing transcription of the α3(IV) and α4(IV) genes. The GBM is characterized by the absence of the α3, α4, and α5(IV) chains and persistence of the fetal distribution of α1 and α2(IV) chains.
  - In patients with autosomal recessive Alport syndrome, primary mutations in the α3(IV) chain prevent the expression of the α3, α4, and α5(IV) chains in GBM.
  - Large deletion or nonsense mutations lead to more severe disease than those with missense mutations.
- Genetic inheritance of Alport syndrome and thin basement membrane:
  - **X-linked (80%),** mutations involving the COL4A5 gene which codes the **α5**(IV) chain. Female heterozygous carriers: almost all have hematuria, but with variable outcome. Only a minority develop ESRD presumably due to "lyonization," a process whereby only one X chromosome is active per cell. Thus, in most women with X-linked Alport, approximately one-half of the cells express the mutant gene while the other half express the normal gene. Lyonization leads to a generally less severe phenotype than that compared with affected males.

- **Autosomal recessive (15%)**, mutations involving either COL4A3 or COL4A4 genes which code for α3(IV) chain (which contains the Goodpasture antigen) and the α4(IV) chain, respectively. Females are as severely affected as males. Clinical manifestations in both sexes are identical to those of classic X-linked Alport's in males.
- **Autosomal dominant (5%)** with heterozygous mutations in either the COL4A3 or COL4A4 genes.
  - Similar clinical and pathologic features as those of X-linked disease, but with slower kidney function decline.
  - While some heterozygous mutations in the COL4A3 or COL4A4 genes cause autosomal dominant Alport syndrome and progressive kidney failure, others only develop **thin basement membrane nephropathy (TBMN)**, a typically more benign condition where patients present with microscopic hematuria without progression to ESRD. Genetic factors other than mutations in these collagen genes have been suggested to affect phenotypes.
- NOTE: Histopathologic finding of TBMN does not necessarily rule out Alport syndrome due to the possibility of inadequate biopsy or early Alport. Clinical evaluations for hearing loss and abnormal optical lens, investigation for family history, and follow-up visits are necessary to rule out Alport syndrome. The diagnosis of TBMN is, in effect, a diagnosis of clinical exclusion.
- Mutations of the α3-5(IV) chains may also occur de novo.

Clinical Manifestations

- Renal manifestations of Alport syndrome:
  - Asymptomatic persistent microscopic or gross hematuria
  - Boys without hematuria by age 10 are unlikely to have Alport syndrome.
  - ESRD:
    - X-linked or autosomal-recessive disease: ESRD usually occurs by age 35, but may be later in life.
    - Autosomal dominant: ESRD occurs later in life, generally by age 45 to 60.
  - In X-linked females, recurrent gross hematuria, proteinuria, hearing loss, and diffuse GBM thickening are associated with worse renal outcomes.
- Extra-renal manifestations of Alport syndrome:
  - Sensorineural hearing loss:
    - Thought to be due to impaired adhesion of the auditory sensory cell containing organ of Corti to the inner ear basilar membrane which lacks the normal α3-4-5(IV) collagen network.
    - Initial hearing loss is in high-frequency range.
    - Rate of hearing loss is similar to the rate of kidney disease progression.
  - Ocular abnormalities:
    - Anterior lenticonus due to abnormal (α3, α4, and α5[IV]) and associated with thinning of the lens capsule
    - Other ocular findings: spherophakia, anterior polar and posterior cortical cataract, corneal changes with recurrent corneal erosions
    - Retinal findings: drusen, perifoveal dot and fleck retinopathy, neovascularization
  - Leiomyomas:
    - Associated with X-linked Alport, but rare
    - Affected patients carry deletions that involve COL4A5 extending into the adjacent COL4A6 gene. Deletions involving both the COL4A5 and COL4A6 are thought to cause misregulation of neighboring genes and resultant smooth muscle overgrowth.

- In addition to leiomyomas, arterial aneurysms have been reported in young males and may involve thoracic, abdominal aorta, and even intracranial artery.

Histopathology

- LM: Interstitial foamy macrophages in the absence of significant proteinuria or nephrotic syndrome. Global and/or segmental glomerulosclerosis may be present in more advanced disease (Fig. 7.13).
- EM: Classic Alport: GBM with irregular thinning and thickening, layered or lamellated "basket-weave" appearance in the thickened area due to GBM injury and remodeling, and subepithelial scalloping. There are no electron dense deposits.
- IF: Pattern of staining depends on chain being stained for and type of mutation.
  - Staining for the α3(IV) or α5(IV) chain will be positive within the normal GBM since the protomers [α3, α4, α5] are distributed within the GBM.
  - In an X-linked Alport male (mutation of the α5(IV) chain), staining for α3,4 and 5 (IV) chains is typically negative due to the lack of [α3, α4, α5] protomer formation.
  - In an X-linked Alport female (mutation of the α5(IV) chain), IF staining for α3,4 and 5(IV) is segmental due to lyonization.
  - In an autosomal recessive Alport, no α3(IV)- α5(IV) labeling may be detected in the GBM, but α5(IV) from the [α5, α5, α6] protomer will be positive in Bowman's capsule and basement membrane of collecting ducts.

Diagnosis

- Clinical syndrome, particularly if known family history
- Kidney or skin biopsy:
  - Kidney biopsy: Note that classic lamellation of GBM may not be present in early disease.
  - Skin biopsy is stained for α5(IV) chain. Absent or segmental staining suggests X-linked Alport. Normal staining may signify:
    - Autosomal-recessive Alport syndrome involving either α3 or α4(IV) chains.

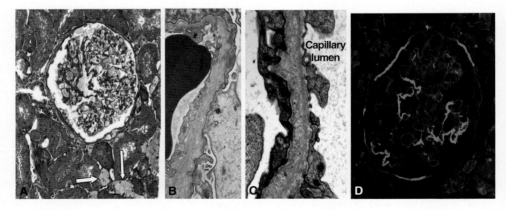

FIGURE 7.13 Alport syndrome. **A.** Normal glomerulus and interstitial foam cells (*arrows*) (Masson trichrome, ×200). **B.** Irregular thick and thin layered glomerular capillary basement membrane (19,000). **C.** Thick glomerular capillary basement membrane with "basket-woven" appearance and subepithelial scalloping (25,000). **D.** Focal Bowman capsular and glomerular capillary basement membrane staining for α 5(IV) collagen chain in a female heterozygote for Alport syndrome (×400).

- • Mutation of α5(IV) that affects the function but not structure of the chain.
    - • Diseases other than Alport
- • Genetic testing (www.genereviews.org)

Management

Slow progression of kidney disease: (ACEI or ARB) reduces proteinuria and rate of disease progression.

Kidney Transplantation

- • Recurrent disease does not occur in the transplanted graft because the donor kidney has a normal GBM.
- • Anti-GBM disease occurs in 3% to 4% of affected males who receive transplants. X-linked females do not develop posttransplant anti-GBM disease because they generally do carry a normal copy of the affected gene and do express the normal counterpart.
- • In males with X-linked disease, antibodies are directed primarily against the α5(IV) chain, but antibodies against the α3(IV) chain are also found in some patients.
- • In patients with autosomal recessive Alport syndrome who develop posttransplant anti-GBM disease, the predominant target of anti-GBM antibodies is the α3(IV) chain.
- • Retransplantation in patients who have developed posttransplant anti-GBM is questionable due to high risk of recurrence.

THROMBOTIC MICROANGIOPATHY/HEMOLYTIC UREMIC SYNDROME

Background

- • TMA is characterized by hyaline thrombi within the microvasculature in association with:
    - • Thrombocytopenia < 150,000 or >25% decline in platelet count from baseline.
    - • Microangiopathic hemolytic anemia (MAHA) which arises from endothelial injury, fibrin deposition, and platelet aggregation. Red blood cells going through the fibrin mesh become fragmented, hence presence of schistocytes.
    - • End-organ dysfunction involving one or more organs (e.g., brain, kidneys, gastrointestines)
- • TMA may be seen in three clinical disorders:
    - • Disseminated intravascular coagulation (DIC)
    - • Thrombotic thrombocytopenic purpura (TTP)
    - • Hemolytic uremic syndrome (HUS), which may be further categorized as:
        - • Shiga-toxin associated with bloody diarrhea (typical HUS), or
        - • Atypical HUS, absence of diarrhea
- • While DIC has reduced platelet survival and increased fibrinolysis and plasminogen activator, TTP-HUS have reduced platelet survival and normal plasminogen and fibrinogen turnover.
- • DIC:
    - • Classic presentation: elevated PT/PTT, increased fibrinogen degradation products (FDP), increased D-dimer
    - • Low grade or chronic DIC: PT/PTT and fibrinogen may be normal, but MAHA will be present and FDP and D-dimer will be increased.

- Conditions associated with DIC: sepsis, liver failure, malignancy, tissue death, pre-eclampsia, septic abortion
- TTP:
  - Classic pentad for TTP (thrombocytopenia, MAHA, kidney failure, neurologic signs, fever) is rare.
  - Pathogenesis: one-third of patients have severe deficiency of **a d**isintegrin and **m**etalloproteinase with a **t**hrombospondin type 1 motif, member **13** (ADAMTS13), a von Willebrand factor (vWF)-cleaving protease and two-third of patients have ADAMTS13 inhibitors (i.e., ADAMTS13 autoantibodies). ADAMTS13 is a protease that normally cleaves ultra-large vWF multimers on endothelial cell surface into smaller fragments to make them "less sticky" to circulating platelets. The absence of normally functioning ADAMTS13 leads to the presence of ultra-large wWF multimers, increased platelet trapping, and subsequent intravascular formation of microthrombi.

> **NOTE** Patients with severe ADAMST13 deficiency are at least three times more likely to relapse. Close monitoring and prompt initiation of therapeutic plasma exchange is indicated at onset of signs/symptoms of relapse.

- HUS:
  - Diarrheal (bloody) HUS:
    - Pathogenesis:
      - Shiga toxin-mediated
      - Associated with enterohemorrhagic *E. coli*: *E. coli* O157:H7, *E. coli* O104:H4
      - Note that 30% of TTP and aHUS may present with diarrhea.
  - Nondiarrheal HUS, a.k.a. atypical HUS:
    - Pathogenesis: Dysregulated activation of the alternative complement pathway due to genetic mutations of or autoantibody formation against various complement regulatory proteins (loss of function of factors H or I or gain of function of C3 convertase or factor B, among others).
- TTP-HUS:
  - TTP and HUS may have overlap clinical symptoms at presentation. Diagnosis for the distinct syndrome may not be obvious at presentation and requires testing for ADAMST13.
  - Only 20% to 60% of patients with TTP have kidney failure.
  - Again, note that 30% of TTP and aHUS may present with diarrhea.
  - Given the significant overlap of signs/symptoms, patients may be classified as TTP-HUS pending ADAMST13 result.
  - NOTE: Immediate initiation of therapeutic plasma exchange (TPE) is recommended if TTP or TTP-HUS is suspected on presentation pending ADAMST13 result.
  - Conditions associated with primary TTP-HUS: Idiopathic/acquired (decreased functional ADAMTS13 or presence of inhibitory anti-ADAMTS13 antibody), hereditary/congenital (severely decreased ADAMTS13 level)
  - Conditions associated with secondary TTP-HUS: autoimmune disease, drugs (ticlopidine, clopidogrel, quinine, valacyclovir, oral contraceptives, chemotherapy, cyclosporine, TAC, sirolimus, mitomycin C), infections (HIV, *S. pneumoniae*), pregnancy/postpartum, pancreatitis, malignancy, systemic sclerosis, malignant hypertension, stem cell transplant, familial, sporadic

- Therapeutic plasma exchange (TPE) indications:
  - TTP
  - aHUS: 50% of aHUS respond to TPE. All respond to eculizumab. However, eculizumab is very expensive. Additionally, pretreatment with meningococcal vaccination and prophylactic antibiotic coverage are MANDATORY due to high risk for life-threatening meningococcemia associated with eculizumab.
  - dHUS with severe neurologic or renal involvement
  - TTP-HUS at presentation unless known association with mitomycin C, stem cell transplant, malignancy, systemic sclerosis, or dHUS without severe neurologic or renal involvement
- Figure 7.14 summarizes the three clinical syndromes associated with TMA.

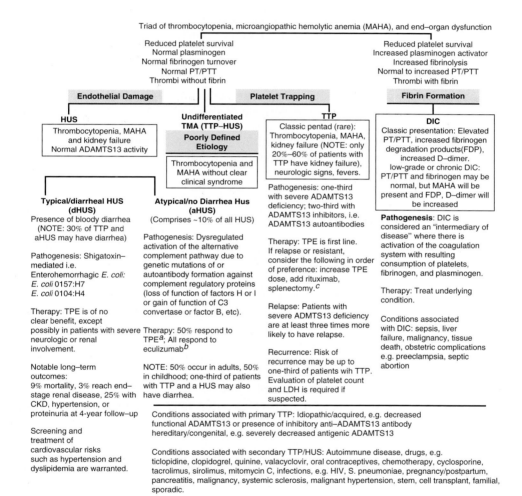

FIGURE 7.14 Evaluation of thrombotic microangiopathy.

[a]For patients in the "Undifferentiated TMA, TTP/HUS" category, initiate TPE *unless* patient has any of the following due to *lack of benefit*: mitomycin C, stem cell transplant, malignancy, systemic sclerosis, malignancy, or dHUS without severe neurologic or renal involvement.
[b]Eculizumab: Very high cost; pretreatment meningococcal vaccination and prophylactic antibiotic coverage (levofloxacin for 2 weeks) are *mandatory* due to high risk for life-threatening meningococcemia.
[c]Maximize TPE by increasing exchange volume and/or frequency (i.e., twice daily exchange). Rituximab may be administered in four weekly doses of 375 mg/m^2 body surface area once the platelet count has increased to >150,000/mL and serum LDH level < 25% of upper limit of normal. TPE is preferably delayed for 1 to 2 days after administration of rituximab due to removal of the drug. Immediate reinitiation of TPE is indicated for recurrent symptoms, platelet count < 50,000/mL, and/or serum LDH more than two times upper-normal limit. On average, eight TPE sessions are required following rituximab therapy.

- Pregnancy-associated TTP-aHUS:
  - Pregnancy-associated TTP due to ADAMTS13 deficiency:
    - May occur early in pregnancy, but typically occurs in the late second and third trimesters, with median gestational age of 23 weeks
    - During pregnancy, plasma vWF including the ultra-large multimers increase steadily up to 200% to 500% of normal at term, while ADAMTS13 activity declines gradually from the end of the first trimester up to the end of early puerperium.
  - Pregnancy-associated aHUS:
    - Typically occurs postpartum (80%), but may occur early in pregnancy.
    - Complement dysregulation has been reported in 75% of patients with pregnancy-associated aHUS.
    - Late (i.e., postpartum) occurrence is thought to be due to the loss of placental protective complement inhibitory factors against mother's underlying complement dysregulation.
    - Patients with complement dysregulation may have a 20% risk of pregnancy-associated aHUS.
    - Pregnancy-associated aHUS is associated with higher incidence of fetal losses (4.6% vs. 2% to 3%) and preeclampsia (7.4% vs. 4% to 5%) compared to the general population.
    - Two-third of affected patients develop ESRD within a month of diagnosis.
  - Other factors such as infections may induce earlier occurrence of pregnancy-associated TTP-HUS.

SLE AND THROMBOSIS

- Arterial thromboembolic events are increased in patients with SLE: increased risks for myocardial infarctions and strokes after adjustments for traditional risk factors.
- Reported risks for arterial thromboembolic events:
  - Traditional factors: age, male gender, smoking, dyslipidemia, hypertension, obesity, hyperhomocysteinemia
  - Nontraditional factors: SLE disease duration, presence of antiphospholipid antibodies (aPLs), higher SLE damage scores, duration and cumulative dose of corticosteroid use
- Reported risks for venous thromboembolic events: male gender, higher body mass index, aPL antibodies, low serum HDL cholesterol, hemolytic anemia, kidney disease
- Leukopenia has been reported to be associated with a decreased risk of both arterial and venous thromboembolic events.
- The coexistence of the 3 aPLs lupus anticoagulant, anticardiolipin, and anti-β_2-glycoprotein I is especially high risk for thromboembolic events.
- The use of antimalarials (hydroxychloroquine) is protective against both arterial and venous thromboembolic events. Adverse effects of antimalarials: retinopathy, cardiotoxicity, neuromyopathy, cutaneous hyperpigmentation, transamititis, and/or increased serum creatinine
- The use of aspirin is inconclusive but warranted due to its low adverse effect profile.
- Routine evaluation for other genetic conditions must also be considered (e.g., factor V Leiden, methylenetetrahydrofolate reductase, fibrinogen γ mutations).

ANTIPHOSPHOLIPID SYNDROME

- Systemic APS is defined as the presence of:
  - ≥1 clinical manifestations: unexplained repeated spontaneous abortions or vascular thrombosis (e.g., deep vein thrombosis, pulmonary embolism, stroke, and myocardial infarction, ±APS nephropathy), *and*
  - Positive antiphospholipid antibodies (aPLs) detected on ≥2 occasions separated by several weeks
    - aPLS are autoantibodies (typically IgG or IgM, but can be IgA) directed against plasma proteins bound to anionic surfaces.
    - aPLs of interest: lupus anticoagulant, anti-β_2-glycoprotein I, anti-vimentin/cardiolipin, antibodies against cell membranes including phosphatidylserine, phosphotidylinositol, phosphatidylethanolamine, phosphatidic acid
    - The prevalence of aPLs is 1% to 5% of general population, but may be as high as 16% to 40% in patients with SLE, and 16% in those with rheumatoid arthritis.
    - The prevalence of APS may be > 20% during long-term follow-up in SLE patients.
- *Renal* APS may present with renal artery or vein thrombosis or APS nephropathy.
- APS *nephropathy* is a vasoocclusive kidney injury due to TMA and is a subset of renal APS. APS nephropathy per se is not generally considered a clinical manifestation required for the diagnosis of systemic APS.
  - APS nephropathy has been reported in 10% of patients with LN and in 20% to 30% of those with SLE.
  - Up to one-third of patients with APS nephropathy does not have systemic APS.
- Systemic APS may be classified as primary or secondary APS. Primary APS has no associated systemic disease, whereas secondary APS is associated with a systemic disease, typically autoimmune (e.g. SLE).

Clinical Manifestations

- Renal APS: renal vascular fibrointimal hyperplasia, renal artery or vein thrombosis with or without associated hypertension, cortical ischemia/necrosis, hematuria, kidney injury, tubulointerstitial fibrosis, glomerulosclerosis, and any glomerular lesions noted below.
- Histopathology of APS nephropathy (Fig. 7.15):
  - Arterial/arteriolar fibrin thrombi ± fibrin extending into the vascular intima and endothelial cell swelling with narrowed lumens
  - Fragmented red blood cells in vessel lumens, or walls, or in areas of glomerular mesangiolysis
  - Concentric thickening (onion skinning) ± mucoid subendothelial widening of arterial/arteriolar walls
  - Glomerular capillary ischemic wrinkling, sometimes with double contours
  - IF: Fibrin in glomerular capillaries and/or vessel walls and lumens
  - EM: subendothelial electron lucent widening between glomerular capillary basement membrane and swollen endothelium
  - Glomerular lesions commonly associated with APS:
    - Primary APS: membranous, MCD, FSGS
    - Secondary APS: typically LN of any World Health Organization class

Pathogenesis

- Inciting event is thought to arise from aPL-mediated blood vessel injury, followed by endothelial disruption, formation of β_2-glycoprotein I IC, activation of endothelial cells, platelets, and circulating monocytes, all leading to a thrombogenic state.

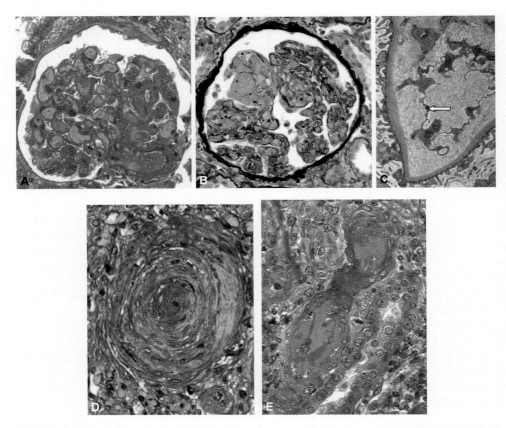

FIGURE 7.15 Antiphospholipid syndrome. **A.** Bland thrombosis of arteriole and glomerular capillaries (Masson tri-chrome, ×400). **B.** Glomerular capillary thrombosis with irregular, ischemically wrinkled capillary walls and segmental double contours (Jones silver, ×400). **C.** Wide subendothelial lucency (which stains for fibrin) corresponding to thick-ened capillaries (*arrow*) on LM (×14,000). **D.** Arteriole with "onion skin" appearance due to muscular hypertrophy, with a thrombus in the very narrowed lumen (Masson trichrome, ×600). **E.** Thrombosed arteriole (Masson trichrome, ×400).

- Other downstream effects that would favor thrombus formation:
  - Release of tissue factor, followed by activation of the extrinsic coagulation path-way, and production of vasoconstrictive thromboxane A2
  - Reduction of endothelial nitric oxide production, leading to increased endo-thelial monocyte adhesion, superoxide generation, and decreased arterial relaxation
  - Activation of classical complement pathway, increased expression of C5a, lead-ing to neutrophil recruitment to area of tissue injury

Management

- Life-time anticoagulation for APS, even APS nephropathy alone, with goal INR 2-3. Aspirin alone is inadequate therapy.
- NOTE: Overanticoagulation (INR > 3.0) may be associated with warfarin-related nephropathy (WRN, AKI associated with glomerular hemorrhage and intratubu-lar red blood cell obstruction). Underlying CKD is thought to be a risk factor for WRN (Fig. 7.16).

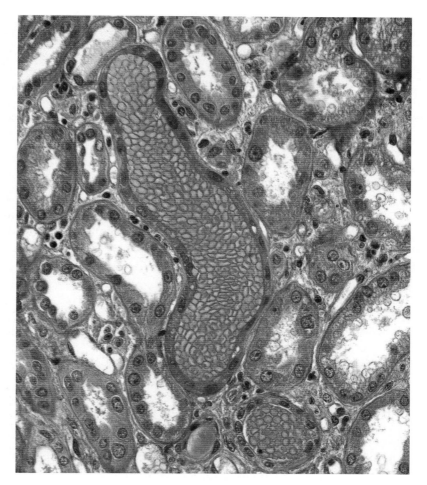

FIGURE 7.16 Warfarin-related nephropathy. Red blood cells are within and occluding the lumen of distal tubules (Masson trichrome, ×400).

SLE AND THROMBOTIC THROMBOCYTOPENIC PURPURA

Epidemiology

- TTP typically precedes the diagnosis of SLE in children. 6% of patients with TTP have SLE.
- SLE typically precedes the diagnosis of TTP in adults. <5% of SLE patients have TTP.
- Differential diagnoses of MAHA other than TTP in patients with SLE:
  - Disseminated intravascular coagulopathy
  - Malignant hypertension
  - (±Catastrophic) antiphospholipid antibody syndrome
  - Active lupus complicated by hemolytic anemia
  - Small-vessel vasculitis with end-organ damage

Clinical Manifestations

- Presence of MAHA, anemia, thrombocytopenia
- Patients with SLE-associated TTP tend to be younger males, have worse kidney function (both proteinuria and serum creatinine), class IV diffuse proliferative LN, lower C3 levels, and other complications such as APS, serositis, pulmonary hypertension, nephritis, and central nervous system involvement.
- Mortality in SLE-associated TTP is approximately 50%, commonly associated with infections

Diagnosis

- Diagnosis is based on clinical assessment, serologic and coagulation tests, and exclusion of all other differential diagnoses above.
- Unclear utility of ADAMTS13 in SLE: reduced ADAMTS13 levels and/or presence of ADAMTS13 antibodies may be detected in SLE patients *without* overt TMA. However, SLE patients with TTP do have severely depressed ADAMTS13 levels or high titers of anti-ADAMTS13 inhibitory antibodies.

Management

- Poor data
- Plasma exchange *plus* immunosuppressive therapy (e.g., corticosteroids and CYC) to control both TTP and active SLE, respectively.
- Rituximab may be considered if above fails. Again, poor data.

DIABETIC KIDNEY DISEASE

Epidemiology

- DKD is the most common primary diagnosis for patients who start dialysis (~50%)
- Kidney diseases in diabetic patients who present with ESRD:
  - 60%: classic DKD (large kidneys, proteinuria > 1 g/d, ± diabetic retinopathy)
  - 25% to 30%: another primary kidney disease in addition to DKD
  - 10% to 15%: atypical presentation with ischemic nephropathy (low level proteinuria)
- Cumulative prevalence of proteinuria is ~50% to 60% at 25 years after diagnosis of diabetes.
- Cumulative prevalence of progression to ESRD is ~60% at 5 years *after onset of proteinuria*.
- Cumulative prevalence of proteinuria and progression to ESRD are similar for DM types 1 and 2.

Risks for the Development of DKD and Progression

- Unmodifiable risks:
  - Genetic susceptibility:
    - Family history of predisposition to abnormal sodium handling and hypertension
    - Genotypes: angiotensin-converting enzyme (ACE), angiotensin II type 2-receptor, aldose reductase
  - Ethnicity: Blacks, Hispanics, Pima Indians with DM type 2
  - Gender: Caucasian males and African American females

- Age: possibly early onset
- Duration of DM
- Modifiable risks: hypertension, early glomerular hyperfiltration, prolonged uncontrolled hyperglycemia, obesity, tobacco smoking, use of oral contraceptives

Clinical Manifestations

- Albuminuria:
  - Moderate increase in albuminuria may predict high risk for eventual DKD
  - The American Diabetes Association recommends screening for microalbuminuria in:
    - All patients with DM type 2 at the time of diagnosis and annually thereafter
    - All patients with DM type 1 five years after the diagnosis and annually thereafter
- (Microscopic) Hematuria:
  - May occur with DKD
  - Red blood cell casts may be present, but other glomerular diseases *must* be ruled out.
- Morbidities and mortality:
  - Increasing albuminuria and decreasing GFR correlate with cardiovascular and renal events in patients with DM type 2.
  - Mortality among diabetics with ESRD is 1.5 to 2.0-fold greater compared to non-diabetics.

Natural History

- Proposed scheme of DKD stages for type 1 DM (less reliable for type 2 DKD):
  - Pre-DKD: 0 to 5 years since disease onset: glomerular hyperfiltration, renal hypertrophy
  - Incipient DKD: 5 to 15 years
    - Microalbuminuria (30 to 300 mg/24 h or overnight albuminuria at 20 to 200 μg/min in at least two of three consecutive nonketotic sterile urine samples) occurs in 20% to 30% of patients, less than 50% of whom will progress to overt nephropathy, hypertension
    - Structural changes: mesangial expansion, moderate glomerular basement thickening, arteriolar hyalinosis
  - Overt DKD: 15 to 25 years:
    - Proteinuria (>300 mg albuminuria/24 hours or overnight albuminuria > 200 μg/min—when severely increased albuminuria occurs, the majority will progress to ESRD), nephrotic syndrome, reduced glomerular filtration
    - Structural changes: severe glomerular basement membrane thickening, mesangial nodules (Kimmelstiel–Wilson lesions), tubulointerstitial fibrosis
  - ESRD > 25 years: 4% to 17% at 20 years from time of diagnosis of type 1 DM

Pathogenesis

- Hyperglycemia:
  - Enhances matrix production, glycation of matrix proteins, formation of advanced glycation end (AGE) products
  - Stimulates VEGF, endothelial injury
  - Increases expression of transforming growth factor β (TGF-β)
- Advanced glycation end products:
  - AGE crosslinking with collagen

- AGE:AGE receptor interaction (AGE:RAGE) leads to oxidative stress, activation of protein kinase C (PKC)
- Activation of PKC pathway leading to:
  - Endothelial dysfunction with decreased NO production
  - Increased expression of ET1, VEGF, NFκB, and plasminogen activator inhibitor-1 (PAI-1) leading to tissue inflammatory response, TMA, vascular injury
- Polyol pathway (via aldose reductase): thought to contribute to diabetic complications including diabetic cataracts, neuropathy, hyperfiltration, albuminuria. Use of aldose reductase inhibitors have been disappointing due to hypersensitivity reactions and liver abnormalities.
- Accumulation of N-acetylglucosamine via hexosamine pathway: N-acetyleglucosamine may lead to increased synthesis of TGF-β1, PAI-1.
- Prorenin activation of mitogen-activated protein kinases
- Reduction of nephrin expression presumably via angiotensin II
- Systemic hypertension
- Metabolic stress leading to mitochondrial dysfunction (which may lead to type B lactic acidosis observed in patients with diabetic ketoacidosis)

Structural Changes

- Gross structural changes: kidney weight increases by ~15% due to glomerular hypertrophy and hyperfiltration
- Histopathology (Fig. 7.17):
  - Glomerular basement thickening (up to three times normal)
  - Mesangial expansion:
    - Due in part to hyperglycemia induced increased matrix production or glycation of matrix proteins, AGE crosslinking with collagen, and decreased matrix degredation.
    - Mild to severe diffuse mesangial expansion without nodules
    - Nodular glomerular intercapillary lesions (Kimmelstiel–Wilson lesion):
      - Associated with mesangiolysis and capillary microaneurysms
      - Differential diagnoses of nodular glomerulosclerosis: dysproteinemias (e.g., amyloidosis and monoclonal Ig deposition diseases, and immunotactoid GN), fibronectin glomerulopathy, collagen III glomerulopathy, chronic hypoxic/ischemic conditions, chronic MPGN, or idiopathic.
      - Patients with Kimmelstiel–Wilson lesions are more likely to have diabetic retinopathy (DR) and worse kidney function.
  - Advanced diabetic sclerosis
  - Vascular lesions including hyalinization of both afferent and efferent arterioles, pathognomonic for diabetic nephropathy, and arterial intimal fibrosis.

Indications for Kidney Biopsy in Patients with DM

- Absence of DR (particularly in DM type 1). Note, however, the absence of DR in DM type 2 does not exclude DKD.

> **NOTE**
> - Patients with DM type 1 and DKD *almost always* have other evidence of diabetic microvascular disease (i.e., DR, neuropathy), but the converse is not true (i.e., not all patients with DR have DKD)
> - DR is present in only ~50% to 65% of patients with DM type 2 and DKD. Albeit the absence of DR does not exclude DKD, patients without DR have a high likelihood of having a non-diabetic glomerular disease.

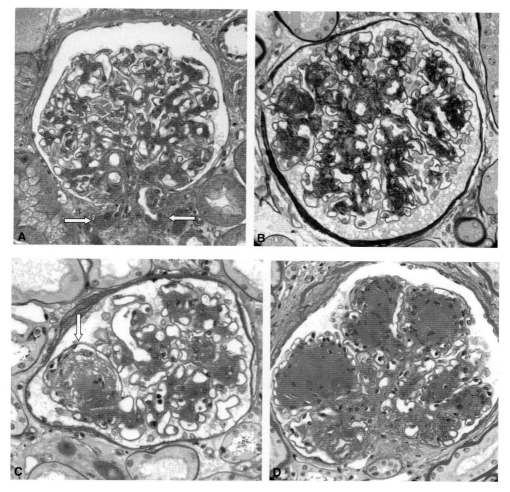

FIGURE 7.17 Diabetic nephropathy. **A.** Mild/early diffuse diabetic glomerulosclerosis with mild expansion of matrix. Note hyalinization of afferent and efferent arterioles (*arrows*) (Masson trichrome, ×400). **B.** Moderate diffuse increase in mesangial matrix (Jones silver, ×400). **C.** Diffuse and nodular matrix expansion with mesangiolysis and microaneurysm formation (*arrow*) (Periodic acid–Schiff, ×400). **D.** Global mesangial matrix nodules with peripheral nuclei (Periodic acid–Schiff, ×400).

- Acute onset of proteinuria, particularly if less than 5 years from diagnosis in DM type 1
- Presence of active urinary sediment (e.g., red blood cell casts) or significant hematuria (gross hematuria)
- Rapid decline in kidney function
- Presence of extrarenal manifestations and/or positive serologies suggestive of another glomerular disease (e.g., positive ANCA, hypocomplementemia)

Management (KDIGO 2012 Unless Specified Otherwise)

Glucose Control

- Maintain hemoglobin A1C ~7% for both DM types 1 and 2
- Renal dose adjustments for pharmacologic therapy:
  - Metformin: contraindicated for eGFR < 30 mL/min/1.73 m^2.

- Dipeptidyl peptidase-4 inhibitors:
  - Linagliptin: no dose adjustment
  - Saxagliptin: half-dose adjustment for creatinine clearance < 50 mL/min
  - Sitagliptin, alogliptin: half-dose adjustment for creatinine clearance 30 to 50 mL/min; quarter-dose adjustment for creatinine clearance < 30 mL/min
- Rationale: Protective effects of intensive glycemic control:
  - Reduction in rates of development of microalbuminuria
  - Partial reversal of glomerular hypertrophy and hyperfiltration
  - Stabilization or decrease protein excretion in patients with albuminuria after apparent normoglycemia > 2 years
  - Slowing of GFR decline
  - Successful pancreas transplantation leads to stabilization of glomerular structure at 5-year follow-up *and* significant reversal of DKD histopathologic changes at 10 year.
- Data:
  - *Studies indicating that strict glycemic control decreased risk for microalbuminuria:*
    - Diabetes Control and Complications Trial (DCCT) (DM type 1): 9-year follow-up, intensive therapy group with mean A1C of 7% had a 35% to 45% lower risk for development of microalbuminuria compared with control group (mean A1C 9%); Renoprotection persists even after return to less intensive therapy, a phenomenon known as "legacy effect." This is presumably due to the effect of euglycemia on long-lasting modification of transcription of genes responsible for DKD.
    - Kumamoto study, DM type 2: 60% rate reduction of microalbuminuria in relatively young non-obese DM type 2 patients in intensive group (mean A1C 7%) compared with conventional therapy group (mean A1C 9.4%)
    - U.K. Prospective Diabetes Study (UKPDS), DM type 2: A1C ~7.0% versus 7.9%
      - Relative risk reduction for development of microalbuminuria
      - Ten-year follow-up after study ended still revealed 24% lower risk of microvascular disease and myocardial infarction. All-cause mortality also remained reduced and attributed to "legacy effect."
  - *Strict glycemic control: effects on cardiovascular disease (CVD):*
    - Action in Diabetes and Vascular Disease, Perindopril and Indapamide Controlled Evaluation (ADVANCE): intensive control (A1C 6.5% vs. 7.3%) resulted in a *10% relative reduction in combined outcome of major macrovascular and microvascularly events*, primarily as a consequence of a 21% relative reduction in nephropathy.
    - Action to Control Cardiovascular Risk in Diabetes (ACCORD): very tight control (A1C 6.5% vs. 7.5%) had *higher mortality,* up by 22%, $p = 0.04$.
    - Veterans Affairs Diabetes Trial (VADT): A1C 6.9% versus 8.4%: *no difference in reduction in cardiovascular deaths or events* at 7.5-year follow-up

> **NOTE** In patients with long-standing DM and known CVD, current data do not support strict glycemic control in reducing risk for further CVD events or mortality.

Blood Pressure Control

- Hypertension occurs in ~40% of DM type 1 and 70% of type 2.
- Higher BP is associated with both development and progression of DKD.
- Progressive lowering of BP to 120 mm Hg was associated with improved renal and patient survival. However, SBP < 120 mm Hg or DBP < 70 mm Hg, are poorly tolerated and associated with increased incidence of myocardial infarction

and mortality. The latter is thought to reflect reduced coronary perfusion during diastole, particularly in patients with underlying coronary artery disease (Irbesartan Diabetic Nephropathy Trial (IDNT)).

- Recommendations (JNC 8):
  - Maintain SBP < 140 mm Hg and DBP < 90 mm Hg
  - If DKD is present, one antihypertensive agent should include ACEI or ARB.

ACEI versus ARB:

- ■ RAAS inhibition with either ACEI or ARB confers renoprotection in patients with DKD independent of BP control via both intraglomerular hemodynamic and nonhemodynamic (i.e., antiproliferative and antifibrotic) effects of angiotensin II.
- ■ RAAS inhibition also blocks aldosterone, thus its effects on sodium retention, potassium and magnesium wasting, and tissue inflammation and fibrosis. 40% to 50% of patients on ACEI or ARB develop "aldosterone escape" by 12 months of therapy. Aldosterone antagonism may be added if safely tolerated.
- Data on DM type 1:
  - ACEI reduces the risk of progression from microalbuminuria to overt nephropathy.
  - In *normotensives* with microalbuminuria, ACEI leads to a 60% reduction in progression to macroalbuminuria and 3 times likelihood in regression to normoalbuminuria.
  - Captopril treatment in patients with macroalbuminuria or overt nephropathy reduces albuminuria and GFR decline and delays onset of kidney failure.
  - Insufficient data for ARB, but expected to be similar to ACEI.
- Data on DM type 2:
  - Irbesartan in Patients with Type 2 Diabetes and Microalbuminuria study (IRMA 2) trial: Irbesartan reduces progression to overt DKD by 70% in hypertensive type 2 patients over 2-year follow-up.
  - Microalbuminuria Reduction with Valsartan in Patients with Type 2 DM (MARVAL) trial: daily valsartan 80 mg reduces urinary albumin excretion better than amlodipine (44% vs. 8%)
  - IDNT and the Reduction in Endpoints in NIDDM with the AII Antagonist Losartan (RENAAL) trials: DM type 2 with macroalbuminuria and reduced GFR, ARBs reduce proteinuria and composite end points of death, dialysis, and doubling of serum creatinine.

> **NOTE** In contrast to DM type 1, data on efficacy of ACEI in type 2 DKD are not as robust.

- Recommendations:
  - DM types 1 and 2: Use ACEI or ARB in normotensive patients with albuminuria ≥ 30 mg/g Cr who are at high risk for DKD or its progression
  - High risk for DKD or its progression is defined as having increasing albuminuria in the microalbuminuria range, macroalbuminuria, declining GFR, increasing BP, presence of DR, elevated lipids and/or uric acid concentrations, or family history of HTN, macrovascular disease, or DKD.
  - In patients with microalbuminuria range and without high risks, follow-up without RAAS inhibition may be appropriate.
  - In patients with macroalbuminuria without retinopathy, especially if present within 10 years of diagnosis of DM, consider evaluation for nondiabetic kidney disease.

- Special notes regarding RAAS inhibition:
  - Combination therapy of RAAS inhibition in DKD: not advised due to unacceptable increase in adverse events (i.e., impaired kidney function and hyperkalemia). Additionally, there was no significant benefit in primary end point (progression of kidney disease), mortality, or cardiovascular events: Veterans Affairs Nephropathy in Diabetes (VA NEPHRON-D) trial.
  - Aliskiren (renin inhibitor): should not be used in combination with either ACEI or ARB due to increased risk of stroke and adverse events (i.e., hyperkalemia, hypotension, and ESRD or death due to kidney disease)—Aliskiren Trial in Type 2 Diabetes Using Cardio–Renal Endpoints (ALTITUDE).

Lipid Management

- "Lowering low-density lipoprotein cholesterol (LDL-C) with statin-based therapies reduces risk of major atherosclerotic events, but not all-cause mortality in patients with CKD including those with DM."
- Recommendations:
  - Use of lipid-lowering agents (statins or statin/ezetimibe combination) is recommended to reduce risk of major atherosclerotic events in patients with diabetes and CKD including kidney transplant recipients. There is no evidence to suggest improvement in kidney disease outcomes with statin therapy.
- *Initiating* statin in patients with diabetes who are about to receive or already receiving dialysis is *not* recommended. Statins provide little or no benefit in death rates due to CVD events in dialysis patients with diabetes and appear to increase risk of hemorrhagic stroke:
  - A Study to Evaluate the Use of Rosuvastatin in Subjects on Regular Hemodialysis (AURORA) revealed no significant benefit on primary cardiovascular outcome (cardiac death or nonfatal MI and fatal or nonfatal stroke); Risk of hemorrhagic stroke increased by greater than fivefold. Twofold increased hemorrhagic stroke risk also noted in Die Deutsche Diabetes Dialyse Studie (4D).
  - Study of Heart and Renal Protection (SHARP) trial (combined simvastatin 20 mg/ezetimibe 10 mg): no significant reduction in primary outcome of major atherosclerotic events in over 3,000 patients on dialysis.
- Other data not yet incorporated into practice guidelines (confirmatory data still needed):
  - Veterans Affairs High-density Lipoprotein Intervention Trial (VA-HIT): gemfibrozil reduces the risk of major cardiovascular events (fatal coronary heart disease, nonfatal MI, and stroke) by 42% in a post hoc analysis of 297 individuals with eGFR < 75 mL/min/1.73 m^2 and diabetes.
  - Diabetes Atherosclerosis Intervention Study (DAIS) and Fenofibrate Intervention and Event Lowering in Diabetes (FIELD) study: fenofibrate lowered the risk of developing new onset microalbuminuria.

Other Therapeutic Candidates

- Bardoxolone methyl:
  - Background:
    - Oxidative stress and impaired antioxidant capacity adversely affect CKD progression.

- Oxidative stress and inflammation are associated with impaired activity of the nuclear 1 factor (erythroid-derived 2)-related factor 2 (Frf2) transcription factor in animals with CKD.
  - Bardoxolone methyl is the most potent known activators of the Nrf2.
- Bardoxolone Methyl Evaluation in Patients with CKD and type 2 DM: the Occurrence of Renal Events (BEACON):
  - Bardoxolone did *not* reduce the risk of ESRD or death from cardiovascular events.
  - Bardoxolone had a higher rate of cardiovascular events compared with placebo.
- Peroxisome proliferator-activated receptor γ (PPAR) agonists:
  - PPARγ modulates numerous effectors of ECM accumulation.
  - Thiazolidinediones (TZD) are PPARγ agonists.
  - TZDs prevent increase in TGF-β and ECM and inhibit mesangial cell and fibroblast proliferation *in vitro*.
  - TZD + ARB losartan may confer better renoprotection than ARB alone, although safety of using TZD needs to be addressed:
    - Prior concerns for coronary artery disease with rosiglitazone (Avandia) but recent trial revealed no increased risk of myocardial infarction;
    - Concerns for possible association with bladder cancer with pioglitazone (Actos).
  - More data still needed for PPARγ agonists.
- AGE-targeted therapies:
  - Aminoguanidine blocks AGE formation and improves mesangial matrix expansion and albuminuria, but its use is limited by side effects.
  - Pyridoxamine dihydrochloride (pyridorin), a derivative of vitamin B_6 and potent inhibitor of AGE formation has been shown slow DKD progression, but only in patients with relatively preserved kidney function (i.e., baseline SCr 1.3 to 1.9 mg/dL).
  - Phenacylthiazolium bromide may be able to cleave AGE-derived protein cross-links.
- Other potential medical interventions:
  - Anti-TGF-β agent: pirfenidone has been shown to be renoprotective in mice.
  - Inhibitor of protein kinase C, β-isoform: ruboxistaurin
    - Small study suggests reduction of albuminuria and eGFR decline.
    - Efficacy in DR is being studied.
  - Pentoxifylline 1,200 mg/d, a nonspecific phosphodiesterase inhibitor commonly used to treat occlusive peripheral vascular disease, has been shown to improve eGFR decline and albuminuria in patients with DM2, DKD stages 3 to 4 at 24-month follow-up.

Other Considerations in the Management of DKD

- Nonmedical strategies to slow down progression of DKD: smoking cessation, weight loss
- Autonomic neuropathy exacerbates uremic symptoms.

SICKLE CELL DISEASE

Renal Manifestations of Sickle Cell Disease

- Cortical manifestations are thought to arise from hemolysis associated endothelial dysfunction:
  - Early alterations: hyperfiltration, glomerular hypertrophy, hypermetabolism

- Supranormal proximal tubular function:
  - Increased reabsorption of sodium, phosphate, β_2-microglobulin
  - Increased secretion of:
    - Uric acid (in early disease with good kidney function, serum uric acid level may be normal despite increased uric acid production)
    - Creatinine (thus eGFR based on serum creatinine may be greatly overestimated. Best equation for eGFR is thought to be CKD-EPI, but even then there may be as much as 45 mL/min overestimation.)
- Late alterations:
  - Proteinuria
  - Glomerulopathy:
    - FSGS is the most common lesion.
    - Others: MPGN (commonly occurs without IC deposits, may be associated with blood borne viral infections from transfusions), "sickle cell glomerulopathy" defined as glomerular hypertrophy with or without mesangial hypercellularity, TMA (associated with history of retinitis)
  - CKD and failure:
    - Genetic variants of MYH9 and APOL1 are associated with proteinuria, CKD, and loss of kidney function in sickle cell disease (SCD).
    - Higher fetal hemoglobin (Hbf) is protective against sickle cell nephropathy and vasoocclusive complications.
    - Coinheritance with α-thalassemia appears to be protective against proteinuria and sickle cell nephropathy in SCD patients.
    - Special considerations of CKD in SCD:
      - Hemoglobin target with erythropoiesis-stimulating agent use should not exceed 10.5 g/dL.
- Medullary manifestations are thought to arise from viscosity-associated vasoocclusion:
  - Structural injury:
    - Micro- to macroscopic hematuria:
      - 10% bilateral, left kidney affected 4 times greater than right due to increased venous pressure in left renal vein.
      - There is increased sickling of red blood cells in vasa recta due to low oxygen tension, low pH, high osmolality in renal medulla. Sickling leads to increased blood viscosity, microthrombus formation, and ischemic necrosis.
      - Management of hematuria:
        - Conservative: bed rest, volume repletion, rule out papillary necrosis
        - For persistent hematuria, consider vasopressin or ε aminocaproic acid (synthetic inhibitor of the plasmin-plasminogen system) 2 to 3 g daily over several days, not to exceed 12 g daily due to risk of thrombosis.
        - For medical therapy failure or life-threatening bleeding, arterial embolization or surgical intervention must be considered.
    - Papillary necrosis (typically asymptomatic) $\pm$ acute obstructive uropathy. NOTE: current data suggest that hematuria and papillary necrosis do *not* portend greater risk for renal failure. Papillary necrosis with sloughing can give the appearance of "egg in a cup" or "golf ball and a club" on contrast computed tomogram urography. See Figure 7.4 in Tubular, Interstitial, and Cystic Diseases chapter.
- Tubular manifestations:
  - Impaired concentrating ability with resultant isosthenuria (urine osmolality < 450 mOsm/kg). May present as polyuria, hypovolemia prone with poor oral

intake, and nocturnal enuresis in young patients. This defect may be reversible with blood transfusion in young patients, but become uncorrectable by age 15.
- Impaired potassium secretion with resultant hyperkalemia. Renin–angiotensin–aldosterone system is intact.
- Incomplete renal tubular acidosis: typically not clinically significant, but can be unmasked with reduction in GFR.
  - Voltage-dependent hyperkalemic distal RTA: patients fail to secrete both H^+ and K^+, thus urine pH > 5.5.
  - Selective aldosterone deficiency distal RTA: patients have hyperkalemia induced suboptimal ammoniagenesis, but can secrete H^+, thus urine pH can be <5.5. These patients respond to fludrocortisone.

Kidney Transplantation in SCD

- One year graft survival ≥ 60 to $80+\%$
- Confers survival benefit: although survival of SCD kidney transplant recipients is inferior to that of matched African American transplant recipients without SCD, survival of SCD transplant recipients is comparable with that of matched diabetic patients.
- Kidney transplant may be complicated by allograft venous thrombosis, deep vein thrombosis, and vasoocclusive crises.

> **NOTE**   Of interest, hydroxyurea, an agent often used in patients with frequent vasoocclusive crises to increase Hbf levels, has been suggested to reduce proteinuria and hyperfiltration. Confirmatory studies are required.

Renal Manifestations of Sickle Cell Trait (SCT)

- Similar abnormalities noted above with SCD but lesser extent of injury
- NOTE: Most notable renal manifestation with sickle cell trait is renal medullary carcinoma:
- Medullary carcinoma: occurs *exclusively in sickle cell trait* and typically presents as an aggressive metastatic disease at the time of diagnosis in young patients (20 to 30 years old).
- Prognosis is poor (median survival is 3 months following diagnosis).
- Hematuria/flank pain/abdominal mass must be taken very seriously in sickle cell trait!
- Whether SCT predisposes to CKD is not clear.
- However, among African American with polycystic kidney disease, cystic hemorrhage is more common and progression to ESRD is more rapid.

VIRAL NEPHRITIDES

Human Immunodeficiency Virus

- HIV may be associated with various renal lesions including HIV-associated nephropathy (HIVAN), HIV-associated immune complex kidney disease (HIVICK), combined antiretroviral treatment (cART) nephropathy, and TMA.

HIV-Associated Nephropathy

Epidemiology

- Predominantly observed in African American
- Associated with advanced HIV (i.e., CD4 < 200 cells/mm^3, high viral load)

Clinical Manifestations

- Nephrotic range proteinuria, hematuria, normal to enlarged kidneys due to microcyst formation

Pathogenesis

- Genetic susceptibility: APOL1
- Both direct and indirect mechanisms involving HIV are thought to be contributory.

Histopathology

- LM: collapsing FSGS, tubular microcystic dilatation with proteinaceous casts, and variable acute tubular injury, tubular atrophy, lymphocytic infiltrates, interstitial fibrosis (Fig. 7.18)
- EM: presence of tubuloreticular inclusions in endothelial cell cytoplasm in untreated patients

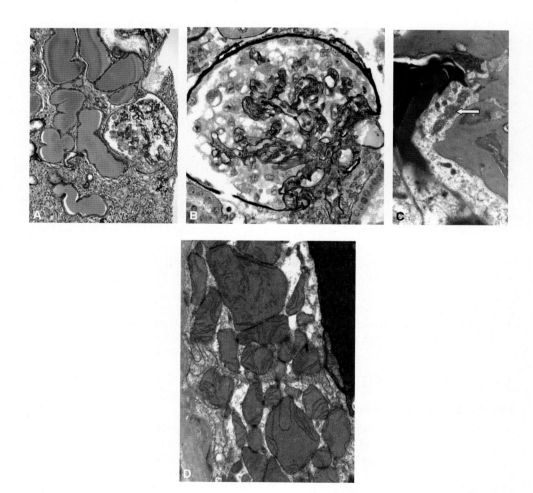

FIGURE 7.18 HIV-associated nephropathy. **A.** Cluster of dilated tubules with plasma protein casts and collapsing glomerulopathy (Jones silver, ×100). **B.** Collapsing glomerulopathy showing capillary collapsing with podocyte hypertrophy, hyperplasia, and cytoplasmic vacuoles (Jones silver, ×400). **C.** Tubuloreticular inclusion (*arrow*) in glomerular endothelial cell. These disappear with HAART (×15,000). **D.** Enlarged atypical proximal tubular mitochondria with broken cristae associated with nucleotide reverse transciptase inhibitor (tenofovir) treatment (×10,000).

Natural History/Prognosis
- Rapid progression to ESRD if untreated

Management
- Combined antiretroviral therapy (cART), renin–angiotensin system inhibition, corticosteroid therapy *if* rapid decline in kidney function despite cART *and* absence of superimposed/opportunistic infections

HIV-Associated Immune Complex Kidney Disease
Background
- Typically occurs in patients with HIV duration ≥ 10 years
- Reported lesions: IgAN, lupus-like GN, MGN, membranous/mesangial proliferative GN, postinfectious GN, immunotactoid/fibrillary GN. NOTE: Since IgAN is rare in African Americans, the presence of IgAN should raise the possibility of concurrent HIV infection.

Clinical Manifestations
- Nephrotic syndrome, hematuria, HTN; Laboratory findings may be positive for ANA, low C3

Histopathology
- IF: notable for variable Ig/complement staining, "full house" of Ig may be present
- EM: presence of cytoplasmic tubuloreticular structures in endothelial cells

Combined Anti-retroviral Treatment (cART) Nephropathy
- Nucleotide analog reverse transcriptase inhibitors: mitochondrial dysfunction, Fanconi syndrome, AKI/ATN:
  - Most well-recognized: tenofovir
  - Others: lamivudine (3TC), abacavir (ABC), didanosine (ddI)
  - NOTE: mitochondrial injury may be seen on EM as giant mitochondria with atypical shapes and broken or absent cristae.
- Protease inhibitors with associated crystal-induced nephropathy/urolithiasis: indinavir, atazanavir, nelfinavir, amprenavir, saquinavir, lopinavir/ritonavir—Indinavir crystals have been described as "plate-like rectangles and fan-shaped or starburst forms"

Thrombotic Microangiopathy
- May be seen with advanced HIV, not treated with cART
- Pathogenesis thought to involve direct HIV attack of endothelial cells
- Affected individuals may have low ADAMTS13 levels, in which case, good response to therapy including corticosteroids and plasma exchange may be expected.

Kidney Transplantation in Patients with HIV
- May be considered if undetectable viral load *and* CD4 > 200 cells/mm^3
- Requirement for immunosuppressive therapy is typically minimal due to drug-drug interactions.
- NOTE: major drug interaction: protease inhibitors (e.g., darunavir, ritonavir) can markedly increase CNI levels. Less than 5% of usual CNI dose is typically required.

Hepatitis A

- Most common kidney presentation is AKI, ATN.
- Other possible lesions: tubulointerstitial disease, IC-proliferative GN
- Renal recovery typically parallels liver recovery.

Hepatitis B

Associated Lesions

- MGN with or without concurrent anti-PLA2R antibodies is most common.
- Other notable associated lesions: MPGN (type I), IgAN (in association with chronic liver disease), PAN (IC deposits formed by HBsAg and anti-HBs antibody (IgM) along vessel walls)

Management

- Antiviral therapy: first-line agents include tenofovir, entecavir, and Peg-IFN alfa-2a. Alternatively, adefovir and telbivudine may be used, but at the risk of high rate of resistance. Lamivudine has high rate of resistance and is not preferred.
- Consider corticosteroids (i.e., prednisone 1 mg/kg/d for 2 weeks) and plasma exchange prior to antiviral therapy in PAN.
- Nonspecific therapies: RAAS inhibition, BP control
- Do *not* use rituximab due to association with hepatitis B reactivation. Rituximab may be used with hepatitis C but *not* hepatitis B.

Hepatitis C

Clinical Extra-hepatic Manifestations of Hepatitis C

- Cryoglobulinemia, IC and lymphoproliferative disorder with associated arthralgias, fatigue, palpable purpura, digital ischemia, renal disease, peripheral neuropathy, CNS vasculitis, hypocomplementemia
- MPGN with or without cryoglobulinemia:
  - Cryoglobulins are immunoglobulins directed against the Fc portion of anti-HCV antibody which defines rheumatoid factor activity.
  - Laboratory findings: positive rheumatoid factor, hypocomplementemia
  - Chronic active HCV infection may be associated with B-cell lymphoproliferative diseases, with the most common monoclonal gammopathy being IgM, κ light chain.
  - Clinical manifestations: asymptomatic hematuria and proteinuria, nephrotic syndrome, slowly progressive CKD, or rapidly progressive GN
  - EM: cryoglobulins resemble "fingerprint" pattern of fibrils of 30 nm.
- Other HCV-associated renal lesions: MGN (two-third of patients have positive anti-PLA2R antibody, significance unknown), fibrillary/immunotactoid GN, PAN

Clinical Impact of Hepatitis C

- Chronic hepatitis C correlates with the incidence of DM type 2 and adverse outcomes.
- Successful antiviral therapy against HCV is associated with improved insulin resistance and reduced incidence of new-onset DM type 2.
- The incidence of ESRD, ischemic stroke, and acute coronary syndrome is reduced among successfully treated HCV patients with DM type 2 in a large prospective cohort from Taiwan.
- Patients with type 2 DM and insulin resistance with hepatitis C are at increased risk for hepatocellular carcinoma.

- HCV in the dialysis patient:
  - Prevalence is 8% to 9%.
  - Seroprevalence of HCV increases with dialysis vintage.
  - HCV-infected hemodialysis patients have decreased quality of life and increased mortality compared to their noninfected counterpart.
  - HCV infection may reduce both patient and allograft survival in the kidney recipient. However, kidney transplantation in HCV infected patients may improve survival compared with remaining on dialysis. The advent of highly effective interferon-free and direct acting antiviral therapy may improve post-transplant outcomes.

Management

- Antiviral therapy: American Association for the Study of Liver Diseases and Infectious Diseases Society of America, http://www.hcvguidelines.org:
  - Antiviral therapy is recommended for all patients with chronic HCV infection, except for those with short life expectancies.
  - For patients with CrCl > 30 mL/min, no dosage adjustment is needed:
    - Daclatasvir, fixed-dose combination of ledipasvir (90 mg)/sofosbuvir (400 mg), or fixed-dose combination of paritaprevir (150 mg)/ritonavir (100 mg)/ombitasvir (25 mg) with (or without for HCV genotype 4) twice-daily dosed dasabuvir (250 mg), simeprevir, or sofosbuvir
  - For patients with CrCl < 30 mL/min who do not have cirrhosis, but for whom the urgency to treat (or retreat) is high and renal transplant is not an immediate option:
    - Daily fixed-dose combination of paritaprevir (150 mg)/ritonavir (100 mg)/ombisasvir (100 mg) with twice-daily dosed dasabuvir (250 mg) (for HCV genotype 1b) or without dasabuvir (for HCV genotype 4) is recommended. NOTE: Recommendation is based on limited data on safety and efficacy.
    - For HCV genotype 1a, daily fixed-dose combination of paritaprevir (150 mg)/ritonavir (100 mg)/ombitasvir (25 mg) plus twice-daily dosed dasabuvir (250 mg) with ribavirin at reduced doses (200 mg thrice weekly to daily) is recommended. Due to the risk of hemolysis with advanced CKD patients, ribavirin should not be used in patients with baseline hemoglobin concentration ≤ 10 g/dL. Additionally, ribavirin should be discontinued if the hemoglobin level declines >2 g/dL despite use of erythropoiesis-stimulating agents.
    - For patients with HCV genotype 2, 3, 5, or 6 and CrCl < 30 mL/min, PEG-interferon and dose-adjusted ribavirin is recommended if treatment is necessary and transplantation cannot be performed.
- For patients with hepatitis C-related renal disease and cryoglobulinemia: Interferon-based regimens have been shown to reverse proteinuria and nephrotic syndrome, but not necessarily ameliorate azotemia.
- Addition of immunosuppressive therapy (e.g., corticosteroids plus either CYC or rituximab) and/or plasmapheresis (if cryoglobulinemia) should be considered if severe renal involvement and poor response to antiviral therapy alone

Parvovirus

- May be associated with collapsing FSGS, MPGN, diffuse proliferative GN

Hantavirus

- Hemorrhagic nephritis; see Tubulointerstitial Diseases

BK Nephropathy
- See Kidney Transplantation chapter.

Cytomegalovirus
- Associated proliferative GN has been reported, but presumed to be very rare. In kidney transplants, CMV infections involving renal tubular cells and macrophages may result in intracytoplasmic inclusions with "owl-like" appearance.

FABRY DISEASE

Background
- Second most prevalent lysosomal storage disease after Gaucher disease
- May be seen in all ethnics and races
- X-linked inborn error with deficiency or defect of lysosomal hydrolase α-galactosidase A (α-Gal A), an enzyme that normally catalyzes the hydrolytic cleavage of the terminal galactose from globotriaosylceramide (Gb3). The enzymatic deficiency/defect leads to lysosomal accumulation of Gb3 in various cells including vascular endothelium and smooth muscle cells, cardiac muscle cells and conduction fibers, kidneys, and nerve root ganglia.

Clinical Manifestations
- Neurologic: neuropathic pain in extremities, stroke in early age
- Dermatologic: telangiectasias, angiokeratomas in groin, hip, periumbilical areas, corneal opacities, thickened lips, bullous nose, hypohidrosis or hyperhidrosis and associated heat/exercise or cold intolerance, respectively
- Cardiac: arrhythmias, left ventricular hypertrophy
- Gastrointestinal: abdominal pain, diarrhea
- Renal: proteinuria (both tubular and glomerular proteinuria possible), progressive CKD, Fanconi syndrome due to proximal tubular injury, polydipsia and polyuria due to distal tubular injury and associated defective urinary concentrating ability, multiple renal sinus, and parapelvic cysts on imaging studies

Histopathology
- LM:
  - Vacuolization/foamy appearance of podocytes and rarely distal tubular epithelial cells due to glycolipid accumulation (Fig. 7.19)
  - Nonspecific findings: FSGS or global glomerulosclerosis, tubulointerstitial fibrosis
- EM: "myeloid" or "zebra" bodies which are concentric lamellated inclusions often with a striped (zebra) appearance formed by Gb3 deposits within enlarged secondary lysosomes.
- NOTE: lamellar inclusions may be seen prominently in podocytes associated with chloroquine or plaquenil administration. Less often they occur in gentamicin toxicity, or silicosis, predominantly in proximal, not distal, tubules.

Diagnosis
- Low α-Gal A activity in leukocytes of plasma in males
- Female carriers may have normal to low levels of α-Gal A, thus require genetic analysis for the α-Gal A gene.

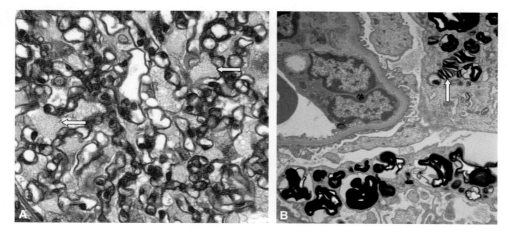

FIGURE 7.19 Fabry disease. **A.** Enlarged foamy podocytes (*arrows*) throughout the glomerulus (Masson trichrome, ×600). **B.** Podocytes contain whorled and clumped electron dense inclusions (myelin figures) composed of accumulated globotriaosylceramide. These inclusions may have a striped or "zebra body" appearance (*arrow*) (×10,000).

- Genetic analysis may also be required in males with marginally low α-Gal A activity levels.
- Tissue biopsy (skin or kidney) reveals characteristic findings but is typically not necessary.

Management
- Genetic counseling
- Enzyme (α-Gal A) replacement therapy:
  - Recommended for all males and females with classic presentations
  - Patient-specific consideration in asymptomatic female carriers or males with atypical presentations
  - Enzyme-replacement therapy effectively reduces deposition of Gb3 in most tissues except for podocytes and vascular smooth muscle. Nonetheless replacement therapy may slow kidney function decline in early disease.
  - Replacement options: agalsidase α 0.2 mg/kg or agalsidase β 1.0 mg/kg infusion every 2 weeks. Notable side effects: infusion reactions, development of antibodies against the enzyme

Kidney Transplantation
- Improves survival compared to nontransplant

Access the eBook for self-assessment questions.

8 Kidney Transplantation

Phuong-Thu T. Pham, Jennifer Q. Zhang, and Cynthia C. Nast

TRANSPLANT IMMUNOBIOLOGY

ABO Blood Group Antigens

- The ABO blood group antigens are expressed on the surface of red blood cells as well as in the kidneys, gastrointestinal, respiratory, and other organ systems. The ABO blood group is the most important tissue barrier to successful kidney transplantation, followed by the Major Histocompatibility Complex (MHC) antigens. Non-MHC molecules, referred to as minor histocompatibility antigens, can also mediate rejection (MHC-matched siblings, unlike identical siblings require immunosuppressive therapy to prevent graft rejection).
- ABO-incompatible kidney transplantation results in hyperacute rejection and graft loss.
- A number of variant A antigens are known, with the A1 antigen providing more potent antigenicity than the antigen A2. Successful transplantation can be performed using A2 kidneys into O recipients and A2 and A2B kidneys into B recipients.
- Within the past decade, various desensitization protocols have allowed successful ABO-incompatible kidney transplantation.

Major Histocompatibility Complex, Human Leukocyte Antigen Molecules

- The major histocompatibility (MHC) genes are located on the short arm of chromosome 6 and represent the most polymorphic genes in human genome. In human, MHC was first discovered in leukocyte; therefore, it is also called the Human Leukocyte Antigens (HLAs).
- In kidney transplantation, HLAs are the predominant antigens that form the targets for the immune response.
- Each parental chromosome 6 provides a linked set of MHC genes (called a haplotype) to the offspring in a Mendelian codominance inheritance. Statistically, there is a 25% chance that siblings share the same two haplotypes (two-haplotype match), a 50% chance they share one same haplotype (one-haplotype match), and a 25% chance they do not share any of their parental haplotypes (zero-haplotype match). By definition, a child is a haplotype match to each parent unless recombination has occurred (Fig. 8.1).
- In two unrelated individuals, it is not possible to identify the haplotypes because it is not known which antigens are linked on each chromosome. Therefore, the term "three-antigen match" or "three-antigen mismatch" is used.

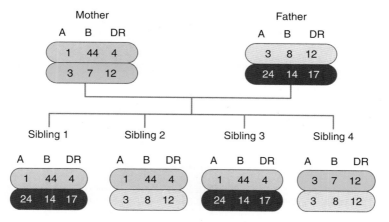

FIGURE 8.1 Inheritance of haplotypes and HLA profiles in four theoretical siblings. Sibling 1 is a one-haplotype match to sibling 2, a two-haplotype match to sibling 3, and a zero-haplotype match to sibling 4.

- Terms used for HLA match (or mismatch):
  - Kidney from parent (father or mother): one haplotype match (1 HLA-A, 1 HLA-B, and 1 HLA-DR match)
  - Kidney from siblings: zero-haplotype match, one-haplotype match, or two-haplotype match (Fig. 8.1).
  - Kidney from deceased donor:
    - 1 out of 6 HLA antigen match (or 5 HLA antigen mismatch)
    - 2 out of 6 HLA antigen match (or 4 HLA antigen mismatch)
    - 3 out of 6 antigen match (or 3 HLA antigen mismatch)
    - 4 out of 6 HLA antigen match (or 2 HLA antigen mismatch)
    - 5 out of 6 HLA antigen match (or 1 HLA antigen mismatch)
    - 6 out of 6 HLA antigen match (or 0 HLA antigen mismatch)
- HLA class I:
  - The classical HLA class I antigens (HLA-A, -B, and -C) are composed of a polymorphic α or heavy chain of 44 kDa and a nonpolymorphic light chain, β_2-microglobulin of 12 kDa.
  - They are expressed on all nucleated cells and generally present peptides derived from intracellular proteins (e.g., viral proteins) to cytotoxic CD8$^+$ T cells (Fig. 8.2)
- HLA class II:
  - The classical class II antigens (HLA-DP, -DQ, and -DR) are composed of polymorphic α and β chains of similar molecular weight (32 kDa), covalently bound to each other (encoded by DPA, DPB, DQA, DQB, DRA, DRB genes).
  - They are constitutively expressed only on professional antigen-presenting cells (APC) including dendritic cells, macrophages, and B lymphocytes. Their expression may be upregulated on epithelial and vascular endothelial cells after exposure to proinflammatory cytokines.
  - Class II molecules present larger peptides derived from extracellular proteins (e.g., bacterial proteins) to CD4$^+$ T cells (Fig. 8.2)
- The degree of HLA mismatch between donor and recipient plays an important role in rejection risk and graft loss.
- Donors and recipients are typed for HLA-A, -B, –DRB and DQB that are used for matching before transplantation. HLA-Cw typing is also mandatory for all deceased donors.

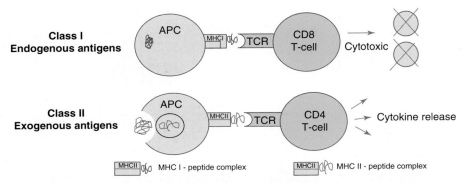

FIGURE 8.2 HLA Class I and Class II Antigens. **Class I Pathway**: Endogenous antigens are digested into peptides and loaded into class I MHC. The MHC-peptide complex is assembled within the cell's endoplasmic reticulum, transported through the Golgi apparatus and expressed on the cell surface where it is recognized by CD8[+] T-cell receptor (TCR), leading to T cell activation. **Class II Pathway**: Exogenous antigens are degraded within endosomes and loaded into class II MHC. The MHC–peptide complex is ultimately expressed on the cell surface where it is recognized by CD4[+] T-cell receptor, leading to T cell activation.

- HLA-DP, and DQA are increasingly typed and used in many transplant centers.
- In the settings of kidney transplant, the number of HLA mismatches on graft survival is more important than HLA matches (i.e., the fewer the mismatches, the better the graft survival).
- One-year graft survival is more related to HLA class II mismatching than to class I mismatching. In the current United Network for Organ Sharing (UNOS) allocation scheme, points are given to patients without class II mismatch: 2 points if there are no DR mismatches and 1 point if there is one DR mismatch.

Minor Histocompatibility Antigens

- Minor histocompatibility antigens are small endogenous peptides that occupy the antigen-binding site of the donor MHC molecules.
- Minor histocompatibility antigens are usually recognized by CD8[+] cytotoxic T cells in the context of self-MHC, leading to graft rejection.
- Class I-like genes (MHC class I-related chain A [MICA] and MHC class I-related chain B [MICB]) are examples of minor antigen expressed on endothelial cells. Antibodies against MICA and/or MICB can cause antibody-mediated rejection (AMR).
- HLA identical siblings require immunosuppression albeit at reduced dose due to differences in minor histocompatibility antigens.

Allorecognition Pathways: Direct, Indirect, and Semidirect Allorecognition

- In the direct pathway, recipient T cells recognize intact allogeneic Human Leukocyte Antigens (HLAs) expressed by donor cells (Fig. 8.3).
- In the indirect pathway, T cells recognize peptides derived from donor HLAs presented by recipient antigen presenting cells (APCs) (Fig. 8.3).
- In the semidirect pathway, intact donor HLAs are presented on the recipient APCs (through either membrane exchange or exosome uptake) to the recipient T cells (Fig. 8.3).
- Acute rejection of an allograft is primarily dependent on direct allorecognition whereas the indirect pathway has been suggested to be more important in chronic rejection. The semidirect pathway also plays an important role in chronic allograft rejection

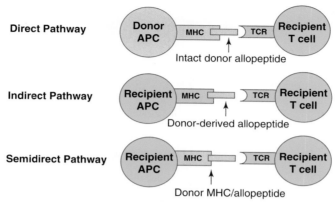

FIGURE 8.3 Direct, indirect, and semidirect allorecognition pathways. (1) In the direct allorecognition pathway, recipient T cells recognize intact allogeneic HLA antigens expressed by donor cells. (2) In the indirect pathway, T cells recognize peptides derived from donor HLAs presented by recipient antigen presenting cells APCs. (3) In the semidirect pathway, the donor MHC is recycled and presents as intact molecule on recipient APCs to recipient T cells (MHC can be recycled through internalized donor extracellular vesicles containing donor MHC or through membrane exchanges between donor and recipient APCs. Detailed discussion is beyond the scope of this chapter.)

Pretransplantation Crossmatch

- Preformed HLA antibodies prohibit successful organ transplantation.
- The crossmatch test is performed prior to transplantation to determine whether patient has antibody directed against a potential donor.
- The potential donor lymphocytes serve as the target cells for the patient's serum.
- Complement–dependent cytotoxicity (CDC) crossmatch test is used to determine high titer of HLA antibodies in patient's serum against donor cells. The presence of preformed cytotoxic IgG antidonor HLA antibodies is a contraindication to transplantation.
- Flow crossmatch test is more sensitive as compared to CDC crossmatch for HLA antibody detection.
- Antibodies directed against HLA class I result in a positive crossmatch with both B and T cells.
- A positive crossmatch against T cells is an indication of anti-class I antibodies in the patient, whereas a positive crossmatch with B cells could be caused by either anti-class I or anti-class II antibodies.
- Antibodies directed against class II will only cause a positive crossmatch with B lymphocytes.
- The different pretransplantation crossmatch methods is summarized in Table 8.1

Cytotoxicity Panel Reactive Antibodies

- Sensitization to allogeneic HLA antigens can occur through pregnancies, prior transplantation, and blood transfusions.
- Anti-HLA antibodies in patient's serum may react with cells from a panel of donors that represent a given donor pool.
- Panel reactive antibodies (PRA), expressed as percentage, is the percentage of potential donors' cells tested that were killed by the patient's serum.
- The PRA estimates the percentage of organ donors who would be crossmatch incompatible with a transplant candidate in a given donor pool tested. A PRA of 80% indicates that patient has 20% of chance to receive a negative crossmatch.

Table 8.1	Different crossmatch methods used for kidney transplantation	
Crossmatch	**Methods**	**Comments**
NIH standard technique (Complement-dependent lymphocytotoxicity-CDC)	(1) Recipient serum mixed with donor lymphocytes (T cells, B cells, or mixed) (2) Complement added If recipient antidonor antibodies bind to the antigens on the donor lymphocytes, added complement will kill donor lymphocytes. Cells that are killed are evaluated using fluorescent dyes that identify live and dead cells. Results are recorded using a semiquantitative score (e.g., negative, weakly positive, strongly positive)	Detect high titer of HLA antibodies that fix complement. Positive T- and/or B-cell crossmatch test is a contraindication to kidney transplantation.
Antiglobulin-enhanced CDC crossmatch	(1) Recipient serum mixed with donor lymphocytes (2) Antihuman Ig potentiating reagent added (3) Complement added	More sensitive than the standard CDC crossmatch Can detect antibodies present in small amount or non–complement-binding antibodies
Flow crossmatch	(1) Recipient serum mixed with donor lymphocytes (2) Fluorochrome-coated antihuman antibodies added (3) Assess with flow cytometer	Most sensitive crossmatch test Can be useful if donor lymphocytes are nonviable

Techniques for Detection of Anti-HLA Antibodies: General Concepts

- The tests used to identify anti-HLA antibodies are based on assessing reactions of antibodies present in the patient's serum with well-characterized panels of donor lymphocytes (cell-based, CDC—see Table 8.1) or purified HLA antigens coupled to microspheres (bead-based, flow cytometry).
  - The use of donor lymphocytes can detect whether a patient has antibodies against donor antigens but does not allow identification of specific antigens to which the patient has antibodies.
  - The use of antigen-coated beads can determine PRA and identify antibodies to specific antigens (discussed under Luminex Technology).
- Bead-based Luminex technology has replaced cell-based technology for detecting anti-HLA antibodies. However, it should be noted that Luminex single antibody (SAB) testing is not a FDA-approved quantitative assay.

Flow Cytometry

- Flow cytometry is used to assess the specificity of anti-HLA antibodies that are not normally detected by the less-sensitive complement–dependent lymphocytotoxicity test.
- Flow PRA value is expressed as the percentage of HLA antigen-coated beads in a pool that react with antibodies in the patient's sera. A high PRA generally indicates that the patient is primed to react immunologically against a large proportion of the population.

Solid-Phase Assays Using Luminex Technology

- Luminex is a solid phase assay that uses single HLA antigen-coated beads to detect and identify preformed HLA antibodies before transplantation as well as to monitor for de novo development of anti-HLA antibodies after transplantation. The Mean Fluorescence Intensity (MFI) is a semi-quantitative measurement of antibody titer (strength of the anti-HLA antibodies) (Fig. 8.4).

- The Luminex technology permits identification of unacceptable donor antigens.
- Unacceptable HLA antigens are defined by the strength of the HLA antibodies present in the patient's serum (measured as mean fluorescence intensity [MFI]).
- Individual centers set their own MFI threshold that would result in a positive cross-match against donors who express the target HLA specificities and enter the information into the national computer. For instance, if a patient has a high MFI titer to HLA-B8, potential donors expressing HLA-B8 would not be acceptable (i.e., HLA-B8 is an "unacceptable HLA antigen"), and kidneys from these donors will not be offered to that patient due to a predicted positive crossmatch (see Virtual Crossmatch).
- UNOS uses a calculated PRA (cPRA) based on "unacceptable antigens."
- cPRA is calculated based on HLA antigen frequencies from actual UNOS donor pool; therefore, it permits a uniform measurement of sensitization.
- Patients with donor-specific antibodies (DSA) or anti-HLA antibodies in the serum have been shown to have poorer graft survival compared with those without DSA or anti-HLA antibodies.

Virtual Crossmatch

- A virtual crossmatch is a crossmatch that involves a determination of the presence or absence of DSA in a patient by comparing the patient's HLA antibody specificity profile to the HLA type of the proposed donor without performing an actual crossmatch (such as CDC or flow cytometry crossmatch).
- A virtual crossmatch requires the following:
  - Complete tissue typing of the donor (HLA-A, -B, -C, -DP, -DQ, -DR)
  - Complete tissue typing of the recipient

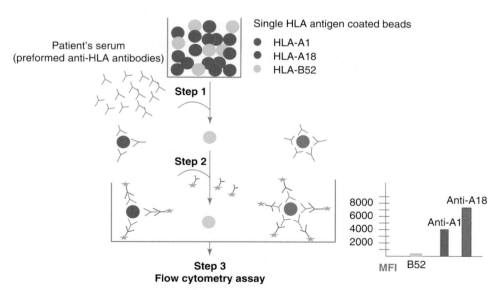

FIGURE 8.4 Bead-based Luminex technology. An array of polystyrene microbeads is labeled with different ratio of two fluorescent dyes. By measuring the composition of the emissions of these beads, up to 100 distinct beads with a unique HLA antigen can be identified concomitantly. **Step 1**: Single HLA antigen-coated beads are incubated with patient's serum. **Step 2**: Flurochrome-tagged antihuman antibodies are added. **Step 3**: Flow cytometry assay: The detection of the emission intensities of the fluorochrome-tagged secondary antibodies correlates with the relative strength of the HLA antibodies (measured as mean fluorescence intensity or MFI).

- Up-to-date solid-phase anti-HLA antibody analysis of the recipient (using recombinant single HLA antigen bead technologies)
- Crossmatch results can now be accurately predicted based on the MFI values of the DSA. Due to interlaboratory variation, each laboratory must establish the MFI values that correlate with positive crossmatch at their centers.
- Virtual crossmatch is important for deceased donor allocation for heart and lung transplant recipients to reduce cold-ischemia time. Accurate virtual crossmatch is also important for import deceased donor for kidney transplantation.

EVALUATION OF THE POTENTIAL KIDNEY TRANSPLANT CANDIDATES

- Kidney transplantation is the treatment of choice for suitable candidates with end-stage renal disease (ESRD).
  - It confers survival advantage over remaining on dialysis across all ages and in both diabetic and nondiabetic transplant recipients.
  - It offers long-term economic benefits compared to dialysis.
  - Although there has been no consensus on the upper age limit at which patients are accepted for kidney transplantation, 80 years of age has been suggested to be a sensible biologic limit. Suitability for transplantation should be assessed on a case-by-case basis.
- The routine assessment of a kidney transplant candidate includes thorough history and physical examination, psychosocial evaluation, and psychiatric evaluation as needed. In addition, patients should attend a patient education session and undergo a number of routine laboratory testing and imaging studies as outlined in Table 8.2
- The absolute and relative contraindications to transplantation are outlined in Table 8.3
- The UNOS listing criteria for deceased donor kidney: chronic kidney disease with glomerular filtration rate (GFR) $\leq$ 20 mL/min or ESRD.
- Transplant candidates with a history of malignancies: Table 8.4 provides general guidelines for minimum tumor-waiting periods for common malignancies.
- Disease recurrence after transplantation: patients should be informed of the risk of disease recurrence after transplantation and the risk of graft loss associated with disease recurrence (discussed under Posttransplant Noninfectious Complications).
- Candidates with specific medical conditions:
  - Hepatitis B and C:
    - Diagnostic tests for hepatitis B virus (HBV) and hepatitis C virus (HCV) are shown in Table 8.5
    - Consider HCV-positive donor for HCV-positive recipient who are viremic (informed consent should preferably be obtained at the time of pretransplant evaluation).
    - Screen for hepatocellular carcinoma particularly in high-risk patients (such as those with high HBV viral load, HBeAg positive, HBsAg positive, Asian or African ethnicity)
    - Patients with hepatitis B and/or C infection should be referred to hepatology.
    - Liver biopsy is often indicated to assess the severity of liver disease (grade and stage) because liver enzymes may be spuriously normal in patients with chronic kidney disease despite advanced liver disease.
    - Advanced liver disease or liver cirrhosis is generally considered as a contraindication to kidney alone transplantation (see also Table 8.3 for relative contraindications). Patients with decompensated liver disease should be referred for simultaneous liver–kidney transplantation.

Table 8.2	Pretransplant routine laboratory testing and imaging studies

Laboratory evaluation

Comprehensive metabolic panel

CBC with platelets

Prothrombin time panel (INR and PTT)

Urinalysis and urine culture

Hepatitis B (surface Ag, IgM and IgG core Ab, and surface Ab)

HCV Ab screening (if positive, check PCR confirmatory test)

HIV1/HIV2 antibody screen

CMV antibody panel

EBV-VCA IgM/EBNA-1 IgG panel

RPR or VDRL (FTA-ABS confirmatory test if positive RPR or VDRL)

Serum immunofixation electrophoresis if age > 60

Iron and iron-binding capacity, ferritin

Type and screen

Coccidioides IgG/IgM EIA (recommended for patients with history of valley fever or those who live in endemic areas)

Special laboratory evaluation

Hypercoagulability panel in patients with history of recurrent thrombosis

PSA screening for men with family history, obstructive voiding symptoms or hematuria[a]

Other evaluation

EKG

Chest X-ray

PPD skin test or QuantiFERON TB Gold test

Renal ultrasound to assess for acquired cystic disease or mass

Abdominal ultrasound in diabetics to evaluate for gallstones

Cardiac evaluation (nuclear stress test and/or echocardiogram to assess wall motion abnormality and ejection fraction—choice of cardiac studies differ among centers)

Colonoscopy screening (appropriate for age similar to the general population)

Pap smear and mammogram screening (appropriate for age similar to the general population)

Urologic evaluation if history of bladder/voiding dysfunction, recurrent urinary tract infections

Immunologic studies

Blood group and HLA typing

Anti-HLA antibodies screening by Luminex technology

Sera for crossmatch

[a] Routine screening may be more harmful than protective because it does not appear to confer a survival benefit and may delay listing and decrease transplantation rates (single-center study, $n = 3,782$ men ≥18 years of age undergoing primary kidney transplant evaluation).

- Interferon-based therapy increases the risk of allograft rejection in the post-transplant period.
- The advent of interferon-free, protease inhibitor-based regimen (e.g., sofobusvir and ledipasvir) may improve outcomes in hepatitis C-positive kidney transplant candidates and recipients.
- All patients with HBV infection should be placed on antiviral therapy after transplantation to avoid HBV reactivation and progression of liver disease associated with the use of immunosuppressive therapy.
- In transplant candidates with active HBV replication, antiviral therapy should be initiated pretransplant.

Table 8.3	Contraindications to kidney transplantation

Absolute contraindications

Recent[a] or active malignancy, metastatic malignancy

Untreated current infection or ongoing nonhealing ulcers

Severe irreversible extrarenal disease (e.g., severe cardiovascular disease not amenable to intervention or severe pulmonary disease)

Life expectancy <2 years

Recalcitrant treatment nonadherence

Poorly controlled psychiatric illnesses

Limited, irreversible rehabilitation potential

Lack of social support that will likely pose a significant threat to medical adherence in the posttransplant period

Decompensated liver cirrhosis (consider simultaneous liver–kidney transplantation)

Advanced liver disease or liver cirrhosis is generally considered as an absolute contraindication to kidney-alone transplantation (see Relative Contraindications).

Primary oxalosis (consider simultaneous liver–kidney transplantation)

Relative contraindications (should be assessed on a case-by-case basis)

Morbid obesity (center-dependent, generally defined as BMI >35)

Advanced age (center dependent—consensus on upper age limit is lacking)

Aggressive native kidney disease and history of rapid recurrence of native kidney disease in previous transplant[b]

Recent alcohol or substance abuse or lack of compliance with substance abuse rehabilitation (center-dependent)

Patients unwilling to accept blood transfusions while taking anticoagulants

Extensive peripheral vascular disease (surgical expertise required)

Compensated liver cirrhosis with hepatic portal venous gradient <10 mm Hg (limited data/investigational protocols)

Primary amyloidosis (in general patients should be discouraged from transplantation due to high morbidity and mortality, although a subgroup of patients without extrarenal disease may be considered acceptable candidates)

Special considerations[c]

ABO incompatibility

Positive T cell crossmatch

Postpercutaneous coronary intervention (PCI) patients

ACC/AHA 2016 updated guidelines for PCI patients on dual antiplatelet therapy: Elective noncardiac surgery should be delayed

- 30 days after bare metal stent implantation
- 6 months after drug eluting stent implantation

[a]See Table 8.4.

[b]See "Non-infectious complications after transplantation" (Table 8.22 Glomerular disease recurrence after transplantation and graft loss from disease recurrence).

[c]Pretransplant preconditioning regimen or desensitization protocols may allow successful transplantation across these barriers (discussion is beyond the scope of this chapter).

BMI, body mass index; ACC/AHA, American College of Cardiology/American Heart Association.

- HIV:
  - Highly active antiretroviral therapy (HAART) regimen has allowed successful transplantation of stable HIV patients, defined as:
    - HIV viral load less than 50 copies/mL (undetectable HIV viral load required by some centers)
    - CD4 lymphocyte count $\geq 200/mm^3$
    - Absence of opportunistic infections in the previous year

Table 8.4	Tumor-free waiting periods for common pretransplant malignancies[a,b]	
Most tumors: wait time ≥ 2 y		
No waiting time:		
Long-standing history of monoclonal gammopathy of undetermined significance (MGUS)		
Hematology consult is advisable in patients with newly diagnosed monoclonal gammopathy.		
No waiting time if cure at the time of transplantation		
Incidental renal cell carcinoma		
In situ carcinoma of bladder		
In situ carcinoma of cervix		
Basal cell carcinoma		
Squamous cell carcinoma (skin)[b,c]		
Waiting time: 2–5 y[b]		
Invasive bladder	2 y	
Uterine body	2 y	
Prostate	2 y	
Wilms tumor	2 y	
Renal cell carcinoma	2 y if <5 cm	
	5 y if >5 cm or <5 cm with invasion	
Breast carcinoma[d]	2–5 y (2-y wait for ductal carcinoma in situ)	
Lymphoma	2–5 y	
Colorectal carcinoma	2–5 y (at least 5 y for Dukes B1 or higher)	
Invasive cervical carcinoma	2–5 y	
Melanoma[b,e]	5 y	

[a] Certain cancers may recur despite a tumor-free waiting period.
[b] Oncology evaluation or consultation with the Israel Penn International Transplant Tumor Registry at https://ipittr.uc.edu may be invaluable.
[c] Surveillance.
[d] Individuals with advanced breast cancer (stage III or IV) should be advised against transplantation.
[e] In situ melanoma may require a shorter waiting period of 2 years (dermatology consultation recommended).

- Specific recommendations may vary from center to center.
- Clinicians should remain vigilant to significant drug–drug interactions between HAART and immunosuppressive drugs metabolized by cytochrome P450 3A4 (calcineurin inhibitors and mTOR inhibitors). Raltegravir is an HIV integrase inhibitor that has no known drug interaction with tacrolimus.
- Latent tuberculosis (TB) (positive purified protein derivative [PPD] skin test or QuantiFERON TB Gold test)
  - Obtain chest X-ray (part of routine pretransplant workup).
  - Patients with untreated latent TB should receive prophylactic isoniazid (INH) and B6 therapy for 9 months.
  - Active TB is a contraindication to transplantation.
- Pregnancy after transplantation:
  - Patient must be at least 1 year posttransplant.
  - Serum creatinine < 2.0 mg/dL, preferably <1.5 mg/dL (higher creatinine level increases the risk of allograft loss).
  - No recent acute rejection episodes
  - Well-controlled hypertension on minimal antihypertensive regimen
  - Minimal or no proteinuria
  - Normal kidney allograft ultrasound
  - See also drug safety in pregnancy.

Table 8.5	Diagnostic tests for hepatitis B and C
Hepatitis type	**Diagnostic tests and interpretation**
Hepatitis B	• HBsAg (hepatitis B surface antigen): HBV infection • IgM Anti-HBc (IgM antibody to hepatitis B core antigen): Acute or recent HBV infection • IgG Anti-HBc (IgG antibody to hepatitis B core antigen): Chronic or remote HBV infection • HBsAb (antibody to hepatitis B surface antigen): Immunity to HBV (prior infection or through vaccination) • HBeAg (hepatitis B e antigen): Can persist in carriers and is usually associated with detectable HBV DNA • HBV DNA: Active replication

Hepatitis C	• Anti-HCV: used for initial screening. The third-generation EIA-3 has excellent sensitivity and high specificity.
	• Nucleic acid test for detection of HCV RNA
	  • HCV qualitative
	    • Confirm HCV infection in anti-HCV (+) patients.
	    • Useful in immunocompromised patients (dialysis patients, transplant recipients)
	  • HCV quantitative
	    • Assess viral load (useful in monitoring response to therapy).
	• HCV genotyping: May predict response to treatment (helpful in treatment decision)

- Male fertility
  - Fertility, as assessed by sperm counts, improves in half of patients.
  - There is no increased incidence of neonatal malformations in pregnancies fathered by kidney transplant recipients.

LIVING DONOR EVALUATION

- Options: Living related, living unrelated, kidney paired donation, altruistic, and living donor–deceased donor exchange
- Approximately 30% of potential live donors are incompatible to their intended recipients due to ABO blood type incompatibility or the presence of preformed donor-reactive antibody, or both.
- Kidney paired donation in which an incompatible donor/recipient pair is swapped with another incompatible donor/recipient pair is a transplant option for transplant candidates who have a living donor who is medically suitable, but cannot donate to their intended recipients due to ABO incompatibility or the presence of preformed donor-reactive antibody, or both.
- Living donor–deceased donor exchange: The donor donates to the wait list in exchange for the intended recipient's receiving priority on the list.
- The Declaration of Istanbul on organ trafficking and transplant tourism and the World Health Organization (WHO) prohibit and condemn the exploitation of vulnerable living donors (defined as illiterate or impoverished individuals, undocumented immigrants, and political or economic refugees).
- General assessment:
  - Complete history and physical examination, and psychosocial assessment.

Table 8.6	Suggested routine evaluation and optional testing[a]

Laboratory tests

Blood group, HLA typing, crossmatch

Urinalysis and urine culture

24-h urine for protein and creatinine clearance or GFR determination by nuclear medicine test

CBC with platelets, INR, and PTT

Comprehensive metabolic panel

Serologies: Hepatitis B (surface Ag, IgM and IgG core Ab, and surface Ab), HCV Ab screening (if positive, check PCR confirmatory test)[b], HIV1/HIV2 antibody screen[b], CMV, EBV, HSV, RPR, or VDRL (FTA-ABS confirmatory test if positive RPR or VDRL)

Other tests

Electrocardiogram

Chest X-ray

Pap smear appropriate for age similar to the general population

Mammogram appropriate for age similar to the general population

Renal imaging: spiral CT, CT angiogram, or MR angiogram

Further testing depending on age, history, abnormal laboratory findings, family history

Cardiac screening: ETT or nuclear medicine stress test, echocardiogram

Twenty-four-hour ambulatory blood pressure monitoring

Renal biopsy

Cystoscopy

PPD skin test or QuantiFERON TB Gold test

PSA screening: Shared decision-making for men aged 55–69. For high-risk patients < 55 y of age (e.g., positive family history, African American race, or those who are symptomatic), screening should be individualized.

Screening for hypercoagulability

Oral glucose tolerance test

[a] Criteria may differ among centers.

[b] Anti-HIV1/HIV2 antibody screen or HIV antigen/antibody (Ag/Ab) combination assays as close as possible but within 28 days prior to organ recovery and HCV ribonucleic acid (RNA) by nucleic acid testing (NAT) as close as possible but within 28 days prior to organ recovery.

- A formal psychiatric evaluation by the transplant center is recommended to evaluate for any significant psychiatric problem and any possibility of coercion. The presence of either of these would preclude donation.
- Suggested routine evaluation and optional testing are listed in Table 8.6
- Absolute and relative contraindications to living kidney donation are listed in Table 8.7
- Evaluation for specific conditions:
  - Diabetes
    - Fasting plasma glucose in all patients
    - 2 hours 75 g oral glucose tolerance test (OGTT) and hemoglobin A1C (HbA1C) if fasting blood sugar (FBS) is between 100 and 125 mg/dL. For prospective donors with normal FBS, OGTT and HbA1C should be considered if risk factors (defined below) are present:
      - History of gestational diabetes or large birth weight (> 9 pounds at delivery)
      - First-degree relative with type 2 diabetes
      - Donors younger than 40 years of age with a second-degree relative with type 2 diabetes
      - HDL level ≤ 35 mg/dL
      - BP > 140/90

Table 8.7	Absolute and relative contraindications to living kidney donation

Absolute Contraindications	Relative Contraindications
Evidence of kidney disease (GFR < 80 mL/min or inappropriately low for age and gender, microalbuminuria or overt proteinuria)	Age < 18 (seldom-performed) or >65 (center-dependent, need to evaluate on a case-by-case basis)
Significant renal or urologic abnormalities	Borderline or mild hypertension
Transmissible infectious disease (HIV, hepatitis B, or hepatitis C infection)	Borderline urinary abnormalities in the absence of renal function impairment
Active malignancy	
Chronic illness that places patient at significant risk of undergoing surgery	Single prior episode of kidney stone without evidence of secondary risk
Poorly controlled psychiatric illness or active substance abuse	
Cognitive deficit	Obesity (center-dependent, generally defined as body mass index > 30 kg/m²)
Current pregnancy	
Hypertension (clinically significant)	
Diabetes mellitus	Young donor with risk factors for future development of diabetes mellitus
Recurrent nephrolithiasis or bilateral stones	
History of thrombotic disorders with risk factors for future events or inherited hypercoagulable states (e.g., the presence of anticoagulant or anticardiolipin antibody, factor V Leiden, or prothrombin gene mutation FII-20210)	Jehovah Witness

- Body mass index (BMI) > 30
- Fasting TG ≥ 250 mg/dL
- Hypertension
  - Blood pressure measurement on three separate occasions
  - Elevated blood pressure requires further evaluation with ambulatory blood pressure monitoring to exclude white-coat hypertension.
  - Echocardiogram may be considered to evaluate for cardiac hypertrophy in patients with borderline high blood pressure, chest X-ray findings suggestive of cardiomegaly, or EKG findings suggestive of left ventricular hypertrophy.
  - A history of mild hypertension may be acceptable for donation if
    - The prospective donor is not African American.
    - >50 years of age without evidence of microalbuminuria or end-organ damage.
    - Normal GFR for age
    - Blood pressure well controlled with lifestyle and behavioral modifications or use of no more than a single antihypertensive agent
- Donor with history of nephrolithiasis. See Table 8.8
- Donor safety
  - Surgical mortality within 90 days of live kidney donation: 3.1/10,000 donors (UNOS database consisting of 80,347 live kidney donors)
  - At long-term follow-up, unilateral nephrectomy reduces renal function by about 20%.
  - Similar to the nondonating population, an additional 5 mL/min loss in GFR per decade occurs after donating.
  - Risk of ESRD is small (<0.5% increase in incidence at 15 years).
  - May increase risk of gestational hypertension and preeclampsia
  - No apparent adverse effect on life expectancy
  - Systematic review, meta-analysis and meta-regression study (n > 5,000 donors from 27 countries): Kidney donation resulted in small increases in urinary

Table 8.8	Prospective donors with history of kidney stones

Kidney Donation Acceptable	Contraindications to Donation if One or More of the Following Risk Factors Are Present
Distant history of stone (>10 y) without metabolic abnormalities associated with stone formation (e.g., hypercalcemia, hyperuricemia, hyperoxaluria, hypocitrauria, or metabolic acidosis)	Cystinuria
	Sarcoidosis
	History of struvite stones
Current asymptomatic single stone if	Inflammatory bowel disease
the stone is small and/or potentially extractable during transplantation, and	Evidence of nephrocalcinosis
	Primary or enteric hyperoxaluria
Further evaluation must reveal no evidence of metabolic abnormalities, urinary tract infection, or nephrocalcinosis.	History of bilateral stones or history of recurrent stones despite preventive therapy
Single-stone episode associated with treated primary hyperparathyroidism and normocalcemia does not necessarily preclude donation (must evaluate on a case-by-case basis).	

A stone initially detected in an individual > 50 years of age is unlikely to recur whereas the risk of stone recurrence is higher in the 25 to 35 age group and must be considered during the evaluation process.

albumin, which increased with the time after donation. An initial decrement in GFR was not followed by accelerated losses over the subsequent 15 years.

- Impact of age on long-term safety
  - **Single-center study**: $n = 539$ consecutive live kidney donors (422 donors were <60 years and 117 were 60 years or older (of which 25 were older than 70)). Older donors had lower mean predonation GFR (80 vs. 96 mL/min for donors aged <60 years), higher BMI, and higher American Society of Anesthesiologists (ASA) classification compared with younger donors
  - **Results**: There were no differences in the mean maximum decline in eGFR between the two groups at a median follow-up of 5.5 years (maximum decline in eGFR was 38% $\pm$ 9%). Furthermore, the percentage maximal decline was comparable between older and younger age groups. At 5 years follow-up, significantly more elderly had an eGFR < 60 mL/min compared with younger donors (80% vs. 94%, respectively ($p < 0.001$)). However, renal function stabilized during follow-up, and no donors had an eGFR of <30 mL/min during follow-up.
  - **Conclusion**: After kidney donation, decline in eGFR is similar in younger and older donors. As kidney function does not progressively decline, live kidney donation by elderly is considered safe.
- For interested readers, a calculator to assess the risk for developing kidney disease in the absence of donation can be found on http://www.transplantmodels.com/esrdrisk/ (However, this should not replace clinical judgment)

KIDNEY ALLOCATION SYSTEM

- UNOS listing criteria: GFR of ≤20 mL/min or on dialysis
- Kidney donor profile index (KDPI)
  - Deceased donor kidneys are given a kidney donor profile index (KDPI) value ranging from 0% to 100% based on longevity-matching concepts.
  - Ten donor characteristics used to calculate KDPI:
    - Donor age
    - Height

- Weight
- Ethnicity
- History of hypertension
- History of diabetes
- Serum creatinine
- Cause of death
- Hepatitis C status
- Donation after circulatory death status
- Lower KDPI values are associated with longer-estimated function, whereas higher KDPI values are associated with shorter-estimated function (e.g., a kidney with a KDPI of 20% is expected to have longer longevity than 80% of recovered kidneys).
- Factors determining kidney allocation
  - Waiting time
    - Time spent after dialysis start date (e.g., wait-listed candidates who have been on dialysis for 2 years have 2 years of waiting time).
    - Candidates not yet on dialysis at the time of registration will still begin to accrue waiting time once they are registered on the waiting list.
  - Highly sensitized candidates, cPRA
    - Kidney candidates are assigned a cPRA score that is based on the "unacceptable antigens" listed for each candidate.
    - Prioritization points will be assigned based on a sliding scale, beginning with a cPRA score of 20% (candidates with cPRA of 20% will receive 0.08 points, which is equivalent to about 1 month of waiting time. Candidates with cPRA 75% to 79% will receive 1.58 points; those with cPRA of 80% to 84% will receive 2.46 points. Candidates with cPRA of 98%, 99%, or 100% will receive 24.4, 50.09, and 202.10 points, respectively).
    - Candidates with cPRA of 98%, 99%, or 100% will also receive local, regional, and national priority.
  - Pediatric status
  - Prior living donor
  - Geographic area: Allocation first to candidates in the area closest to the donor
  - Survival benefit
    - Estimated posttransplant survival (EPTS) score: The EPTS score is designed to achieve better longevity matching and is based on four factors: candidate age, length of time on dialysis, prior transplant of any solid organ, and current diabetes status. The candidates with the top 20% EPTS scores will receive offers for kidneys from donors with KDPI scores of 20% or less before other candidates at the local, regional, and national levels of distribution. Candidates will not be prioritize based on EPTS for allocation of kidneys from donors with KDPI scores greater than 20%.

IMMUNOSUPPRESSIVE AGENTS

The Three-Signal Model of Alloimmune Responses

- T-cell activation requires three signals (Fig. 8.5).
  - **Signal 1** is initiated by the binding of the alloantigen on the surface of antigen presenting cell (APC) to the T-cell receptor (TCR)–CD3 complex.
  - **Signal 2** is a nonantigen specific costimulatory signal provided by the engagement of B7 on the surface of APC with CD28 on T cell. These dual signals

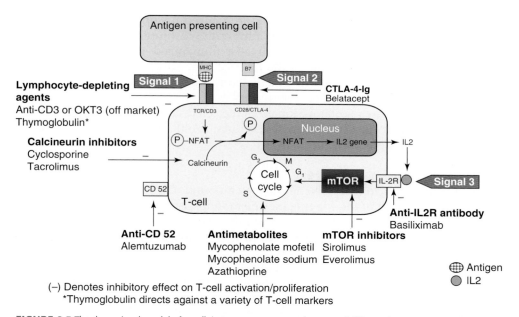

FIGURE 8.5 The three-signal model of an alloimmune response and targets of different immunosuppressive agents.

activate the intracellular pathways that trigger T cells to activate Il-2 and other growth-promoting cytokines.

- **Signal 3**: Engagement of IL-2 to its receptor activates the mammalian target of rapamycin (mTOR) pathway to provide signal 3, which leads to cell proliferation. If a TCR is triggered without the accompanying costimulatory signal 2, the T cell is driven into an anergic state.
- Lymphocyte proliferation, which requires the synthesis of purine and pyrimidine nucleotides, is inhibited by the antimetabolites mycophenolate mofetil, enteric-coated mycophenolate sodium, and azathioprine (AZA).
- T cells also express cytotoxic T-lymphocyte associated antigen-4 (CTLA-4), a cell surface molecule that is homologous to CD28. However, the binding of B7 to CTLA-4 produces an inhibitory signal that inhibits T-cell proliferation and helps terminate the immune response.

Targets of Various Immunosuppressive Agents

- The targets of various immunosuppressive agents are shown in Figure 8.5.
- Cyclosporine and tacrolimus (also termed "calcineurin inhibitors" [CNIs] due to the similarity in their mechanism of action). *Calcineurin* is a phosphatase that dephosphorylates and facilitates the translocation of the nuclear factor of activated T cells–NFAT (and other nuclear factors) to the nucleus. Hence, inhibition of *calcineurin* impairs the expression of IL-2 and several cytokines that promote T-cell activation.
- Thymoglobulin is a polyclonal antibody preparation made by immunization of rabbits with human lymphoid tissue. The purified immunosuppressive product contains cytotoxic antibodies directed against a variety of T-cell markers.
- Alemtuzumab is a humanized monoclonal antibody targeting against CD52 on the surface of both B and T lymphocytes leading to a rapid and profound depletion of peripheral and central lymphoid cells.

- Agent targeting signal 2: Belatacept is a humanized fusion protein of CTLA-4Ig that binds to B7 with high affinity and inhibits the costimulatory pathway.
- Agent targeting signal 3: Basiliximab is a humanized monoclonal antibody that targets against the α chain of the IL-2 receptor (also known as anti-IL2R or anti-CD25 antibody), blocking IL-2 mediated responses.
- mTOR inhibitors: sirolimus and everolimus
  - The mTOR is a key regulatory kinase in the cell division process. Hence, its inhibition reduces cytokine–dependent cellular proliferation at the G1 to S phase of the cell division cycle.
- Antimetabolites:
  - Mycophenolate mofetil (MMF)
    Mycophenolic acid (MPA) is the active compound of MMF. MPA is a reversible inhibitor of the enzyme inosine monophosphate dehydrogenase (a rate-limiting enzyme in the de novo synthesis of purines). Depletion of guanosine nucleotides by MPA has a relatively selective antiproliferative effect on lymphocytes.
  - Mycophenolate sodium is an enteric-coated formulation of MPA.
  - Azathioprine (AZA) is a precursor of 6-mercaptopurine. It inhibits gene replication and consequent T-cell activation.
  - MMF and mycophenolate sodium have largely replaced AZA.

Basic Principles of an Immunosuppressive Protocol

- A standard immunosuppressive protocol consists of induction and maintenance immunosuppression.
- **Induction therapy** refers to intense immunosuppression in the first few days or week after transplantation. Induction therapy can be classified into lymphocyte-depleting and nonlymphocyte-depleting agents (Table 8.9).
- **Maintenance immunosuppression**: A standard maintenance immunosuppressive regimen consists of triple therapy with CNI (cyclosporine or tacrolimus) + adjunctive agent + steroid. The side-effect profiles of cysclosporine and tacrolimus are shown in Table 8.10.

Table 8.9	Induction therapy: lymphocyte-depleting versus non–lymphocyte-depleting agents	
Lymphocyte Depleting[a]	**NonLymphocyte Depleting**	**Comments**
Thymoglobulin	Basiliximab	Thymoglobulin vs. basiliximab induction
Alemtuzumab	Daclizumab[b]	Thymoglobulin: commonly used in high immunologic risk patients (e.g., highly sensitized or reallograft transplant recipients, DSA positive) or anticipated delayed graft function to avoid early exposure to cyclosporine or tacrolimus (nephrotoxic)
Atgam[b] (equine polyclonal antibody)		
OKT3[b] (mouse monoclonal antibody targeting against CD3)		Basiliximab: commonly used in low to moderate immunologic risk transplant recipients
		Alemtuzumab: used at a small number of institutions in the United States

[a] Lymphocyte-depleting agents can cause first-dose reaction or cytokine-release syndrome including chills, fever, arthralgia, and rarely serum sickness.
[b] No longer used, withdrawn from market.
DSA, donor-specific antibody

Table 8.10	Side-effect profiles of cyclosporine and tacrolimus	
Cyclosporine (CSA)	**Tacrolimus (Tac)**	**Comments**
Nephrotoxicity	Nephrotoxicity	CSA > Tac
HTN and sodium retention	HTN	CSA > Tac
Hyperlipidemia	Hyperlipidemia	CSA > Tac
Diabetes mellitus	Diabetes mellitus	Tac > CSA
Neurotoxicity (headache, tremors, confusion, paresthesia)	Neurotoxicity (headache, tremors, confusion, paresthesia, insomnia)	Tac > CSA
Thrombotic microangiopathy	Thrombotic microangiopathy	
Gastrointestinal side effects (e.g., decreased appetite, abdominal pain, nausea, vomiting)	Gastrointestinal side effects (e.g., diarrhea, abdominal pain, nausea, vomiting, decreased appetite)	
Hepatotoxicity	Hepatotoxicity	
Hyperkalemia	Hyperkalemia	
Hypomagnesemia	Hypomagnesemia	
Hyperchloremic acidosis	Hyperchloremic acidosis	
Hirsutism	Pancreatitis	
Gingival hyperplasia	Alopecia	
Hyperuricemia	Hyperuricemia	CSA > Tac

Table 8.11	Side-effect profiles of mycophenolate mofetil and mycophenolate sodium
Mycophenolate Mofetil (MMF) CellCept	**Mycophenolate Sodium (Enteric-Coated MMF) Myfortic**
Diarrhea, nausea, vomiting, abdominal pain, flatulence, dyspepsia	Presumably less gastrointestinal toxicity compared with CellCept
Hematologic effects: leukopenia, anemia, thrombocytopenia	Hematologic effects: leukopenia, anemia, thrombocytopenia
Comments: more than 2 g/d usually not tolerated	Comments: myfortic 180 mg = CellCept 250 mg (similar efficacy)

- MMF (or the enteric-coated mycophenolic sodium formulation) is the most commonly used adjunctive agent. The side-effect profiles of MMF and mycophenolate sodium are shown in Table 8.11.
- AZA, sirolimus, or everolimus is generally used in place of MMF for special indications:
  - AZA
    - AZA use is safe in pregnancy (MMF is teratogenic and it must be discontinued in anticipation of pregnancy)
    - Avoid use with allopurinol (a xanthine oxidase inhibitor) because of the inhibition of AZA metabolism by xanthine oxidase inhibitors.
    - Febuxostat is a nonpurine selective inhibitor of xanthine oxidase. Hence, it should also be avoided (or used with caution) in patients taking AZA.
  - Sirolimus or everolimus:
    - Potential beneficial effect in patients with history of malignancy particularly skin cancer, renal cell carcinoma, or Kaposi sarcoma

Table 8.12	Side-effect profiles of mTOR inhibitors (sirolimus and everolimus)
Side effects	**Comments**
Delayed recovery of acute tubular necrosis	Not recommended in the early postoperative period
Impaired wound healing	
Increased risk of lymphocele formation	Calcineurin inhibitor target level should be lowered when used in combination with mTOR inhibitors.
May potentiate calcineurin inhibitor nephrotoxicity	
Oral ulcers	
Diabetogenic	
Proteinuria	
Dyslipidemia (↑cholesterol, ↑↑triglyceride)	
Peripheral edema	
Pulmonary toxicity	
Thrombotic microangiopathy	
Others: acne, rash, anemia, thrombocytopenia, decreased testosterone	

- Not recommended in the early postoperative period (may impair wound healing and delay recovery of ATN)
- Sirolimus and everolimus have been shown to be teratogenic in animal models. Their use should be avoided in pregnancy (Pregnancy Category C)
- The side effect profiles of sirolimus and everolimus are shown in Table 8.12.
- Steroid-free or CNI-free maintenance immunosuppression protocol:
  - Clinicians must be familiar with its use.
  - Must be individualized based on immunologic risk
    - Steroid withdrawal (CNI + MMF): safe in short-term in low immunologic risk patients
    - Belatacept in CNI-free protocol (belatacept + MMF + steroid): Belatacept is contraindicated in Epstein–Barr virus (EBV) naïve kidney transplant recipients due to increased risk of posttransplant lymphoproliferative disease (PTLD).

Treatment of Acute Rejection

See Kidney Allograft Biopsy Findings section for classification of the different types of acute rejection.
- Acute cellular rejection (ACR):
  - High-dose intravenous steroids (usually referred to as "pulse steroid")
  - The antilymphocyte antibody thymoglobulin is commonly used for type IIA ACR (also known as vascular rejection) or more severe rejection as defined by Banff classification, and in ACR refractory to steroid therapy.
  - Increase maintenance immunosuppressive drug target levels (tacrolimus or cyclosporine).
  - Maximize antimetabolite therapy as tolerated (if patient is not already on maximum dose of MMF or mycophenolate sodium).
- Acute antibody-mediated rejection (AMR). The potential mechanisms of action of various treatment modalities are shown in Table 8.13.
  - Plasmapheresis

Table 8.13	Potential mechanisms of action of various treatment modalities used in the management of acute antibody-mediated rejection	
Treatment	**Potential Mechanism(s) of Action**	**Comments**
Plasmapheresis	Removes circulating alloantibodies	May stimulate rebound immunoglobulin production
Intravenous immunoglobulin (IVIG)	Anti-idiotypic antibodies (inhibits anti-HLA antibody) Produces long-term suppression or elimination of anti-HLA reactive T and B cells Induces apoptosis of B cells Downregulates antibody production by plasma cells Inhibits complement-mediated damage Inhibits cytokine signaling pathway and alloimmunization via blockade of the T-cell receptor Immune modulation	Removed by plasma exchange (must give after plasmapheresis)
Agent targeting B cells: Rituximab	Anti CD20 monoclonal antibodies May induce naïve and memory B-cell depletion Plasma cells lack CD20 and are unaffected by rituximab	Clinical use: Treat acute antibody-mediated rejection (AMR) Use as part of a conditioning regimen in patients with preformed anti-HLA antibodies or ABO incompatibility
Agent targeting plasma cells: Bortezomib	Proteasome inhibitor Induces plasma cell apoptosis Reduces donor-specific antibody (DSA) production by plasma cells	Rescue therapy for AMR refractory to IVIG and/or rituximab (based on small studies)
Agent targeting the complement system: Eculizumab	Terminal complement inhibitor (binds to C5, preventing cleavage of C5 into C5a and C5b, and the formation of C5b and membrane attack complex) Protects endothelium from injury caused by existing antibodies	Preventive or rescue therapy (based on small studies) Treatment of acute AMR (ongoing clinical trials) Increased risk of meningococcal infections Meningococcal vaccination recommended at least 2 wk prior to eculizumab therapy. If vaccination is given <2 wk prior to first dose, must start levofloxacin (continue for 2 wk)
Antilymphocyte antibodies	May downregulate B-cell response via a decrease in the activity of helper T cells	
Pulse steroids	May downregulate B-cell response via a decrease in the activity of helper T cells	

- Intravenous immunoglobulin (IVIG)
- Agents targeting B cells: rituximab
- Agents targeting plasma cells: bortezomib
- Agents targeting the complement system: eculizumab
- Pulse steroid and antitlymphocyte antibodies may also be beneficial in the treatment of AMR.

Drug–Drug Interactions
- Important drug–drug interactions are shown in Table 8.14.

Table 8.14	Drug–drug interactions

Drugs that increase CNI level by inhibition of the P450 (CYP3A4/5) enzyme system or by competition for the enzyme binding sites

- Calcium channel blockers[a]: Diltiazem, verapamil > nicardipine
- Antifungal agents[b]: The "azole" (fluconazole, ketoconazole, itraconazole, voriconazole)
- Antibiotics: Erythromycin > other macrolide antibiotics[c] (clarithromycin, josamycin, ponsinomycin)
- Antiretroviral agents (protease inhibitors): Essentially all currently available protease inhibitors (e.g. ritonavir, ritonavir/lopinavir combination therapy (a.k.a. kaletra), darunavir).
- Others (less well-established): Amiodarone, carvedilol, allopurinol, bromocriptine, chloroquine

Drugs that decrease CNI level by induction of P450 (CYP3A4/5) activity

- Antituberculous drugs: Rifampin > rifabutin. Pyrazinamide and ethambutol may reduce drug levels
- Anticonvulsants: Barbiturates > phenytoin > carbamazepine. Oxcarbazepine (trileptal) may decrease cyclosporine level
- Antidepressant herbal preparation: *Hypericum perforatum* (St John's wort)
- Others (less well established/case reports): Nafcillin, IV trimethoprim, imipenem, cephalosporins, terbinafine

Drugs or food that increase the absorption of CNIs

- Metoclopramide
- Grapefruit juice (also inhibits P450 3A4)

Commonly used herbals that may have an immune-stimulating effect

- Ginseng, licorice, alfalfa sprouts, astragalus

Nephrotoxic drugs or drugs that may potentiate CNI toxicity

- NSAIDS, mTOR inhibitors, tenofovir, amphotericin, aminoglycosides, cidofovir, foscarnet

Cholesterol-lowering agents

- The concomitant use of CNI and statins (HMG-CoA reductase inhibitors) can cause rhabdomyolysis and acute kidney injury[d] (NOTE: most cases reported occurred between cyclosporine and statins. Rhabdomyolysis associated with tacrolimus and statin use is generally seen in patients on concomitant diltiazem therapy).
- Pharmacokinetic studies have demonstrated that cyclosporine increases statin drug levels due in part to competitive inhibition of cytochrome P450.

*This table provides a general guideline. Clinicians should refer to drug packet inserts for full drug-drug interaction. Sirolimus and everolimus interact with calcium channel blockers, antifungal agents, anticonvulsants, proteinase inhibitors, antituberculous agents, St John's wort and grapefruit juice in a manner similar to the CNIs.

[a]Nifedipine, amlodipine, isradipine, and felodipine have minimal effects on CNI levels.

[b]The newer antifungals "echinocandins" are poor substrates for cytochrome P450 enzymes. Drug-to-drug interaction of micafungin with CNIs are minimal. Anidulafungin has no significant drug–drug interaction with the CNIs or mTOR inhibitors. **Caspofungin** may interact with tacrolimus and reduce its AUC by 20%.

[c]Azithromycin does not increase CNI levels.

[d]The lowest dose should be introduced, any increase in dose requires close monitoring.

CNI, calcineurin inhibitor; NSAIDS, nonsteroidal anti-inflammatory drugs; HMG-CoA, 3-hydroxy-3-methylglutaryl coenzyme A.

Note: This table provides a general guideline. Clinicians should refer to drug packet inserts for full drug–drug interaction. Sirolimus and everolimus interact with calcium channel blockers, antifungal agents, anticonvulsants, proteinase inhibitors, antituberculous agents, St John wort, and grapefruit juice in a manner similar to the CNIs.

KIDNEY ALLOGRAFT BIOPSY FINDINGS

Acute Tubular Necrosis

- Most common cause of delayed graft function (DGF)
- Although the terms DGF and acute tubular necrosis (ATN) are often used interchangeably, not all cases of DGF are caused by ATN. Unless an allograft biopsy is performed, posttransplant ATN should be a diagnosis of exclusion.
- Pathogenesis: Posttransplant ATN is largely due to ischemic injury that may be synergistically exaggerated by both immunologic and nephrotoxic insults (generally due to CNI-induced renal afferent arteriolar vasoconstriction).
- Histopathology (Fig. 8.6):
  - Tubular cells show flattening, loss of proximal cell brush border staining, and may be degenerated or necrotic.

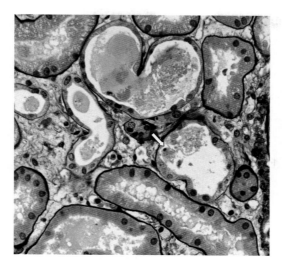

FIGURE 8.6 Acute tubular necrosis. Tubular cells are flattened with relative dilatation of tubular lumina and proximal cells have lost brush borders. Focally, necrotic cells are sloughed into tubular lumina (*arrow*) (Periodic acid methenamine silver, ×400).

- Tubular lumina are relatively dilated with or without sloughed tubular cells.
- There is variable interstitial edema without inflammation.

Allograft Rejection

Allograft rejection can be classified into hyperacute, acute, and chronic rejection:
- Hyperacute rejection:
  - Can occur immediately following vascular anastomosis or within minutes to hours after graft revascularization and uniformly results in graft loss
  - Pathogenesis:
    - Caused by preformed antidonor HLA antibodies
    - Preformed antidonor HLA antibodies bind to graft endothelial antigens and activate complement leading to severe vascular injury, thrombosis, coagulative necrosis, and obliteration of the graft vasculature.
  - With the current cytotoxic crossmatch, hyperacute rejection has become virtually nonexistent.
  - Histopathology (Fig. 8.7):
    - Thrombosed arteries, arterioles, and glomerular capillaries, often with neutrophils incorporated into the thrombi
    - Ischemic acute tubular injury
    - No interstitial or tubular inflammation
- Acute rejection: can be classified into acute T-cell mediated or acute antibody-mediated rejection. Diagnosis requires allograft biopsy.
  - Acute T-Cell-mediated rejection (also known as acute cellular rejection or ACR)
    - Generally occurs after the first posttransplant week and most commonly within the first 3 to 6 months after transplantation.
    - In unsensitized patients with low levels of preformed anti-HLA antibodies, ACR rarely occurs in the first week.
    - Clinical manifestations: Most patients present with asymptomatic acute rise in serum creatinine. In the era of potent immunosuppression, fever, malaise, oliguria, and graft tenderness are usually absent unless immunosuppression is completely discontinued.

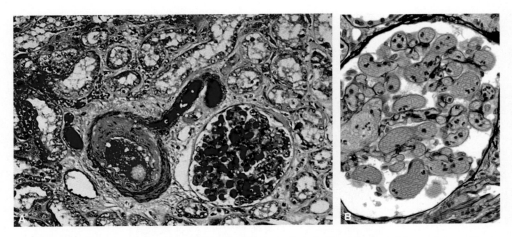

FIGURE 8.7 Hyperacute rejection. **A.** There is thrombosis of vessels, including arteries, arterioles, and glomerular capillaries, without tubulointerstitial inflammation (Masson trichrome, ×100). **B.** There are neutrophils incorporated into the thrombi, indicative of an antibody-mediated process (Periodic acid methenamine silver, ×400).

- Pathogenesis: caused by T-cells reacting to donor histocompatibility antigens expressed in the tubules, interstitium, vessels, and glomeruli to various extent
- Histopathologic terminologies:
  - Tubulitis: lymphocytes within tubular walls between epithelial cells
  - Intimal arteritis, endarteritis, or endothelialitis: lymphocytes underneath the endothelium in the arterial intima
  - Arterial transmural inflammation (transmural arteritis): involving both the intima and media
  - Transplant glomerulitis: leukocytes within glomerular capillary lumens
  - Transplant glomerulopathy: subendothelial lucencies with new deposition of subendothelial basement membrane and capillary double contours
  - Mononuclear interstitial infiltrate consists predominantly of lymphocytes. Plasma cells, macrophages, eosinophils, and/or rare neutrophils may be seen.
- Banff classification of ACR
  - Borderline changes (suspicious for rejection): focal, mild tubulitis, and at least 10% to 25% interstitial mononuclear infiltrate; severe tubulitis with any interstitial inflammation
  - TYPE 1:
    - Type 1A: mononuclear infiltrate in ≥25% of parenchyma, focal tubulitis (>4 lymphocytes/tubule).
    - Type 1B (Fig. 8.8A): mononuclear infiltrate in ≥25% of parenchyma, any tubule with severe tubulitis (>10 lymphocytes/tubule)
  - TYPE 2
    - Type 2A (Fig. 8.8B): mild to moderate intimal arteritis (<25% of luminal area)
    - Type 2B: severe intimal arteritis (>25% of luminal area)
  - TYPE 3: arterial transmural inflammation and/or necrosis of media
- Histopathology:
  - Tubular and vascular inflammation as described above, often with associated tubular cell necrosis
  - Interstitial edema and variable inflammation

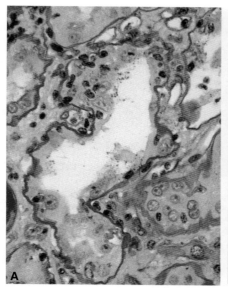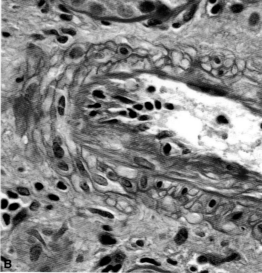

FIGURE 8.8 Acute cell-mediated rejection. **A.** Tubule with more than 10 lymphocytes in the wall (Banff 1B) and associated tubular cell necrosis. **B.** Artery with swollen endothelial cells and undermining lymphocytes, which are present in the vascular intima (endarteritis, endothelialitis). There is less than 25% involvement of the artery, indicating a Banff 2A lesion (Both Periodic acid–Schiff, ×600).

- ■ Isolated vascular rejection is rare, but may occur.
- ■ Glomerular inflammation is not commonly seen.
- • Acute AMR:
  - • Clinical manifestations: allograft dysfunction frequently more severe than that of ACR
  - • AMR with concomitant features of ACR may be seen.
  - • Pathogenesis: caused by DSA against HLA. Rarely, other DSA have been implicated in AMR, including MHC class I-related chain A [MICA] and MHC class I-related chain B [MICB], antiendothelial antibodies, or antiangiotensin receptor 1 antibodies.
  - • AMR is a risk factor for chronic rejection.
  - • 2013 Revised Banff criteria for AMR: All three features must be present for diagnosis:
    - ■ Serologic evidence of DSAs against HLA (or other antigens)
    - ■ Histologic evidence of acute tissue injury, including *one or more* of the following:
      - • ATN
      - • Acute thrombotic microangiopathy (TMA) in the absence of any other cause
      - • Microvascular inflammation (glomerular or peritubular capillaries)
      - • Intimal or transmural arteritis
    - ■ Evidence of current/recent antibody interaction with vascular endothelium, including *one or more* of the following:
      - • Immunofluorescence (IF): diffuse C4d staining in peritubular capillaries (PTCs)
      - • Immunohistochemistry (IHC): focal or diffuse C4d staining in PTCs
      - • At least moderate microvascular inflammation
      - • Increased expression of gene transcripts in the biopsy indicative of endothelial injury, if thoroughly validated

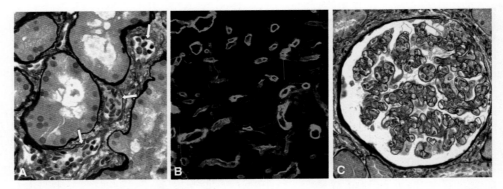

FIGURE 8.9 Active antibody-mediated rejection. **A.** Peritubular capillaries (*arrows*) are filled with leukocytes, typically monocytes and/or neutrophils (peritubular capillaritis) (Periodic acid methenamine silver, ×450). **B.** Immunofluorescence for C4d showing bright staining of peritubular capillary walls (×400). **C.** Glomerulus with capillary lumina occluded by leukocytes and swollen endothelial cells (acute glomerulitis) (Periodic acid methenamine silver, ×400).

- • Histopathology (Fig. 8.9):
    - ■ PMNs, monocytes, less often lymphocytes in glomerular and/or peritubular capillaries with swollen endothelial cells
    - ■ May be interstitial edema, acute tubular injury
- • Chronic rejection:
    - • Various terminologies have been used (multiple etiologic factors): chronic rejection, transplant glomerulopathy, chronic allograft nephropathy, chronic allograft injury (CAI)
    - • Occurs months to years after transplantation
    - • Clinical manifestations: progressive decline in graft function. Proteinuria of varying degrees and hypertension may be present.
    - • Pathogenesis: caused by both alloantigen-dependent and alloantigen-independent factors
        - • Alloantigen-dependent: Acute rejection episodes, antibody-mediated immune response, poor HLA matching, prior sensitization, inadequate immunosuppression
        - • Alloantigen-independent: for example, chronic cyclosporine nephrotoxicity, BK nephropathy, cytomegalovirus (CMV) infection, CMV nephropathy, donor or recipients factors such as age, diabetes, or hypertension
    - • Pathologic changes: The pathologic changes are primarily cortical with interstitial fibrosis and tubular atrophy (IFTA), vascular and glomerular scarring. The glomerular changes may show features of transplant glomerulopathy with glomerular capillary walls displaying double contours (AMR). The arterial walls are thickened and the lumen narrowed as a result of intimal fibrosis, leading to concentric fibrointimal thickening (discussed further under Histopathologic Findings in Chronic Allograft Injury).

C4d Stain in Kidney Allograft

- • C4d is a marker of AMR in ABO compatible kidney transplant.
- • C4d negative AMR was added to the 2013 revised Banff classification schema as a separate category of AMR. C4d negative AMR is characterized by the presence of microvascular injury in the presence of DSA but without PTC C4d staining.
- • C4d negative AMR may occur early or late after transplantation.
- • Both C4d positive and C4d negative AMR may adversely impact graft survival.

- C4d positivity without histologic tissue injury *cannot be used* as a diagnostic tool for AMR in the setting of *ABO-incompatible* kidney transplantation.

Histopathologic Findings in Chronic Allograft Injury

CAI denotes chronic allograft dysfunction that involves both alloantigen-dependent and -independent factors. The biopsy features of CAI vary with the underlying etiologic factors.

- Banff classification based on severity of IFTA
  - IFTA Grade I (mild): mild interstitial fibrosis (6% to 25%) and tubular atrophy with or without changes suggesting chronic rejection
  - IFTA Grade II (moderate): moderate interstitial fibrosis (26% to 50%) and tubular atrophy with or without changes suggesting chronic rejection
  - IFTA Grade III (severe): severe IF (>50%) and tubular atrophy and tubular loss with or without changes suggesting chronic rejection
- Chronic transplant glomerulopathy (Fig. 8.10)
  - Common cause of CAI
  - Associated with chronic AMR
  - There is currently no effective therapy for Chronic Transplant Glomerulopathy (CTG)
- Chronic cell-mediated vascular rejection (Fig. 8.11)
- Chronic calcineurin-inhibitor nephrotoxicity (Fig. 8.12)
  - Occurs months to years after transplantation
  - Clinical presentation: insidious rise in serum creatinine and varying degrees of hypertension and proteinuria
  - Histopathologic features: outer nodular arteriolar hyalinosis, striped fibrosis without inflammation (tubular cell injury with isometric vacuolization generally seen in acute CNI toxicity)
- Chronic hypertension: Systemic hypertension may exaggerate and perpetuate the vascular injury associated with CAI, which has pathologic features in common with hypertensive nephrosclerosis.
- Viral infection
  - BK nephropathy
    - Most commonly presents with an asymptomatic rise in serum creatinine. A definitive diagnosis requires allograft biopsy (discussed in Posttransplant Infectious Complications section).

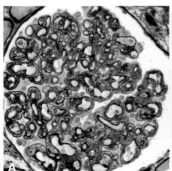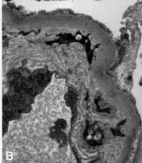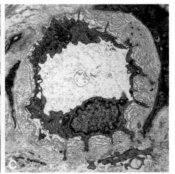

FIGURE 8.10 Chronic antibody-mediated rejection. **A.** Glomerulus with many capillary wall double contours (transplant glomerulopathy) (Periodic acid methenamine silver, ×400). **B.** Glomerular capillary wall showing subendothelial new layers of basement membrane material by electron microscopy (×14,000). **C.** Multilayered peritubular capillary basement membrane seen on electron microscopy (×10,000).

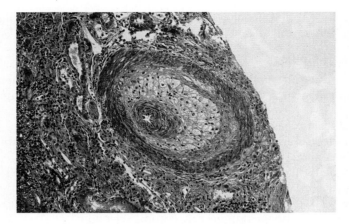

FIGURE 8.11 Chronic cell-mediated vascular rejection. The artery is thickened with intimal fibrosis, and many intimal foam cells and few lymphocytes, resulting in luminal narrowing (Masson trichrome, ×250).

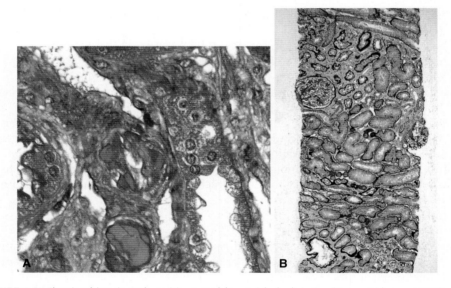

FIGURE 8.12 Chronic calcineurin nephrotoxicity. **A.** Nodular arteriolar hyalinization (Masson trichrome, ×600). **B.** Cortical "striped" fibrosis without inflammation (Periodic acid methenamine silver, ×100).

- Histopathology (Fig. 8.13A): Light microscopy: viral inclusions in renal tubu-lar cell nuclei and rarely in glomerular parietal epithelium. Interstitial mono-nuclear inflammation, often with many plasma cells, degenerative changes in tubules, and focal tubulitis may mimic acute rejection. IHC staining: An-tibodies to SV40
- CMV nephropathy
  - CMV infection is common after solid-organ transplantation (discussed in Posttransplant Infectious Complications section)
  - Diagnosis requires allograft biopsy.
  - Histopathology (Fig. 8.13B): usually characterized by tubulointerstitial ne-phritis. Cytoplasmic and/or nuclear inclusions may be seen in tubular cells, macrophages, or glomerular infiltrating or endothelial cells. IHC stain for CMV is necessary to confirm the diagnosis.

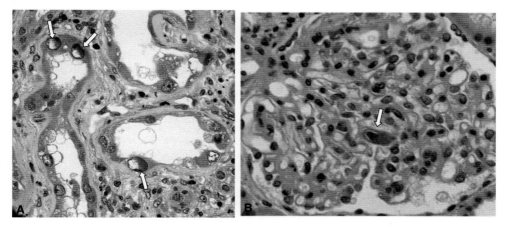

FIGURE 8.13 A. Polyomavirus infection in tubular epithelial cells with "ground glass" nuclear inclusions and focal nuclear clearing (*arrows*) (Hematoxylin and eosin, ×400). **B.** Cell in glomerular capillary showing intranuclear and cytoplasmic CMV inclusions (*arrow*). Immunohistochemical staining is required for confirmation of the viral type (Hematoxylin and eosin, ×400).

POSTTRANSPLANT INFECTIOUS COMPLICATIONS

Infectious Diseases

- Infection follows cardiovascular disease as the second most common cause of death with a functioning graft in kidney transplant recipients.
- Both the type and occurrence of infections in the immunocompromised transplant recipient follow a timetable pattern (Table 8.15).
- All kidney transplant candidates should receive immunization for hepatitis B, pneumococcus, and other standard immunization appropriate for age.
- Live vaccines are contraindicated posttransplant and should be administered before transplant.
- A minimum of 4 weeks should elapse between live virus vaccine administration and transplantation.
- Vaccinations should be administered ≥4 to 6 weeks before transplant to achieve optimal response and to minimize the possibility of live vaccine-derived infection in the posttransplant period.
  Recommended immunizations before and after transplantation is shown in Table 8.16.
- Posttransplant antimicrobial prophylaxis is shown in Table 8.17.

Risk Factors for Posttransplant Infectious Complications

- Net state of immunosuppression: intensity and duration of immunosuppression
- Surgical instrumentation, wound, abdominal fluid collections (see Table 8.15)
- Donor-derived
- Epidemiologic exposure
- Metabolic conditions (e.g., diabetes, uremia)
- Infections with immunomodulating viruses
- Hypogammaglobulinemia: Although prospective controlled trials are lacking, currently available literature suggests that posttransplant monitoring of IgG levels and immunoglobulin replacement therapy may reduce infection rates in patients with hypgammaglobulinemia.

Table 8.15	Timetable of infections	
Month 1 Common nosocomial bacterial pathogens and *Candida* species predominate	**Months 1–6** Unconventional or opportunistic infections due to immunosuppression	**After 6 months** Infection risks associated with duration and intensity of immunosuppression and epidemiologic exposures
Bacterial (sites and sources) Urinary tract Respiratory Bacteremia Surgical wound or intra-abdominal sources (lymphoceles, hematomas, urine leak) Vascular access or instrumentation (catheters, drains, urinary stents) Anatomic or functional genitourinary tract abnormalities (ureteral stricture, vesicoureteric reflux, neurogenic bladder) Clostridium difficile or center-specific multidrug resistant species **Viral** Uncommon except for HSV **Fungal** Candida species predominate (recipient pretransplant colonization or donor-derived) **Organisms transmitted with donor organs**	**Viral** CMV, HSV, VZV, EBV, HBV, HCV, BK (exogenous infection or reactivation of latent disease due to immunosuppression) Others: HHV-6, influenza, RSV, adenovirus **Fungal** Aspergillus species, Cryptococcus, agents of Mucormycosis **Bacterial** Recurrent urinary tract infections or pyelonephritis Nocardia, Listeria, Mycobacterium species, Legionella, tuberculosis **Parasitic** Pneumocystis jiroveci, Toxoplasma and Strongyloides species, leishmaniasis, Trypanosoma cruzi	**Stable patients on low-dose immunosuppressants** Community-acquired respiratory and GI viral pathogens **History of multiple rejection episodes requiring intensification of immunosuppression (or reactivation in patients with previous exposure)** Late opportunistic infections: Cryptococcus, invasive CMV (e.g., CMV retinitis or colitis), VZV, parvovirus B-19, Listeria, tuberculosis **Persistent infections:** HBV, HCV[a], fungal disease, BK virus **Geographically-restricted** (e.g., coccidiodomycosis, histoplasmosis, blastomycosis, paracoccidioidomycosis) **Deep-seated infections** (e.g., osteomyelitis, paravertebral abscess). Predisposing risk factors: chronic skin infections, longstanding poorly controlled diabetes, peripheral vascular disease **Associated with malignancies:** EBV (PTLD), papillomavirus (squamous cell carcinoma), HSV (cervical cancer), HHV-8 (Kaposi sarcoma)

[a] Incidence may decrease with the use of the newer interferon- and ribavirin-free anti-HCV protease inhibitor combination therapy.

CMV, Cytomegalovirus; HSV, Herpes simplex virus; VZV, Varicella zoster virus; EBV, Epstein–Barr virus; HBV, Hepatitis B virus; HCV, Hepatitis C virus; HHV-6, Human herpes virus-6; HHV-7, Human herpes virus-7; HHV-8, Human herpes virus-8; RSV, Respiratory syncytial virus; PTLD, Posttransplant lymphoproliferative disease.

- Neutropenia and leukopenia
  - Drug-induced: thymoglobulin, MMF, AZA, sirolimus, acyclovir, valganciclovir, trimethoprim-sulfamethoxazole, dapsone, or possible idiosyncratic drug–drug reaction
  - The use of granulocyte colony-stimulating factor (GCSF) is safe and effective in kidney transplant recipients.

Cytomegalovirus

- CMV infection categorization:
  - Primary infection: donor seropositive (D+), recipient seronegative (R−)
  - Reactivation of endogenous latent virus: D+/R+ or D−/R+
  - Superinfection with a new virus in a seropositive recipient: D+/R+
- Primary CMV infection is usually more severe than reactivated infection or superinfection.

| Table 8.16 | | | Recommended immunizations before and after transplantation |

Vaccine	Before TX	After TX (2–3 mo Post-Tx)	Comments (Vaccinations before 2–3 mo Posttransplant May Result in Suboptimal Response and Protection)
Measles–mumps–rubella	Y	XXX	
Diphtheria–tetanus–pertussis	Y	See comments	Diphtheria and tetanus: booster every 10 y
Varicella-live	Y	XXX	Should be administered ≥4 wk prior to transplant
Poliovirus	Y	Inactivated polio	For travelers to endemic areas (e.g., some parts of Asia, Africa)
Hemophilus *influenza* type b	Y	Y	
Inactivated influenza vaccine: Influenza A	Y	Y	Annually All patients who are >1 mo posttransplant should receive seasonal influenza vaccine. May be administered in the immediate posttransplant period during an outbreak
Live-attenuated influenza (Nasal spray flu vaccine)	XXX	XXX	
Pneumococcal conjugate PCV13	Y	Y	
Pneumococcal polysaccharide PPSV23	Y	Y	Recommended posttransplant if not administered pretransplant
Hepatitis A	Y	Y	Recommended posttransplant if not administered pretransplant For travelers to endemic areas
Hepatitis B	Y	Y	Recommended posttransplant if not administered pretransplant Monitor titers
Human papillomavirus (HPV)	Y	–	Nonpregnant female candidates aged 9–26
Neisseria *meningitides*	Y	Y	Recommended for patients with properdin–terminal component–deficiencies or receiving *eculizumab* therapy, or those with functional or anatomic asplenia *Others*: military members, travelers to high-risk areas, college freshman living on campus
Zoster-live (Zostavax)	Y	XXX	Should be administered ≥4 wk prior to transplant[a]

Live-attenuated and live virus vaccines are contraindicated after transplantation.

[a] If inadvertently given within 4 weeks before transplant, consult infectious disease specialist and administer acyclovir to prevent recurrence.

TX, transplant; Y, Yes; XXX, contraindicated.

- CMV infection generally refers to asymptomatic CMV seroconversion detected during CMV surveillance.
- CMV disease refers to acute symptomatic CMV infection associated with various signs and symptoms including the following:
  - CMV syndrome (fever, fatigue, leukopenia, and/or thrombocytopenia and evidence of CMV viremia)

Table 8.17	Posttransplant antimicrobial prophylaxis	
Prophylaxis	**Regimen**	**Comments**
Pneumocystis jiroveci	**First line** Trimethoprim–sulfamethoxazole (TMP-SMX) × 12 mo **Second line** (sulfa allergies), dapsone, atovaquone, or aerosolized pentamidine	TMP-SMX also reduces the incidence of *Toxoplasma gondii*, *Listeria monocytogenes*, and *Nocardia asteroids* and reduces the incidence of UTI in kidney transplant recipients. For sulfa-allergic patients, consider adding fluoroquinolones or other agents for antibacterial activity Check glucose-6-phosphate dehydrogenase prior to initiation of dapsone
Fungal	Nystatin or fluconazole	Fluconazole recommended in high-risk recipients (e.g., history of valley fever, patients who live in endemic areas, recipients of simultaneous liver–kidney or pancreas–kidney transplants)
CMV	Acyclovir, valganciclovir, ganciclovir	Acyclovir • CMV negative recipient of a CMV negative organ Acyclovir or valganciclovir (center-dependent) • CMV (+) recipient, CMV (−) donor organ[a] • CMV (+) recipient, CMV (+) donor organ[a] Valganciclovir or ganciclovir (if NPO) • CMV (−) recipient, CMV (+) donor organ

[a] Valganciclovir (or ganciclovir if NPO) recommended for patients treated with lymphocyte-depleting agents.

- Invasive CMV disease involving various organ systems including the liver, GI tract, lung, the kidney allograft, or the transplanted organ. Clinically patients may present with hepatitis, esophagitis, colitis, pneumonitis, pancreatitis, or acute kidney injury.
- CMV diagnosis:
  - CMV DNA assay is highly specific and sensitive for the detection of CMV viremia, whereas pp65 antigenemia is a semiquantitative fluorescent assay in which circulating neutrophils are stained for nonspecific uptake of CMV early antigen (pp65).
  - Screening for CMV is best performed using PCR-based methods.
  - With the widespread availability of nucleic acid testing (NAT), antigen-based method has largely been replaced by CMV DNA testing.
  - PCR results may vary significantly among laboratories. CMV quantitative NAT (QNAT) calibration based on the WHO International Reference Standard is recommended.
  - Serum quantitative CMV assays in patients with invasive colitis and gastritis or neurologic disease including chorioretinitis are often negative. Patients suspected to have tissue-invasive CMV disease but with negative QNAT or pp65 antigenemia should have tissue biopsy and histopathology to confirm the clinical suspicion of CMV disease.
- CMV prevention can be achieved by prophylaxis or preemptive therapy.
  - Prophylactic therapy involves antiviral beginning in the immediate postoperative period.
  - Preemptive therapy entails close CMV surveillance and initiation of treatment only in patients who are found to seroconvert.
  - **2009 KDIGO clinical practice guidelines:** CMV prophylactic therapy is recommended over initiation of preemptive therapy.

- Treatment:
  - For mild clinical symptoms: oral valganciclovir 900 mg twice daily (adjusted for GFR)
  - For severe disease, GI disease, or life-threatening disease or in those intolerant to oral medication, IV ganciclovir 5 mg/kg every 12 hours, adjusted for GFR should be used (2010 International Consensus guidelines).
    - Treatment duration:
      - Traditional paradigm: 2 to 4 weeks
      - New paradigm based on The AST Infectious Diseases Community of Practice Guidelines published in 2013: Therapy should be continued until clearance of viremia. Generally, CMV disease should be monitored once weekly using CMV QNAT (or pp65 antigenemia) to assess virologic response.
  - Patients with CMV disease should remain on full therapeutic dose of antiviral therapy until CMV DNA load (or antigenemia) is undetectable. After completion of full-dose treatment, consider a 1- to 3-month course of secondary prophylaxis.
  - Cautious reduction of immunosuppression should be considered in moderate to severe disease, in slow or nonresponders, and in those with high viral load or leukopenia.
  - The beneficial effect of adding IVIg or CMV Ig to existing antiviral therapy is unclear but may be considered for patients with life-threatening disease, CMV pneumonitis, or other severe forms of disease.
  - Ganciclovir-resistant strains: cidofovir or foscarnet (potential for nephrotoxicity and synergistic nephrotoxic effect with CNIs). Obtain genotypic resistance testing (UL97 or UL54 gene mutations).
- Monitor graft function closely during CMV disease. Late-onset CMV disease occurring >2 years after transplant has been shown to be associated with poor transplant outcome.
- Preemptive therapy: weekly CMV QNAT (or pp65 antigenemia) to predict risk of CMV disease (AST Infectious Diseases Community of Practice Guidelines, 2013)
- Measuring anti-CMV cell-mediated immunity (using QuantiFERON-CMV assay to measure the level of T cell IFN-γ production after CMV antigen exposure) to assess the risk of CMV infection or disease and to guide therapeutic response is a subject of ongoing clinical research.

BK Polyomavirus

- BK virus is a ubiquitous human virus with a seroprevalence rate of >60% to 90% among the adult population. After primary infection, BK virus preferentially establishes latency within the genitourinary tract and frequently reactivates in the setting of immunosuppression
- Clinical manifestations: asymptomatic viruria with or without viremia, ureteral stenosis and obstruction, tubulointerstitial nephritis, and BK allograft nephropathy (BKN)
- BKN most commonly presents with an asymptomatic acute or slowly progressive rise in serum creatinine between 2 and 60 months after engraftment (median 9 months). Urinalysis is usually unremarkable but may reveal pyuria, hematuria, and cellular casts similar to those seen in tubulointerstitial nephritis. A definitive diagnosis requires allograft biopsy.
- BKN is an important cause of allograft dysfunction and graft loss.
- Posttransplant BK screening
  - Currently most centers routinely screen kidney transplant recipients for BK viruria or viremia or both by quantitative PCR for BK viral DNA.
  - BKN is unusual in the absence of BK viremia but has been reported (anecdotal case report).

- **The 2009 KDIGO clinical practice guideline** suggests screening all kidney transplant recipients with quantitative plasma NAT:
  - Monthly for the first 3 to 6 months after transplant then
  - Every 3 months until the end of the first posttransplant year
  - Whenever there is an unpexplained rise in serum creatinine and
  - After treatment of acute rejection
- Treatment
  - Reduction in immunosuppression has been accepted as the mainstay of therapy.
  - The effectiveness of currently available antiviral agents are of uncertain benefit (cidofovir, leflunomide, IVIG, fluoroquinolones, and sirolimus alone or in combination therapy with leflunomide have been used with variable success).
  - Tacrolimus to cyclosporine or sirolimus conversion therapy resulted in resolution of BKN and viremia/viuria in anecdotal case reports and cannot be routinely recommended.
  - Routine BK screening and early intervention (i.e., reduction in immunosuppression) may prevent the development of BK nephropathy.
- Patients with graft loss due to BK nephropathy can safely undergo retransplantation (preferably following BK viral clearance).

Herpes Simplex Virus 1, 2

- KDIGO guidelines treatment suggestions:
  - Superficial herpes simplex virus 1,2 (HSV 1,2) infection: oral antiviral agent (e.g., acyclovir, valacyclovir, or famciclovir) until all lesions are crusted
  - Systemic HSV 1, 2 infection: IV acyclovir and reduction in immunosuppression. IV acyclovir should be continued until the patient has a clinical response, then switch to an appropriate oral antiviral agent to complete a total treatment duration of 14 to 21 days.
  - In patients with frequent recurrences of HSV 1, 2 infection, prophylactic antiviral agent is recommended.

Varicella Zoster

- KDIGO guidelines treatment suggestions:
  - Primary varicella zoster virus (VZV) infection (chicken pox): Intravenous or oral acyclovir or valacyclovir and temporary reduction in immunosuppression. Treatment should be continued at least until all lesions have scabbed.
  - Uncomplicated herpes zoster (shingles): oral acyclovir or valacyclovir, at least until all lesions have scabbed.
  - Disseminated or invasive herpes zoster should be treated with IV acyclovir and temporary reduction in immunosuppression, at least until all lesions have scabbed.
  - Prevention of primary varicella zoster should be instituted to varicella-susceptible patients after exposure to individuals with active varicella infection.
  - Varicella zoster immunoglobulin within 96 hours of exposure.
  - If immunoglobulin is not available or more than 96 hours have passed, a 7-day course of oral acyclovir begun 7 to 10 days after varicella exposure.

Hepatitis C

- Kidney transplantation from hepatitis C-positive donors is offered to hepatitis C-positive transplant candidates (who are viremic) and who have consented to receive such kidney.

- Active viral replication at the time of transplant has been shown to be associated with a higher incidence of long-term clinical liver disease and worse allograft function and graft survival compared with HCV positive recipients with persistently negative viremia.
- Patients who were not viremic at the time of transplant but who became viremic posttransplant have inferior outcomes compared with those who remain free of viral replication.
- Interferon-based therapy increases the risk of allograft rejection and should be used only if the benefits clearly outweigh the risks.
- The advent of direct acting antiviral agents (i.e., protease inhibitors) such as sofobusvir and ledipasvir may improve outcomes in hepatitis C positive kidney transplant recipients.

Adenovirus

- Adenoviral infections occur in 4% to 5% of kidney transplant recipients.
- Risk factors: intensity of immunosuppression. Supporting evidence:
  - Higher incidence in the first 3 months after transplantation
  - Infection occurs in association with treatment of acute rejection
  - Resolution of the infection with immunosuppression reduction
- Clinical manifestations:
  - Vary with the transplanted organ, with the allograft itself being the most frequent organ involved.
  - Kidney transplant recipients frequently present with hemorrhagic cystitis, fever, dysuria, frequency, urgency, and gross hematuria.
  - Hemorrhagic cystitis is frequently accompanied by graft dysfunction and kidney function generally returns to baseline after resolution of the adenovirus disease.
  - Histopathology shows viral inclusions and necrosis of the tubulointerstitium.
- Treatment:
  - Reduction of immunosuppression is the mainstay of therapy.
  - Cidofovir is considered standard treatment of adenovirus disease by many centers, although its use is not supported by any prospective randomized clinical trials.

Pneumocystis jirovecii (Previously Known as *Pneumocystis carinii*)

- *Pneumocystis jirovecii pneumonia (PJP)* commonly occurs 2 to 6 months after transplantation or following augmentation of immunosuppression.
- *P. jirovecii* outbreaks and person-to-person spread have been reported to occur >6 to 12 months after transplant.
- Common clinical presentation and radiographic findings: nonproductive cough, fever, arterial–alveolar mismatching, and diffuse interstitial infiltrate or focal airspace consolidation
- Recommended prophylactic therapy in order of efficacy/preference: trimethoprim sulmamethoxazole (TMP-SMX), dapsone, atovaquone, pentamidine. Treatment duration: 12 months. Patients should be tested for glucose-6-phosphate dehydrogenase deficiency prior to initiation of dapsone.
- Prophylactic therapy should be reinstituted following intensification of immunosuppression (e.g., pulse steroids to treat acute rejection).
- All exposed susceptible individuals should receive PJP prophylaxis.

Diarrhea

- Drug-related complications (most common cause of diarrhea in the early post-transplant period):
  - MMF commonly causes GI side effects, including nausea, vomiting, dyspepsia, anorexia, flatulence, and diarrhea.
  - Dose reduction, transient discontinuation of the drug often ameliorates or resolves GI symptoms.
  - Mycophenolate sodium (the enteric-coated formulation of MPA) has not been consistently shown to be better than the original formulation in ameliorating GI symptoms. Nonetheless, MMF to enteric-coated mycophenlate sodium conversion therapy can be considered in patients with GI intolerance associated with mycophenolate mofetil use.
  - Sirolimus, tacrolimus, and cyclosporine have all been suggested to cause diarrhea to variable extent.
- Infectious causes of diarrhea:
  - Commonly encountered bacterial pathogens: *Clostridium difficile*
    - Diagnostic testing: stool PCR
    - Treatment:
      - First episode: metronidazole 500 mg three times a day for 10 to 14 days. For severe disease oral vancomycin 125 mg four times a day for 10 to 14 days or fidaxomicin 20 mg twice a day for 10 days
      - First relapse: treatment same as for first episode
      - Second relapse: oral vancomycin
      - Third or more relapses: prolonged oral vancomycin course. May consider fecal microbiota transplantation
  - Commonly encountered viral pathogens: CMV
    - Diagnostic testing: serum CMV PCR
    - Treatment (see CMV section)
  - Norovirus is increasingly recognized as a cause of diarrhea after solid-organ transplantation:
    - Often causes acute self-limited illness in immunocompetent individuals
    - Can cause both acute and chronic diarrhea in solid-organ transplant recipients
    - Diagnostic testing: norovirus PCR
    - Treatment: supportive (volume repletion), antimotility agents, reduction in immunosuppression (inconclusive evidence)

Posttransplant Infections of the Gastrointestinal Tract

- Posttransplant infections of the GI tract may be viral, fungal, or bacterial in etiology.
- Viral infections are most commonly caused by CMV and HSV
- Common opportunistic fungal infections *Candida albicans* and *Candida tropicalis*
- Commonly encountered bacterial pathogens include *Clostridium difficile* and *Helicobacter pylori*.

Routine Infectious Disease Donor Screening

- Deceased donor testing:
  - Blood and urine cultures
  - Anti-HIV-1 and -2, or HIV antibody/antigen (Ab/Ag) combination assays

- HBsAg, HBcAb, and anti-HCV or HCV NAT
- Cytomegalovirus antibody (anti-CMV)
- Epstein–Barr Virus antibody (anti-EBV)
- Syphilis screening
- Donor screening in endemic settings
  - TB
  - Strongiloides
  - *Trypanosoma cruzi* (Chagas disease)
  - West Nile virus
- Living donor testing:
  - Anti-HIV-1 and -2 or HIV antigen/antibody (Ag/Ab) combination assays as close as possible, but within 28 days prior to organ recovery
  - HBsAg, HBcAb, HBsAb, and anti-HCV
  - HCV ribonucleic acid (RNA) by NAT as close as possible, but within 28 days prior to organ recovery
  - anti-CMV
  - anti-EBV
  - Syphilis screening
  - Donor screening in endemic settings:
    - TB
    - Strongiloides
    - *Trypanosoma cruzi* (Chagas disease)
    - West Nile virus
- If a donor is identified as being at increased risk for HIV, HBV, and HCV transmission according to the US PHS Guidelines, testing must also include HIV RNA by NAT or HIV Ab/Ag combination assays.
- The infectious window period reduced by NAT is shown in Table 8.18

Routine Recipient Infectious Disease Screening

- Routine serologic testing:
  - Anti-HIV-1 and -2 antibody
  - HBsAg, HBcAb (IgM and IgG), HBsAb, and anti-HCV
  - anti-CMV
  - anti-EBV
  - HSV and VZV IgG antibodies
  - Syphilis screening
  - PPD or Quantiferon Gold TB (recommended for patients with history of BCG vaccine)
- Serologic testing based on risk factors (endemic mycoses or travel history)

Table 8.18		Infectious window period reduced by nucleic acid testing	
Etiologic Agent	**Standard Serology**	**Enhanced Serology (Fourth-Generation or Combination Tests)**	**Nucleic Acid Testing**
HIV	17–22 d	~7–16 d	5–9 d
HCV	~70 d	~40–50 d	3–7 d
HBV	35–44 d	NA	20–22 d

- Coccidiodes IgM and IgG antibody, histoplasma immunodiffusion antibody or urine antigen, *Strongyloides stercoralis* antibody, *Leishmania* spp., *Trypanosoma cruzi* antibody, human T-cell lymphotrophic virus (HTLV-1/2) antibody

Posttransplant Serology Monitoring for Recipients Accepting Public Health Services-Increased Risk Organs

- Public Health Services (PHS) risk organs are defined as follows:
  - Male homosexual contact
  - Promiscuous sexual relations in exchange for money or drugs
  - Persons who have had sexual contact with persons known or suspected to have HIV/HBV/HCV infection (through percutaneous inoculation or through contact with an open wound, nonintact skin, or mucuous membrane)
  - Nonmedical intravenous, intramuscular, or subcutaneous use of drugs
  - Inmates of correctional systems
  - Persons with known or suspected sexually transmitted disease (e.g., syphilis, genital herpes simplex)
  - Persons who are receiving dialysis treatments
  - Persons with known HIV, hepatitis B or C infection
  - Persons who are hemodiluted as per OPTN/UNOS policy
- Informed consent must be obtained prior to transplantation of PHS-increased risk organs
- Monitoring of recipients of PHS-increased risk donor organs should include the following (Table 8.19):
  - Pretransplant baseline serologic testing
    - For HIV testing: HIV-1 RNA
    - For HBV testing: HBsAg and HBV DNA quantitative PCR
    - For HCV testing: HCV RNA quantitative PCR testing
  - Posttransplant surveillance:
    - For HIV testing: HIV-1 RNA 6 weeks posttransplant
    - For HBV testing:
      - HBsAg and HBV DNA quantitative PCR test 6 weeks posttransplant
      - HBsAg, anti-HBs and anti-HBc at 12 months posttransplant
    - For HCV testing: HCV RNA quantitative PCR testing at 6 weeks posttransplant
- Additional testing may be performed based on patient's clinical characteristics, symptoms, immunosuppression, or at the discretion of the transplant team.
- In the event a recipient seroconverts, a treatment plan will be developed by the transplant team in conjunction with transplant infectious disease consultation.

Table 8.19 Protocol surveillance for PHS increased risk donor kidney recipient

Pretransplant	Posttransplant
At baseline • HIV-RNA • HBsAg, HBV DNA quantitative PCR • HCV RNA quantitative PCR	At 6 wk posttransplant: • HIV-RNA quantitative PCR • HBsAg, HBV DNA quantitative PCR • HCV RNA quantitative PCR At 12 mo posttransplant: • HBsAg or HBV NAT, Anti-HBsAb, and anti-HBcAb

NONINFECTIOUS COMPLICATIONS AFTER KIDNEY TRANSPLANT

Surgical Complications (Usually Occur Early after Transplantation)

- Wound infections:
  - Obese transplant recipients are at greater risk.
  - Sirolimus may delay wound healing and increase the incidence of lymphocele formation. Its use should be avoided in the early posttransplant period.
- Perinephric fluid collections:
  - Lymphoceles:
    - Most common type of peritransplant fluid collection
    - Usually occur several weeks to months after surgery
    - Incidence higher with sirolimus
    - Small lymphoceles are usually asymptomatic (conservative management), but larger lymphoceles can cause obstruction (management include percutaneous drainage or surgical repair).
  - Hematomas:
    - Usually occur in the immediate postoperative period
    - May be extrarenal or subcapsular, usually resolve spontaneously
    - May occur after allograft biopsy
  - Urinomas:
    - Urine leaks typically occur within the first few days after transplantation or at the onset of diuresis in patients with DGF.
    - Clinical presentation: increasing wound drainage, decreasing urine output, graft tenderness, abdominal or scrotal pain or swelling
    - Diagnosis: significantly elevated fluid to serum creatinine ratio
    - Management: If there is clinical suspicion, a Foley catheter should be placed immediately. Prolonged bladder drainage and ureteral stenting may stop the leakage. Percutaneous antegrade nephrostomy may be used to diagnose the leak and control the urine flow. Surgical repair may be required, and the type of surgery depends on the level of the leak and the viability of the tissues.
- Obstructive uropathy: etiologies: ureteral blood clots, stones, ureteral kinking, neurogenic bladder, benign prostatic hypertrophy causing bladder outlet obstruction, ureteral strictures due to ischemia or BK infection

Medical Complications (May Occur Early or Late after Transplantation)

- Posttransplant cardiovascular disease is the most frequent cause of death with a functioning graft: risk factors for posttransplant cardiovascular events:
  - Conventional risk factors:family history, pretransplant diabetes, male gender, age, white race, hypertension, dyslipidemia, obesity, smoking
  - Unconventional or transplant-related risk factors: posttransplantation diabetes mellitus (PTDM), anemia, proteinuria, impaired graft function, low albumin, hyperuricemia, left ventricular hypertrophy
- Posttransplant hypertension:
  - Etiologic or risk factors: preexisting hypertension, cyclosporine and to a lesser extent tacrolimus, corticosteroids, quality of donor organ, hypertensive donor, delayed graft function, high body mass index, excess weight gain or salt intake, acute rejection episodes, renal transplant artery stenosis, effects of native kidneys
  - There is no conclusive evidence that one class of antihypertensive agent is superior to another in the transplant setting.

- Diltiazem and verapamil increase CNI and mTOR inhibitor levels. Their use permits reduction in CNI and mTOR inhibitor drug dosages.
- Dyslipidemia:
  - Common after transplantation due in part to the hyperlipemic effect of corticosteroids, cyclosporine, tacrolimus, sirolimus, and everolimus. Severe hypertriglyceridemia may occur with the use of sirolimus and everolimus due to decreased catabolism of apoB-100-containing lipoproteins (dose dependent, generally reversible upon discontinuation of mTOR inhibitors).
  - Other potential etiologic factors: age, diet, rapid weight gain, hyperinsulinemia, preexisting hypercholesterolemia, allograft dysfunction, proteinuria, genetic predisposition, β-blocker, and diuretic use.
- Posttransplantation diabetes mellitus (PTDM), also known as new-onset diabetes mellitus after transplantation (NODAT)
  - In 2014, the International Expert Panel consisting of transplant nephrologists, diabetologists, and clinical scientists recommended changing the terminology NODAT back to PTDM.
  - The American Diabetes Association (ADA) diagnostic criteria for prediabetes and diabetes is shown in Table 8.20
  - Risk factors for PTDM (Fig. 8.14)
  - Both preexisting diabetes and PTDM have an adverse impact on patient survival.
- Anemia:
  - Peri- or early postoperative period: dilutional anemia due to aggressive volume expansion, surgical postoperative bleeding
  - Mild anemia is common in the early postoperative period when erythropoietin is discontinued but usually improves within several weeks.
  - Drug-induced: MMF, sirolimus, everolimus, AZA, angiotensin-converting enzyme inhibitors (ACEIs), angiotensin-receptor blockers (ARBs), dapsone
  - ACEIs and ARBs are used to treat posttransplant erythrocytosis.
  - Sirolimus inhibits erythropoiesis at the level of EPO receptor.
  - Other etiologic factors: iron deficiency, impaired graft function, acute rejection episodes
- Posttransplant erythrocytosis (8% to 15%):
  - Commonly occurs within the first 2 years after transplantation
  - Incidence appears to decrease, ascribed to more frequent use of ACEIs and ARBs

Table 8.20	The American Diabetes Association diagnostic criteria for prediabetes and diabetes		
Diagnostic test/criteria	Normoglycemia (mg/dL)	Prediabetes IFG or IGT (mg/dL)	Diabetes (mg/dL)
Casual plasma glucose with diabetic symptoms[a]			>200
Fasting plasma glucose	<100	100–125[b]	≥126
Oral glucose tolerance test	<140	140–199[b]	≥200
HbA1C		5.7–6.4%[b]	≥6.5%

[a]Diabetic symptoms defined as polyuria, polydipsia, weight loss. In the absence of unequivocal hyperglycemia, diagnosis should be confirmed by repeat testing on a different day.

[b]The risk is continuous and becomes disproportionately greater at higher glucose or A1C levels.

IFG, impaired fasting glucose; IGT, impaired glucose tolerance.

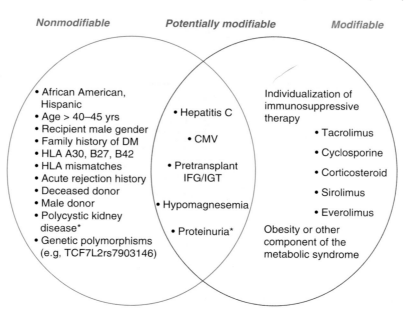

Nonmodifiable   Potentially modifiable   Modifiable

- African American, Hispanic
- Age > 40–45 yrs
- Recipient male gender
- Family history of DM
- HLA A30, B27, B42
- HLA mismatches
- Acute rejection history
- Deceased donor
- Male donor
- Polycystic kidney disease*
- Genetic polymorphisms (e.g, TCF7L2rs7903146)

- Hepatitis C
- CMV
- Pretransplant IFG/IGT
- Hypomagnesemia
- Proteinuria*

Individualization of immunosuppressive therapy
- Tacrolimus
- Cyclosporine
- Corticosteroid
- Sirolimus
- Everolimus

Obesity or other component of the metabolic syndrome

FIGURE 8.14 Risk factors for PTDM. Restoration of insulin metabolism by a functioning graft may unmask pretransplant IFG or diabetes mellitus. CMV, cytomegalovirus; IFG, impaired fasting glucose; IGT, impaired glucose tolerance.
*The association between polycystic kidney disease (or proteinuria) and PTDM has not been consistently observed

- Treatment: ACEIs or ARBs. Phlebotomy may occasionally be necessary.
- Treatment is generally recommended for a hemoglobin level > 17 to 18 g/dL or hematocrit > 52% because of the associated risk of thromboembolic complications, hypertension, and headaches.
- Chronic allograft injury:
  - Chronic allograft injury (CAI) is a nonspecific histopathologic description and does not distinguish immune from nonimmune injury.
  - Banff 2005 classification of immunologic and nonimmunologic causes of CAI are shown in Table 8.21
  - Clinical manifestations:
    - Gradual decline in graft function occurring months to years after transplantation
    - Proteinuria of various degrees may be present. Nephrotic range proteinuria can be seen with Chronic transplant glomerulopathy (CTG).
    - Hypertension
  - Management:
    - The optimal management of CAI remains to be defined.
    - If an element of acute rejection is suspected or documented on allograft biopsy, a steroid pulse may be given. Polyclonal antibodies should not be given for chronic rejection or CAI.
    - If chronic CNI toxicity is demonstrated on biopsy, consider CNI minimization while providing adequate immunosuppression to prevent rejection.
    - CNI to sirolimus conversion therapy may be of little beneficial effect or futile when there is evidence of moderate allograft dysfunction or significant proteinuria at the time of intervention.
    - Treat comorbidities known to slow the progression of CKD (aggressive management of hypertension and proteinuria).

Table 8.21	Banff 2005 classification of chronic allograft injury
Alloimmune Causes	**Nonalloimmune Causes**
Chronic allograft rejection	Specific chronic kidney diseases
Chronic active antibody-mediated rejection	Calcineurin inhibitor toxicity
Chronic active T-cell mediated rejection	Chronic hypertension
	Chronic obstruction
	Bacterial pyelonephritis
	Viral infection
	Recurrent or de novo glomerular or vascular diseases
	Recurrent or de novo diabetic changes

- ACEI or ARB are commonly used due to their well-established antiproteinuric and cardioprotective effects in the nontransplant settings, although the beneficial effects of these agents on posttransplant patient and graft survival have not been consistently demonstrated.
- Histopathologic features (see Kidney Allograft Biopsy Findings section)
- Posttransplant proteinuria:
  - Prevalence: Approximately 10% to 45% (wide range reported due in part to the threshold used to define proteinuria and time after transplantation)
  - Urine-albumin-to-creatinine ratio and urine-protein-to-creatinine ratio are reasonable screening tests. Significant proteinuria warrants confirmation with 24-hour urine collection particularly if allograft biopsy is being considered.
  - Both elevated albumin/creatinine and protein/creatinine ratios have been shown to predict long-term prognosis.
  - Proteinuria from native kidneys generally resolves within the first month after transplantation. Persistent or worsening proteinuria is usually indicative of graft pathology.
  - Consider allograft biopsy for unexplained proteinuria.
  - Etiologies of posttransplant proteinuria:
    - Transplant-related: Recurrent disease particularly primary FSGS, chronic rejection or transplant glomerulopathy, secondary focal segmental glomerulosclerosis, acute allograft rejection (proteinuria usually <500 mg/d), chronic CNI nephrotoxicity, or use of mTOR inhibitors. Proteinuria has also been reported to be associated with de novo DSA detection.
    - Nontransplant-related: de novo glomerular disease or glomerulonephritis similar to that seen in the nontransplant settings
  - Posttransplant proteinuria is associated with an adverse impact on patient and graft survival, and an increased risk of cardiovascular events and PTDM (a.k.a NODAT) development.
  - ACEIs or ARBs reduce proteinuria, but the beneficial effect of these agents on long-term patient and graft survival has not been consistently demonstrated.
- Recurrent diseases:
  - Specific glomerular disease recurrence is summarized in Table 8.22
  - Primary hyperoxaluria type 1 (PH1): Lack of the liver-specific peroxisomal enzyme alanine-glyoxylate aminotransferase in patients PH1 results in decreased transamination of glyoxylate to glycine and increased production of oxalate and glycolate. Because oxalate is eliminated unaltered by renal excretion, isolated kidney transplantation can result in rapid deposition of oxalate in the

Table 8.22	Glomerular Disease Recurrence after Transplantation and Graft Loss from Disease Recurrence[a]	
Primary Glomerular Disease (Comments)	**Recurrence Rates (Graft loss due to recurrence)**	**Treatment**
Primary focal segmental glomerulosclerosis (FSGS) • Rapid-onset heavy proteinuria	20%–50% • 30%–50% graft loss due to recurrence; >75% in subsequent graft if first graft lost was due to recurrence Risk factors: Heavy proteinuria, ESRD within 2–3 years of onset, age < 15, mesangial hypercellularity on biopsy, recurrence in previous graft	Plasma exchange; Rituximab adjunctive therapy[b] (500 mg IV weekly × 4)
Membranous glomerulonephropathy (MGN) • Minimally elevated proteinuria to full blown nephrotic range • Proteinuria may increase with duration of active disease.	10%–30%: Histologic recurrence may be more common. • [10%–30% graft loss due to recurrence]	Supportive (ACEI or ARB, BP control, diuretics); Rituximab[c] (consider if heavy proteinuria and/or worsening renal function); Cyclophosphamide[d]
MPGN-I DDD (a.k.a. MPGN-II) • Hematuria with subnephrotic to nephrotic range proteinuria, often with worsening graft function	MPGN-I 15%–50% DDD 80%–100% Risk factors for MPGN-I recurrence: HLA-B49 and -DR4 (limited data) • Graft loss due to recurrence is common particularly with DDD.	
IgA nephropathy (IgAN) • Microscopic hematuria, mild proteinuria (often <0.5 g/d)	30%–50%, increases with longer duration of follow-up • 2%–16% graft loss due to recurrence	Supportive (ACEI or ARB for proteinuria; BP control)
Lupus nephritis (LN) • Mild proteinuria and microscopic hematuria • Systemic manifestations are rare • Minimal evidence to support predictive role of serologies	3%–10% Defer transplant until SLE is clinically quiescent on <10 mg prednisone without cytotoxic agent for 6–12 months • <5% graft loss due to recurrence	Pulse steroids; Increase MMF dose (or cyclophosphamide)[e]
Granulomatosis with polyangiitis (GPA); Microscopic polyangiitis	10%–20% Clinical remission for >6 months before transplant may reduce recurrence risk. Pretransplant ANCA titers not predictive of recurrence in asymptomatic patients[f] • 20%–50% graft loss due to recurrence	Cyclophosphamide-based regimen
Anti-GBM disease	Recurrence is rare when transplant performed >6 months after antibody disappearance; • 50% graft loss due to recurrence Histologic recurrence in 50% when circulating anti-GBM antibody is positive at the time of transplant.	Plasma exchange, cyclophosphamide, and corticosteroids
Henoch–Schonlein Purpura (HSP)	Clinical recurrence is rare despite 50% histologic recurrence. • Graft loss due to recurrence is rare.	

(continued)

Table 8.22	Glomerular Disease Recurrence after Transplantation and Graft Loss from Disease Recurrence[a] (continued)	
Primary Glomerular Disease (Comments)	**Recurrence Rates (Graft loss due to recurrence)**	**Treatment**
Hemolytic uremic syndrome (HUS)	HUS recurrence risk is associated with underlying causative factors.	
Causative factors		
Childhood Shiga toxin-associated HUS	Recurrence is rare	
Atypical HUS (a.k.a. HUS-TTP or TTP-HUS) At least 1 year of clinical quiescence before transplantation is recommended.	20–25% (approximately 50% of subsequent grafts) • >80% graft loss due to recurrence	Plasmapheresis
Familial HUS (mutations of factor H, factor I, membrane cofactor protein, factor B, or C3) Pretransplant evaluation for genetic mutations recommended	60%–80% • >90% graft loss due to recurrence	Eculizumab
Acquired factor H deficiency (anti-factor H autoantibodies)	• Kidney transplantation is safe when combined with plasma exchange and high-dose steroid to lower the antibody titer; recurrent risk prevention	Monitor autoantibodies and administer rituximab if persistently elevated levels posttransplant.
Alport syndrome (X-linked) • Recurrent Alport syndrome does not occur in the transplanted graft because the donor kidney has a normal GBM. De novo anti-GBM may manifest as rapidly progressive crescentic GN with linear deposits of anti-GBM IgG	De novo anti-GBM glomerulonephritis occurs in 3%–4% of males (the introduction of normal collagen in the basal membrane of the donor allograft may induce antibody formation to the donor kidney collagen) X-linked females do not develop posttransplant anti-GBM because they generally carry a normal copy of the affected gene Retransplantation in patients who developed posttransplant anti-GBM is associated with high risk of recurrence (up to 90%).	De novo anti-GBM: Plasmapheresis and cyclophosphamide (of limited benefit)
Fabry disease	<5%	
Primary oxalosis	80%–100% • High rate of graft loss due to oxalate deposition.	Simultaneous liver–kidney transplantation recommended for type I
Diabetic nephropathy	80%–100% (by histology) • Rare cause of graft loss	

[a]Recurrent rates may vary widely due in part to differences in follow-up period, and protocol biopsies versus biopsy for cause.

[b]Ongoing clinical research; pre-emptive treatment may be considered in planned living donor transplant.

[c]Recommendations based on small case series, clinical response may be delayed for months.

[d]May consider in those not responding to rituximab (clinical experience is anecdotal)

[e]Treatment same as for native kidneys

[f]Successful transplantation in the face of persistent ANCA positivity is well-recognized.

MPGN, Membranoproliferative glomerulonephritis; DDD, Dense deposit disease; TTP, Thrombotic thrombocytopenic purpura; Anti-GBM, Anti-glomerular basement membrane; GN, Glomerulonephritis

allograft and subsequent stone formation, nephrocalcinosis, and graft failure. Liver transplantation corrects the underlying hepatic-based metabolic disorder. Hence, in patients with ESRD due to PH1, simultaneous liver-kidney transplantation is recommended.

- Bone and mineral disorders (discussed under Posttransplant Bone and Mineral Disorders)

POSTTRANSPLANT BONE AND MINERAL DISORDER

Hypophosphatemia

- Frequently encountered in the first months after transplantation
- Concomitant hypercalcemia suggests posttransplantation hyperparathyroidism
- In the absence of hypercalcemia, renal phosphate wasting syndrome or malnutrition should be considered.
- Early after transplantation, hypophosphatemia has been attributed to a massive initial diuresis, defective renal phosphate reabsorption due to ischemic injury, glucosuria (due to hyperglycemia-induced osmotic diuresis), and corticosteroid use (by inhibiting proximal tubular reabsorption of phosphate).
- Fibroblast growth factor-23 (FGF-23) may play a major contributory role in the development of early posttransplantation hypophosphatemia independent of PTH level.
- Pretransplant FGF-23 has been shown to be the main predictor of posttransplant phosphate levels.
- In contrast to hypophosphatemia occurring in the early posttransplant period, persistent hypophosphatemia beyond 1 year posttransplant has been attributed mainly to persistent hyperparathyroidism rather than to increased FGF-23 levels.

Hypercalcemia

- Hypercalcemia is common after transplantation and is generally due to persistent secondary hyperparathyroidism.
- The concomitant presence of severe hypophosphatemia particularly in patients with excellent graft function may exacerbate hypercalcemia through stimulation of renal proximal tubular 1α-hydroxylase.
- Resolution of soft tissue calcifications and immobilization are potential contributing factors.
- In about two-third of cases, hypercalcemia resolves spontaneously within 6 to 12 months.
- In kidney transplant recipients with hypercalcemic hyperparathyroidism, treatment with the calcimimetic cinacalcet can reduce serum calcium and PTH levels and improve hypophosphatemia.
- Whether the beneficial effect of cinacalcet on mineral metabolism translates into improvement in long-term clinical outcomes in kidney transplant recipients remains to be studied.
- Severe hypercalcemia or persistent hypercalcemia ($\geq$12 months) requires further evaluation.
  - Initial assessment should include an intact PTH level.
  - Neck ultrasound or parathyroid technetium 99mTc-sestamibi scan are required to determine if the clinically observed hyperparathyroidism arises from parathyroid adenoma or parathyroid gland hyperplasia, or hyperplastic nodular formation of the parathyroid glands.

Hyperparathyroidism

- Common after kidney transplant
- Generally attributed to continued autonomous production of PTH from nodular hyperplastic glands, reduced density of calcitriol receptors, and decreased expression of the membrane calcium sensor receptors that render cells more resistant to physiologic concentrations of calcitriol and calcium.
- Persistently elevated FGF-23 levels posttransplant has been suggested to contribute to persistent hyperparathyroidism through inhibition of 1α-hydroxylase activity. The latter may contribute to low levels of calcitriol observed in the early posttransplantation period and persistent hyperparathyroidism.
- The risk of developing persistent hyperparathyroidism is increased with the duration of dialysis and the severity of pretransplant hyperparathyroidism.
- Parathyroidectomy should be considered in patients with
  - Tertiary hyperparathyroidism
  - Persistent severe hypercalcemia (>11.5 to 12 mg/dL) for >6 to 12 months
  - Symptomatic/progressive hypercalcemia:
    - Nephrolithiasis
    - Persistent metabolic bone disease
    - Calcium-related allograft dysfunction
    - Progressive vascular calcification
    - Calciphylaxis
  - Whether the advent of calcimimetics to traditional medical therapy confers better normalization of biochemical parameters and obviates the need for parathyroidectomy remains to be studied.

Vitamin D insufficiency or deficiency

- Both vitamin D 25(OH) insufficiency (levels between 20 and 30 ng/mL) and deficiency (levels < 20 ng/mL) are common in kidney transplant recipients.
- Should replete as needed

Posttransplant bone disease

- Osteopenia/Osteoporosis: Posttransplant decline in bone marrow density is most pronounced in the first 6 months and correlates with higher corticosteroid exposure.
- The early rapid decrease in BMD is usually followed by a slower rate of bone loss.
- Avascular necrosis (AVN):
  - Most commonly affects the femoral head and neck but may affect other joints including knees, shoulders, ankles, elbows, and wrists.
  - Risk factors: greater exposure to intravenous corticosteroid pulse therapy, low bone mass, increasing dialysis duration, excessive weight gain, hyperlipidemia, microvascular thrombosis, and history of local trauma.
- Early steroid withdrawal has been shown to reduce fracture risk.

POSTTRANSPLANT MALIGNANCY

Malignancy after Solid-Organ Transplantation

- Recipients of organ transplants are at increased risk for developing certain neoplasms compared with the general population.

- Posttransplant malignancy is an important cause of death in long-term kidney transplant recipients
- Suggested risk factor:
  - Duration and intensity of immunosuppressive agents and their ability to promote replication of oncogenic viruses
  - Infection-associated cancers
    - EBV: PTLD, Hodgkin lymphoma
    - Human Herpes Virus (HHV)-8: Kaposi sarcoma
    - Hepatitis B and hepatitis C: hepatocellular carcinoma
    - Human papillomaviruses (HPV): vulva, vagina, cervix, penis, anus, oral cavity, and pharynx
    - Possibly HPV-related: nonmelanocytic-related skin cancer
  - Others: older age, male gender, Caucasian race, pretransplant dialysis duration, smoking history, deceased donor organ, cumulative exposure to radiation from repeated medical imaging studies, antecedent use of immunosuppressive agents to treat primary kidney diseases

Skin Cancers

- Most common de novo posttransplant malignancy in the adult transplant population
- Incidence of squamous cell >> basal cell skin cancers
- Risk factors:
  - Duration of follow-up after transplant
  - Light skin color (easily sunburned)
  - Intensity of sun (ultraviolet radiation) exposure
  - Older age at transplant
- Dermatology surveillance (guidelines drawn from evidence-based skin cancer surveillance program, United Kingdom):
  - High risk (age > 55 at transplant and light skin color): annually for the first 2 years then every 6 months thereafter
  - Low risk (Asian or Black): every 2 years
  - Increased surveillance recommended after first cancer
- Sirolimus-containing regimen (de novo sirolimus or CNI to sirolimus conversion therapy) is associated with decreased nonmelanoma skin cancer risks (1° and 2° skin cancer prevention).
- The Sirolimus Renal Conversion Trial (CONVERT) in which patients were randomized to sirolimus conversion or CNI continuation demonstrated that:
  - Sirolimus-based, CNI-free immunosuppression was associated with a significant reduction in nonmelanoma skin cancers at 2-years postconversion (1.2 vs. 4.3, $p < 0.001$).
  - Sirolimus-treated patients had a significantly lower incidence of melanoma, although the incidence of melanoma was low (1.1% in the CNI continuation group and 0% in the sirolimus conversion group, $p = 0.06$).
  - There was a nonstatistically significant lower rate of all other cancers (1.0 vs. 2.1, $p = 0.058$).

Posttransplant Lymphoproliferative Disorder

- PTLD encompasses a wide spectrum of lymphoid proliferations ranging from reactive polyclonal lesions to frank malignant monoclonal lymphomas.
- The 2008 modified WHO classification of PTLD can be divided into four subtypes including (1) early lesions, (2) polymorphic PTLD, (3) monomorphic PTLD, and (4) classical Hodgkin lymphoma-type PTLD.

- Most common type of posttransplantation malignancy in children
- Second most common posttransplantation malignancy in adults (follows only nonmelanoma skin cancers)
- Incidence: varies with the type of organ transplanted: kidney (1% to 2%), liver (1% to 4%), simultaneous kidney pancreas (2% to 3%), heart-, lung-, and heart–lung transplants (2% to 10%), small bowel and multivisceral transplantation (up to 33%)
- The majority of PTLD are non-Hodgkin lymphoma of B-cell origin and are CD20$^+$.
- More than 80% to 90% are linked to EBV infection. However, an increased incidence of EBV negative PTLD has been reported and in some series may occur in up to 30% of PTLD.
- Occurs at a median of 18 months after transplantation
- Bimodal distribution with time after transplant has been reported: the first peak occurs in the first year posttransplant, and the second peak > 8 years posttransplant.
- Although typically considered to result from EBV infection of recipient B cells, PTLD may be of donor origin.
- Mortality is greater with PTLD than with lymphomas in the general population.
- Risk factors:
  - EBV donor–recipient mismatch is the most well-established risk factor (recipient seronegative status at transplant).
  - Overall degree of immunosuppression
  - Induction with T cell-depleting antibodies or degree of T-cell immunosuppression. However, studies showed no consistent association between PTLD and any individual immunosuppressive agent.
  - Clinical trials showed an increase in the incidence of PTLD with central nervous system (CNS) involvement among EBV seronegative transplant recipients who received belatacept. Its use is contraindicated in recipients with pretransplant EBV naïve or unknown status.
  - CMV seronegative status at transplant (conflicting data)
  - CMV disease (conflicting data, may be a risk factor)
  - Older age
  - White compared with African-American race
  - Miscellaneous: fewer HLA matches, pretransplant malignancy, infections with HHV-8, and simian virus 40
- It is speculated that EBV (−) PTLD has a different pathogenic mechanism than that of EBV (+) PTLD. The former is often monomorphic, presents with later onset, and has a more aggressive clinical course.
- Clinical Manifestation:
  - May present with constitutional symptoms (e.g., fevers, night sweats, malaise, and weight loss), or localized symptoms of the respiratory tract (infection, mass, tonsillitis, or even gingival involvement), GI tract (diarrhea, pain, perforation, bleeding, mass), or CNS such as headache, seizure, or confusion
  - Extranodal involvement is common, and multiple sites are often involved.
  - Other clinical manifestations: lymphadenopathy or symptoms related to allograft dysfunction or compression of surrounding structures. Extranodal involvement is common.
- Treatment:
  - Reduction or discontinuation of immunosuppression is the mainstay of therapy. Patients with polyclonality are most likely to respond to immunosuppression

reduction. For those with monoclonal tumors, immunosuppression should be drastically reduced or discontinued.

- Rituximab, a chimeric monoclonal antibody targeting against CD20 on the surface of B cells has been used with variable success in patients who fail to respond to manipulation with immunosuppression alone.
- Chemotherapy for those refractory to reduction in immunosuppression and/or rituximab, in those with aggressive disease at presentation, and in those not amenable to surgery. CHOP-based chemotherapy with or without rituximab is the most widely use regimen.
- Surgical resection with or without local radiation for localized disease
- Local radiation is the treatment of choice for PTLD involving the CNS.
- Disease-free for at least 2 years prior to reallograft transplantation is recommended.

MULTIORGAN TRANSPLANTATION

- Kidney and pancreas transplantation in patients with type 1 diabetes
  - Simultaneous pancreas–kidney (SPK) transplantation:
    - Pancreas transplantation performed simultaneously with a kidney transplantation from the same deceased donor (most common surgical procedures done)
    - Advantage: one surgical intervention and one source of foreign HLA
    - Among pancreas recipients, those with an SPK transplantation were found to have the best pancreas graft survival rates.
  - Pancreas after kidney (PAK) transplantation (PAK):
    - Pancreas transplantation performed after a successful kidney transplantation from a living or deceased kidney donor
    - Advantage: important option for patients with a living donor kidney
    - Disadvantage: intensification of immunosuppression (particularly in the early postoperative period) after pancreas transplantation can adversely impact kidney allograft function due to CNI toxicity.
  - Pancreas transplantation alone (PTA)
    - Least common surgical procedures done
    - Therapeutic option for diabetic patients with good native kidney function who have brittle diabetes particularly those with hypoglycemic unawareness
    - Main risks: surgical procedure and long-term effects of immunosuppression
- Simultaneous liver-kidney transplantation (SLKT)
  - SLKT is a well-established therapeutic option for liver transplant candidates with simultaneous end-stage kidney failure.
  - Preemptive kidney transplantation immediately after liver transplantation can be performed in patients with severe CKD in anticipation of further worsening of kidney failure in the postoperative period due to CNI nephrotoxicity.
  - Discussion of special indications for SLKT is beyond the scope of this chapter.

Access the eBook for self-assessment questions.

Pharmacology

Anita Kamarzarian, Phuong-Mai T. Pham, Phuong-Thu
T. Pham, and Phuong-Chi T. Pham

PHARMACOKINETICS

Key Concepts

Bioavailability, volume of distribution, plasma clearance, half-life

Bioavailability

- Percentage or portion of administered drug that reaches systemic circulation
- Intravenous route: bioavailability is 100%
- Nonintravenous route: bioavailability depends on ease of absorption (i.e., through gut, skin, or mucosal membrane), first-pass metabolism (i.e., hepatic metabolism prior to release into systemic circulation).
- Factors that can alter bioavailability in renal patients:
  - Increased salivary urea in uremia reduces salivary acidity, thus reduced absorption of drugs better absorbed in acidic PH.
  - Loss of oral drugs due to nausea/vomiting
  - Slowed absorption and delayed plasma peak concentration due to gastroparesis and reduced bowel peristalsis
  - Increased stomach pH with antacids and proton pump inhibitors can reduce absorption of drugs that are better absorbed in acidic pH (e.g., iron, mycophenolate mofetil [Cellcept] but not mycophenolate sodium [Myfortic])
  - Some drugs form nonabsorbable complexes with phosphate binders (e.g., quinolones)
  - Bowel wall edema (e.g., nephrosis) reduces gut absorption.

Volume of Distribution

- The total amount of drug in the body, expressed as an imaginary volume with the same drug plasma concentration:
  - Volume of distribution (Vd) = Total amount of drug in the body/Plasma concentration of drug. Vd is traditionally expressed as L/kg of ideal body weight.
  - Vd is large for drugs with a high degree of lipid solubility, compartmentalization, and low-plasma-protein binding.
  - Vd is low for drugs with high water solubility and high-plasma-protein binding.
- Plasma-protein binding:
  - Primary drug-binding proteins include albumin and α1-acid glycoproteins:
    - Organic acids generally bind to albumin.
    - Organic bases generally bind to glycoproteins. Increased synthesis of α1-acid glycoproteins may occur in inflammatory states and may alter free drug levels.

- Factors that alter plasma-protein binding in renal patients:
  - Reduced serum proteins due to renal loss, malnutrition, and/or reduced synthesis. NOTE: Reduced serum proteins may increase clearance of free drugs.
  - Competitive binding of uremic toxins to plasma proteins displaces protein-bound drugs into plasma. This leads to more unbound drugs in plasma and lower Vd (e.g., salicylates, warfarin, sulfonamides, phenytoin).
  - Alterations in blood pH

Loading dose is directly proportional to Vd:

$$\text{Loading dose} = (\text{Desired peak drug concentration} \times \text{Vd} \times \text{Ideal body weight})/\text{Bioavailability}$$

where bioavailability = 1 for intravenous drug infusion.

- In the absence of a loading dose, maintenance doses alone will not achieve steady-state level until five drug half-lives later.
- Factors that can alter Vd in renal patients:
  - Increased Vd: edema, ascites/effusions
  - Reduced Vd: muscle wasting, amputations, loss of body fat, volume depletion, reduced plasma-protein binding

> **NOTE** A patient's actual Vd of drug A may be calculated as Vd = Loading dose of A/(post[A] − pre[A]), where pre and post[A] are plasma concentrations of drug A pre- and post-drug loading. When a patient's actual Vd of a drug is greater than that published in the drug insert, a higher dose may be needed. Similarly, if the patient's actual Vd is smaller than that published, dose reduction is necessary.

Plasma Clearance

- Most drugs are cleared/metabolized by the liver and/or kidneys. Plasma clearance is the sum of clearance of a drug by both renal and nonrenal routes.
- There is evidence that renal impairment may also reduce nonrenal (i.e., hepatic) metabolism of drugs, presumably via an increase in a circulating inhibitor of hepatic metabolic pathways (cytochrome P450). This factor is thought to be dialyzable.
- Drug clearance = *maintenance dose*
- Dose adjustment based on altered drug clearance in a patient with kidney failure:

Example: A drug is 40% cleared by liver and 60% by kidneys. Normal maintenance dose is 100 mg. If kidney function is now 40% of normal, what should be the new maintenance dose?

Clearance of the drug is still 40% by liver, but now clearance by kidney is only 40% of 60%, which is, 24%. Total drug clearance would now be 40% by liver *plus* 24% by kidneys, or 64% total clearance. Maintenance dose should be reduced to 64% of normal dose, 64 mg.

Half-life (t½)

- A drug t½ is the time needed for the plasma level of the drug to decrease by 50%.
- Generally, for an oral drug, four to five half-life duration are needed to reach steady state. Example: For a drug with t½ of 12 hours, it takes up to 5 × 12 hours = 2½ days to reach steady state. If an immediate therapeutic level is needed, a bolus dose must be given.
- Half-life determines *dosing frequency*.

> **NOTE** The *pharmacokinetic* t½ of a drug is not the same as its pharmacologic "*effect*" half-life. A drug may be cleared from the blood, but its *pharmacologic effect* may still persists (e.g., glucocorticoids, immunosuppressive agents).

Renal Handling of Drugs

- Renal drug clearance = UV/P of drug, where UV = total amount of drug in urine, and P = plasma concentration of drug
- Renal drug clearance is dependent on the drug characteristics (molecular size, charge, protein binding), glomerular filtration rate (GFR), tubular secretion and reabsorption, and renal epithelial cell metabolism.
- Drug t½ is directly proportional to Vd and inversely proportional to renal drug clearance.
- Drug adjustment in patients with renal insufficiency:
  - Dose reduction in patients with chronic kidney disease (CKD) is generally indicated when ≥30% of a drug or its active metabolite appears unchanged in the urine.
  - Estimation of kidney function for dose adjustment is traditionally done with the Cockroft-Gault (CG) equation. Read drug information provided by the pharmaceutical company regarding method of kidney function estimate used for renal adjustment.
  - Acute and severe kidney injury: Assume <10% kidney function and dose accordingly.
  - Rapidly improving kidney function: dose drug as if patient had normal kidney function
  - There are three methods for maintenance dose adjustment in patients with renal insufficiency:
    - Decrease dosage: This is the preferred method when maintaining constant drug level is more critical than achieving high peak levels for therapeutic effect (e.g., anticonvulsants, antiarrhythmics). Modified maintenance dose for renal insufficiency may be calculated as the (ratio of patient's to normal creatinine clearance) × standard maintenance dose. Example: patient with CrCl 69 mL/min, normal CrCl 120 mL/min, standard maintenance dose 100 mg q8h. Modified dose = (69/120) × 100 = 58 or ~60 mg q8h.
    - Reduce drug administration frequency: Preferred method if peak level is critical for therapeutic effect (e.g., antimicrobials such as aminoglycosides [AG]). Modified drug administration frequency for renal insufficiency may be calculated as the (ratio of normal to patient's CrCl) × current frequency. The modified frequency for above example would be (120/69) × 8 h = 14 h. For simplicity, the drug can be given as 100 mg q12h.
    - Combination of above: Preferred method for drugs with narrow therapeutic index (e.g., digoxin). For same patient above, the drug can be given as 80 mg q10h.

> **NOTE** Dose adjustment in patients with CKD or end-stage renal disease (ESRD) may be needed regardless of alterations in plasma clearance because the *pharmacologic effects* of a drug may be exaggerated due to increased target organ sensitivity (e.g., exaggerated sedation with narcotics in patients with ESRD despite appropriate dose reduction).

Principles of Dialytic Drug Removal

- Dialysis drug clearance may occur via both diffusion and convection.
- Clearance is dependent on characteristics of the drug and dialysis.
  - Drug characteristics: molecular size (<500 Da for hemodialysis [HD], up to 5,000 Da for continuous renal replacement therapy [CRRT]), water solubility, protein binding, Vd, degree of compartmentalization of drug, plasma clearance.

- Dialysis characteristics: membrane pore size, blood and dialysate flow rates, dialysis frequency and duration, ultrafiltration rate, replacement solution location in CRRT (pre vs. postdialysis); See below.
- Drug clearance by dialysis is considered clinically significant if drug clearance is increased by 30% or more with dialysis.
- Whenever feasible, close drug monitoring is recommended.
- Special considerations for different modes of dialysis:
  - Hemodialysis (HD):
    - Drug clearance is dependent on dialysis membrane characteristics, blood and dialysate flow rates, dialysis frequency and duration.
    - "High-efficiency," "high-flux," and "high-permeability" dialysis membranes can lead to significantly higher drug clearance, particularly for highly water-soluble drugs. Example: Vancomycin clearance is significantly increased with high-flux membranes.
    - "High-permeability" membrane is defined as having Kuf > 12 mL/mm Hg/h.
  - Peritoneal dialysis (PD):
    - Protein-bound drugs may be better cleared with PD compared with HD due to larger peritoneal membrane pore size.
    - Drug clearance by PD is typically approximated at 10 mL/min.
    - Drug clearance by PD may increase with the following:
      - Peritonitis due to increased blood flow
      - Increase number of daily exchange
  - Continuous renal replacement therapy: hemodiafiltration
    - Drug is removed by both diffusion (dialysis) and convection (hemofiltration), where drug clearance by convection = sieving coefficient of drug × ultrafiltration rate, where sieving coefficient = drug concentration in ultrafiltrate/drug concentration in arterial line (prefilter blood).
    - A sieving coefficient of 1 implies that a drug is freely filterable across the dialysis membrane, whereas a sieving coefficient much less than 1 implies poor drug dialyzability. Dialysis membrane pore size is the key determinant of sieving coefficient. Sieving coefficients are published in the literature for various drugs.
    - Effect of fluid-replacement location:
      - Prefilter-replacement fluid increases ultrafiltration rates, hence higher proportion of drug removal by convection.
      - Postfilter-replacement fluid increases the drug filtration fraction, hence higher proportion of drug removal by diffusion.
  - Continuous renal-replacement therapy: hemofiltration: Drug removal is via convection.
  - NOTE:
    - For CRRT dose of 25 to 35 mL/kg/h, antibiotics can be easily underdosed. Maintenance dosing on the higher rather than lower side is recommended. Loading dose is unchanged.
    - Renal dose adjustment for CRRT is based on CRRT drug clearance, estimated as CRRT clearance = unbound drug fraction × effluent rate

Example: 100 kg anuric patient receiving 25 mL/kg/h continuous venovenous hemodiafiltration (CVVHDF), dosing of a drug with 80% free fraction, should be

$0.8 \times 100 \times 25$ mL/h = 2,000 mL/h, which is 2,000 mL/60 min = 33 mL/min.

Dosing for the drug should be equivalent to that given to a patient with a GFR of 33 mL/min.

- Plasmapheresis:
  - Literature on drug removal with plasmapheresis is lacking.
  - Plasmapheresis may significantly remove lipophilic and highly protein-bound drugs.

DRUG SELECTION IN KIDNEY DISEASE

Antimicrobial Agents

Many agents are small (<500 Da), water soluble, not highly protein bound, and appear unchanged in the urine. Dosage reduction is thus usually necessary in patients with CKD and dialysis dependency.

- Aminoglycosides (AG):
  - AG are excreted by glomerular filtration and tubular secretion unaltered.
  - AG can cause nephrotoxicity and ototoxicity due to intracellular accumulation and associated injury to lysosomes, Golgi apparatus, mitochondria, and endoplasmic reticulum in proximal tubular cells and inner ear hair cells, respectively. AG nephrotoxicity is typically evidenced by a rise in serum creatinine within 7 to 10 days of exposure.
  - Electron microscopy reveals "myeloid bodies" in proximal tubular cells. Myeloid bodies are thought to arise from drug trapping, followed by a gradual accumulation of drug–phospholipid complexes within the internal lysosomal membranes. The increase in undigested materials interferes with normal membrane activity and results in the accumulation of concentric multilamellar lipid layers known as myeloid bodies which may have similar appearance as those seen in Fabry disease (See Figure 7.19.B in Glomerular/Vascular Diseases).
  - Nephrotoxicity risks: older age, underlying CKD, diuretics, concurrent use of nephrotoxic agents or intravenous radiocontrast agents, hypokalemia, hypovolemia
  - Bactericidal activity of AG is dependent on the initial rapid intracellular accumulation followed by significant tissue release postantibiotic administration. The latter is termed "postantibiotic effect." Drugs with "postantibiotic effect" depends on the bolus dose, but require less-frequent dosing.
  - In general, daily dosing or even q36h to q48h dosing of AG is thought to minimize nephrotoxicity in patients with GFR less than 60 mL/min.
  - In HD, predialysis dosing of AG allows for higher maximal plasma concentration and theoretically better efficacy. Postdialysis dosing of half dose has also been suggested, but potential for higher toxicity must be noted.
  - AG drug removal is thought to be greatest with CVVHDF (significant solute removal by both diffusion and convection), followed by continuous venovenous hemofiltration (CVVH) (significant solute removal by convection) and intermittent HD (predominantly diffusion).
  - In peritonitis, AG should be given intraperitoneally. Dose should be increased by 25% in patients with residual kidney function (e.g. having urine output > 100 mL/day).

> **NOTE** AG and tetracycline can lead to proximal renal tubular acidosis (RTA) or Fanconi syndrome. Additionally, their ability to bind the CaSR can lead to Bartter-like syndrome where patients develop metabolic alkalosis and urinary K^+, Ca^{2+}, Mg^{2+}, and Na^+ wasting.

- Vancomycin and Teicoplanin:
  - Both are predominantly excreted by kidneys.
  - When given intravenously, both agents are nephrotoxic and ototoxic, but teicoplanin is less nephrotoxic.
  - Nephrotoxicity is thought to involve oxidative stress. Use of vitamin E and N-acetylcysteine has been suggested to ameliorate vancomycin-induced nephrotoxicity.
  - Nephrotoxic risks include underlying kidney injury, concurrent use of nephrotoxic drugs, prolonged therapy, and high plasma levels.
  - Dialysis vancomycin dosing of 1 g can maintain plasma level above minimum inhibitory concentration (>15 μg/mL) for 3 to 5 days.
- β-lactams:
  - Most (penicillins, cephalosporins, carbapenems, monobactams) require dose reduction in CKD. β-lactams are commonly combined with β-lactamase inhibitors (e.g., clavulanate, sulbactam, tazobactam) to minimize antibiotic resistance and improve activity spectrum. Dose adjustment for combination drugs must take into account different metabolism rates of both agents. Whereas rates of metabolism of both agents in ampicillin/sulbactam and piperacillin/tazobactam are similar, clavulanate metabolism is much faster than that for ticarcillin in the ticarcillin/clavulanate combination.
  - Unlike AG, most β-lactams have short half-life and no postantibiotic effect. Dose reduction is generally preferred over frequency reduction.
  - CNS toxicity leading to lower seizure threshold is not uncommon with β-lactams (e.g., penicillins, imipenem) when used in high unadjusted dose in advanced CKD patients.

> **NOTE**
> - Penicillin can lead to either hypo- or hyperkalemia depending on its formulation.
>   - Hypokalemia: This is due to excess K^+ excretion that occurs with the high content of nonabsorbable anions in the penicillin formulation.
>   - Hyperkalemia: This is due to the high content of K^+ in some formulations in association with inadequate kidney K^+ excretion.

- Linezolid and tetracyclines can lead to type B lactic acidosis. See Acid-Base/Potassium chapter.
- Sulfonamides and trimethoprim:
  - Sulfonamides are typically combined with trimethoprim. Both are renally excreted.
  - Sulfonamides are excreted following acetylation. Acetylated sulfonamides may crystallize in tubular lumen and cause kidney injury, particularly with accumulative dose > 84 g. Crystallization is enhanced in acidic urine. Good hydration and alkalinization may be both preventive and therapeutic.
  - Sulfonamides may also cause tubulointerstitial nephritis.
  - Trimethoprim may inhibit tubular secretion of creatinine and may cause a rise in serum creatinine without actually causing kidney injury.
  - Trimethoprim may block the epithelial sodium channel (ENaC) and cause both hyperkalemia and metabolic acidosis.
- Rifamycins:
  - Rifamycins are predominantly hepatically metabolized. No renal adjustment is needed.
  - Rifamycins may cause orange–reddish discoloration of body fluids such as urine, effusions, and PD fluids.

- Rifampin may cause various renal lesions including acute tubular necrosis (ATN), acute tubulointerstitial nephritis (AIN), light-chain proteinuria, and even rapidly progressive glomerulonephritis (RPGN). The type of lesion appears to be associated with how the drug is given. Intermittent use (e.g., noncompliant patient) is associated with ATN, with or without interstitial infiltrations, hemolysis, and thrombocytopenia. Continuous use is associated with the other lesions.
- Fluoroquinolones:
  - Ciprofoxacin, norfloxacin, and gatifloxacin are significantly renally excreted and must be dose reduced for GFR below 30 mL/min. For the treatment of urinary tract infection, however, dose adjustment is not advisable unless symptoms of toxicity because high bladder concentrations are needed for effective treatment.
  - Moxifloxacin is only 20% renally excreted and does not require dose adjustment.
  - Quinolones may cause nonspecific CNS symptoms including headaches, dizziness, restlessness, tremors, and kidney injury from interstitial nephritis, crystalluria.
  - Quinolones absorption is reduced with metal-containing compounds and phosphate binders.
- Nitrofurantoin: Avoid in patients with GFR < 40 mL/min or elderly due to toxic metabolite accumulation and potential for pulmonary and hepatic toxicity and peripheral neuropathy.

Antifungals

- Amphotericin:
  - Renal failure typically occurs after 2 weeks of therapy.
  - Risks: older age, underlying CKD, hypovolemia, hypokalemia
  - Amphotericin may induce distal tubular injury, distal renal tubular acidosis (RTA), magnesium and potassium loss, nephrogenic diabetes insipidus, and arteriolar vasoconstriction (afferent greater than efferent arterioles).
  - Other noted adverse effects: anemia with or without thrombocytopenia presumably due to bone marrow suppression, hyperphosphatemia presumably due to high inorganic content in liposomal formulations and possibly measurement interference/error
  - Liposomal or lipid-based formulations confer lower-electrolyte disturbances and are preferred in patients with any degree of residual kidney function. Acute allergic reactions may be seen with lipid-based formulations.
  - Amphotericin is highly protein bound with a large Vd and is thus not well dialyzable.
  - Management of intravenous amphotericin-B–induced nephrotoxicity:
    - Routine preventive measures: normal saline, use of liposomal amphotericin-B, reduce administration frequency if possible.
    - Other suggested measures:
      - Continuous infusion may be less nephrotoxic compared to infusions given over 4 hours.
      - Theoretical benefits of low-dose calcium channel blockers (e.g., diltiazem) to reduce renal vasoconstriction if safely tolerated
- Azoles:
  - With the exception of fluconazole, most agents (keto-, itra-, vori- conazole) are metabolized by the liver and do not require dose reduction.
  - Fluconazole is significantly excreted in the urine and is preferred for the treatment of urinary tract infections. 50% dose reduction is necessary for GFR below <60 mL/min.

- Azoles are potent inhibitors of CYP34A and P-glycoproteins. P-glycoproteins normally serve to secrete various drugs into the gastrointestinal (GI) tract and renal tubular lumen, thus effectively reduce blood levels of the affected drugs. Diarrhea/enterocolitis can reduce P-glycoprotein levels and significantly increase blood levels of drugs that are substrates of P-glycoproteins. It is well-observed that patients receiving tacrolimus, a P-glycoprotein substrate, can present with toxic tacrolimus levels during episodes of diarrhea or enterocolitis.
  - Itraconazole and voriconazole are mixed with cyclodextrin in the intravenous formulation. Accumulation of cyclodextrin in renal patients can lead to increased serum creatinine and CNS toxicity (e.g., agitation, myoclonus, visual and auditory hallucinations, colored or flashing light). Intravenous formulations should be avoided for GFR < 50 mL/min.
  - Flucytosine is predominantly excreted in the urine and requires dose adjustment for patients with CKD. Flucytosine has a high rate of fungal resistance and is typically not used as a sole agent, but in combination with amphotericin for severe fungal infections.
- Echinocandins (caspofungin, micafungin, anidulafungin):
  - Echinocandins are inhibitors of the synthesis of β-D-glucan, a fungal cell wall component. These agents are effective against *Candida* species and azole-resistant *Aspergillus*.
  - No dose adjustment is necessary in patients with renal failure.
  - Unlike azoles, echinocandins typically do not affect CNI levels. NOTE: However, caspofungin has been shown to reduce tacrolimus levels.
- Terbinafine, an agent used to treat onychomycosis, is metabolized by CYP450 and 70% renally excreted. Plasma clearance is reduced by 50% in patients with CrCl < 50 mL/min. There are no safety data for terbinafine in CKD.

Antiviral Agents

- Acyclovir, valacyclovir, and famciclovir:
  - Renally excreted and may crystallize in tubules leading to AKI. Hydration is critical if given in high doses intravenously.
  - Associated with leukopenia, neurotoxicity
  - Dose adjustment for GFR < 20%
- Pegylated interferons α-2a and -2b require dose adjustment for CrCl < 50 mL/min.
- Hepatitis B-specific treatments: Lamivudine, telbivudine, and entecavir require dose adjustment for CrCl < 50 mL/min. Lamivudine is not dialyzable, whereas entecavir and telbivudine are and should be administered postdialysis.
- Hepatitis C-specific treatments: Ribavirin is renally excreted and should be avoided in patients with CrCl < 50 mL/min. Ribavirin is associated with hemolytic anemia, thrombotic thrombocytopenic purpura, and red cell aplasia. For newer agents against hepatitis C, see Hepatitis C in Glomerular/Vascular Diseases chapter. Safety data for newer agents in patients with advanced CKD are limited.
- Anti-influenzal agents (neuraminidase inhibitors): Oseltamivir (Tamiflu) and peramivir (Rapivap) are renally excreted and requires dose reduction for reduced GFR. Oseltamivir should be given once daily instead of twice daily. Zanamivir (Relenza) does not require dose reduction.

Antiretroviral Agents

- Drug class not generally require dose reduction:
  - Integrase inhibitors (raltegravir)
  - Fusion inhibitors (enfuvirtide)—enfuvirtide may be associated MPGN.

- CCR5 antagonists (maraviroc)
- Protease inhibitors (atazanivir, nelfinavir, ritonavir, saquinavir, and tipranavir)
- Nonnucleoside reverse transcriptase inhibitors (delavirdine, efavirenz, etravirine, nevirapine)
- Drug class that requires dose reduction with CKD:
  - Nucleoside and nucleotide reverse transcriptase inhibitors (NRTIs) (zidovudine, lamivudine, emtricitabine stavudine, didanosine, and tenofovir)
  - NRTIs reported to cause Fanconi syndrome: lamivudine (3TC), abacavir (ABC), didanosine (ddI), and tenofovir. Tenofovir is also associated with hypophosphatemic osteomalacia.
  - NRTIs reported to cause nephrogenic DI: abacavir, didanosine, tenofovir
  - NRTIs may cause type B lactic acidosis.
- Drugs that crystallize and cause urolithiasis:
  - Protease inhibitors (nelfinavir, amprenavir, saquinavir, lopinavir/ritonavir, indinavir)
  - Indinavir crystals have been described as "plate-like rectangles and fan-shaped or starburst forms"
  - Saquinavir is also associated with hypocalcemia and lactic acidosis.
- Cobicistat, a component of a fixed-dose four drug combination of elvitegravir, cobicistat, emtricitabine, and tenofovir (Stribild), and dolutegravir (HIV integrase inhibitor) can increase SCr via inhibition of tubular secretion of creatinine without affecting GFR.

Antihypertensive Selection in the Patient Receiving Hemodialysis

- Angiotensin-converting enzyme inhibitor (ACEI): dialyzable: captopril, lisinopril; nondialyzable: benazepril, fosinopril, quinapril
- Angiotensin-receptor blockers (ARB) are generally not dialyzable.
- β-blockers: dialyzable: atenolol and metoprolol; nondialyzable: carvedilol, labetalol
- Calcium channel blocker: amlodipine and nifedipine are not dialyzable.

NEPHROTOXICITY OF MEDICATIONS

Principles/Mechanisms of Nephrotoxicity

- Reduced renal perfusion:
  - Hypovolemia: excessive diuretics
  - Predominant afferent vasoconstriction: nonsteroidal anti-inflammatory drugs (NSAIDS), amphotericin B, CNI, interleukin-2, radiocontrast media
  - Predominant efferent vasodilatation: ACEI, ARB
- ATN:
  - Direct toxicity: cisplastin, AG, particularly combination of cisplastin and AG, cephalosporins, amphotericin-B, rifampin, pentamidine, NSAIDS, radiocontrast media, CNI
  - Rhabdomyolysis-induced ATN: statins, drugs that cause neuroleptic malignant syndrome (e.g., phenothiazines, antipsychotics, narcotics, antidepressants), cocaine, methamphetamine
- Acute tubulointerstitial nephritis: Most antibiotics, thiazides, allopurinol, proton pump inhibitors, cimetidine, many others. See Acute Tubulointerstitial Nephritis in Tubular, Interstitial, and Cystic Diseases chapter.

- Proximal tubular epithelial cell injury resulting in Fanconi syndrome: lead, L-lysine supplement (used for antiviral, wound-healing properties), AG, tenofovir, lamivudine (3TC), abacavir (ABC), didanosine (ddI), valproic acid.
- Obstructive uropathy:
  - Microtubular obstruction due to drug crystallization: sulfadiazine, methotrexate, methoxyflurane, acyclovir, indinavir, nelfinavir, acetazolamide, triamterene, topiramate, zonisamide
  - Methenamine/sulfonamide combination may lead to the precipitation of sulfonamides with formaldehyde. Methenamine is hydrolyzed to formaldehyde in acidic urine. Sulfonamides may also acidify the urine, rendering methenamine less effective. The combination of methenamine/sulfonamide is thus contraindicated and should not be given to the same patient.
  - Retroperitoneal fibrosis: methysergide, hydralazine, methyldopa
- Small-vessel vasculitis (hypersensitivity angiitis):
  - Common antibiotics: penicillin G, ampicillin, sulfonamides
  - Diuretics: thiazides, metolazone
  - Antineutrophil cytoplasmic antibody (ANCA)-associated glomerulonephritis: propylthiouracil, methimazole, allopurinol, hydralazine, levamisole, D-penicillamine, antitumor necrosis factor-α-agents (e.g., etanercept, infliximab, adalimumab), phenytoin, sulfasalazine, clozapine
- Thrombotic microangiopathy (See Thrombotic Microangiopathy in Glomerular/Vascular Diseases):
  - Transplant settings: CsA, tacrolimus, sirolimus
  - Others: mitomycin-C, 5-fluorouracil, quinine, cocaine, ticlopidine, clopidogrel
- Proteinuria, nephrotic syndrome:
  - Common agents: gold, captopril (This is thought to be specific to captopril, not other ACEI, due to the thiol group in captopril), NSAIDS, D-penicillamine, IFN-α
  - Histopathologic patterns associated with drug-induced nephrotic syndromes include membranous glomerulonephropathy, minimal change disease, and focal segmental glomerulosclerosis.
- Chronic tubulointerstitial disease: NSAIDS, thiazides, lithium, aristolochic acid (AA), germanium
- Hemoglobinuria-induced AKI: sulfonamides, dapsone, rifampin, methyldopa, quinidine, procainamide, melphalan, isoniazid, penicillins, cephalosporins, nitrofurantoin, phenacetin
- Myoglobinuria: Drug-induced rhabdomyolysis (see above). NOTE: The risk of statin-induced rhabdomyolysis is increased with concurrent use of CNI or gemfibrozil.
- Amphotericin B:
  - Disruption of endothelial cells leads to both afferent and efferent vasoconstriction (afferent vasoconstriction is more severe than efferent vasoconstriction).
  - Afferent vasoconstriction due to enhanced tubuloglomerular feedback
  - Disruption of tubular cells leads severe hypomagnesemia, hypokalemia, and RTA.
  - Injury of medullary collecting tubules leads to poor response to ADH, poor renal concentrating defect, polyuria, nephrogenic diabetes insipidus.
- NSAIDS: See Acute Tubulointerstitial Diseases in Tubular, Interstitial, and Cystic Diseases chapter.

Antineoplastic Agents

- Cisplatin:
  - Nephrotoxicity is thought to involve free radicals/oxidative stress leading to renal epithelial cell apoptosis and necrosis. Vascular and glomerular injuries may also be seen (thrombotic microangiopathy).

- Toxicity risks: Dose-related, typically >25 to 33 mg/m^2/wk, concurrent use of AG.
- Kidney injuries include ATN, ATIN, proximal (S3 segment) tubular damage with salt wasting (K$^+$, Mg^{2+}, Ca^{2+}, PO$_4^{2-}$), Fanconi syndrome, nephrogenic diabetes insipidus. Hypomagnesemia can be severe.
- Preventive: Fluid and diuretic as needed to maintain urine output > 100 mL/h. Other measures include use of intravenous sodium–thiosulfate (if >200 mg/m^2 of cisplatin will be administered), methylprednisolone, N-acetylcysteine, and antioxidants.
- Management: electrolyte replacement as needed
- Cyclophosphamide:
  - Associated with hyponatremia, premature ovarian failure, hemorrhagic cystitis, bladder cancer
  - Toxic metabolite: acrolein
  - Management:
    - Hydration with normal saline
    - Administration of mesna to detoxify acrolein and reduce hemorrhagic cystitis risk.
    - Use of agonist of pituitary gonadotropin–releasing hormone receptors leuprorelin for gonadal protection in women of childbearing age
    - Limit cumulative dose < 36 g total lifetime exposure if possible to minimize malignancy risk
  - NOTE: Significant interactions with other commonly used drugs:
    - Allopurinol reduces cyclophosphamide metabolism.
    - Cyclophosphamide increases bleeding risks with most anticoagulants due to unknown mechanisms.
- Ifosfamide:
  - Toxic metabolite: chloroacetaldehyde
  - Associated with proximal tubular injury, proximal RTA, Fanconi syndrome, nephrogenic diabetes insipidus, ATN
  - Risks for nephrotoxicity: cumulative dose > 90 g/m^2, underlying CKD, concurrent use of other nephrotoxic drugs
  - Management: supportive, consider mesna
- Methotrexate:
  - Kidney injury likely due to intratubular crystallization and obstruction
  - High dose of folinic acid has been shown to revert nephrotoxicity.
- Bevacizumab: anti-vascular endothelial growth factor (anti-VEGF)
  - Anti-VEGF agent inducing endothelial injury (endotheliosis, swollen vacuolated endothelial cells occluding capillary lumen), disruption of glomerular filtration barrier
  - Clinical manifestations are similar to preeclampsia: proteinuria, hypertension, AKI, thrombotic microangiopathy
- Cetuximab, panitumumab:
  - Antiepithelial growth factor receptor monoclonal antibody used to treat epithelial malignancies
  - Associated with hypomagnesemia
- Sunitinib, imitanib (tyrosine kinase inhibitors): transient hyperparathyroidism

Iodinated Contrast and Other Imaging Agents

See Contrast-induced AKI in Acute Kidney Injury/ICU nephrology chapter.

Calcineurin Inhibitors

- Acute vasoconstriction leading to HTN and significant afferent vasoconstriction:
  - Thought to be due to increased production of vasoconstrictive thromboxane A2 relative to vasodilatory prostaglandin E2.
  - Calcium channel blockers have been shown to reduce CNI toxicity, both short and long terms
- Chronic CNI toxicity:
  - Obliterative arteriolopathy, tubular atrophy, and classic "striped" interstitial fibrosis

Diuretics

- Volume depletion (all diuretics, worst with loop diuretics)
- Hypokalemia nephropathy (seen with all agents except potassium-sparing diuretics)
- Tubulointerstitial nephritis (thiazides, furosemide)
- Vasculitis (thiazides)
- Nephrolithiasis (triamterene, acetazolamide at low urine pH)
- Electrolyte abnormalities, hyponatremia (particularly thiazides), hypokalemia, hyperuricemia (particularly thiazides)

Supplements/Herbs (Toxic Agents): Renal/Urological Manifestations

- *Aristolochia* species (AA): Progressive chronic interstitial nephritis, proximal tubular injury, uroepithelial malignancies
- Balkan endemic nephropathy resembles aristolochic acid nephropathy (AAN) in terms of CIN and association with uroepithelial malignancies, but its rate of disease progression spans over 20 to 30 years compared to a much more rapid course of months to 2 years with AAN. The inciting agent is unknown, but has been suggested to be AA or other regional toxins (e.g., mycotoxins, heavy metals, viruses).
- Bladder wrack, a large brown algae used as food or flavoring agent in Japan and Europe (associated toxins are thought to be heavy-metal contamination): chronic interstitial nephritis
- Cat's claw: acute allergic tubulointerstitial nephritis
- Chaparral tea made of leaves from the Native American shrub creosote (nordihydroguaiaretic acid): renal cysts and renal cell carcinoma
- Cranberry: oxaluria, oxalate stones
- Djenkol (djenkolic acid): nephrolithiasis
- *Echinacea* species, a.k.a. coneflower (arabinogalactan): RTA
- Germanium: tubular degeneration with minor glomerular abnormalities
- Licorice (glycyrrhizic acid): hypertension, hypokalemia, hypokalemic nephropathy
- L-lysine: Fanconi syndrome and tubulointerstitial nephritis
- Ma huang (ephedraz): HTN, nephrolithiasis secondary to ephedra, norephedrine, and pseudoephedrine stone
- Pennyroyal: hemorrhagic kidneys, hepatorenal syndrome, and associated ATN
- Rhubarb (anthraquinone): chronic interstitial nephritis, kidney failure
- Star fruit, cranberry (oxalic acid): nephrolithiasis, interstitial nephritis
- Willow bark (salicin, the precursor of salicylate): renal papillary necrosis
- Wormwood oil: AKI secondary to rhabdomyolysis
- Yellow oleander: renal tubular necrosis with vacuolization in glomerular spaces in the setting of hepatorenal syndrome
- Yohimbe (yohimbe): lupus nephritis

NEPHROTOXICITY OF ILICIT DRUGS

- Heroin and other IV drug use:
  - Nonspecific histopathologic findings: arteriosclerosis, calcifications, interstitial fibrosis, tubular atrophy.
  - Heroin-specific causes for kidney injury: renal amyloid, FSGS, rhabdomyolysis
- Ecstasy (methylenedioxymethamphetamine [MDMA]), N-benzylpiperazine (BPZ), a.k.a. "party pills":
  - Both produce stimulant, euphoric effects.
  - Users may develop hyperthermia, rhabdomyolysis, kidney failure, interstitial nephritis, hyponatremia, and cerebral edema.
  - Other renal/electrolyte effects: hyperkalemia, metabolic acidosis, urinary retention, mesangial proliferative glomerulonephritis
- Cocaine: may cause renal ischemia, infarction, ANCA-associated vasculitis, rhabdomyolysis, accelerated atherosclerotic disease. See ANCA Vasculitis.
- Synthetic marijuana (cannabinoids):
  - Associated with AKI, hypertension, and hypokalemia
  - Toxicologic analysis from many cases revealed presence of (1-(5-fluoropentyl)-1H-indol-3-yl)-(2,2,3,3-tetramethylcyclopropyl) methanone, also known as XLR-11.
- "Bath salts":
  - White powder containing 3,4-methylenedioxypyrovalerone
  - May be inhaled, ingested, or injected
  - May cause fulminant liver failure, rhabdomyolysis and kidney failure, disseminated intravascular coagulopathy
  - Supportive therapy

NEPHROTOXICITY OF ENVIRONMENTAL AND OCCUPATIONAL AGENTS

- Lead (Pb) nephropathy:
  - Mechanism of disease:
    - Pb is absorbed in proximal tubular cells where it binds to specific Pb-binding proteins which facilitate entry into mitochondria. Pb–protein complexes may be seen as intranuclear inclusions in acute lead nephropathy.
    - Pb-protein complexes lead to mitochondrial dysfunction including reduced ATP production, thus affecting normal tubular transports (Fanconi syndrome) and inhibition of various enzymes including aminolevulinic acid (ALA) synthase and ferrochelatase, a heme-containing hydroxylase. The latter interferes with conversion of vitamin D 25 to D 1,25.
    - Major metabolic effects of chronic Pb exposure include hypertension and hyperuricemia. The former is thought to be due to alterations in the balance of vasoactive arachidonic acid metabolites favoring vasoconstriction and the latter to enhanced tubular reabsorption and reduced tubular secretion of uric acid.
  - Acute lead exposure:
    - Multiorgan involvement including headaches, malaise, peripheral neuropathy, poor memory, encephalopathy, seizures, coma, colicky abdominal pain, nausea/vomiting, constipation, anemia, muscle weakness, Fanconi syndrome.
  - Chronic exposure:
    - Chronic interstitial nephritis, gout, hypertension
    - Kidneys are typically contracted with granular surface appearance.

- Note that although hyperuricemia is common in CKD, gout is not a common manifestation of CKD. All patients with CKD and gout should be tested for Pb. Bone Pb levels may better correlate with HTN than blood Pb levels.
- Notable physical finding: gingival lead line
- Differential diagnosis: uric acid nephropathy, arsenic exposure, chronic interstitial nephritis, radiation nephritis, chronic glomerulosclerosis
- Diagnosis:
  - Nonspecific laboratory findings: anemia or chronic disease, microcytic hypochromic anemia, basophilic stippling of red blood cells, nongap metabolic acidosis, hypophosphatemia, Fanconi syndrome, elevated serum creatinine
  - Pb-specific testing:
    - Increased blood and urinary ALA due to inhibition of erythrocyte aminolevulinic acid dehydratase (ALAD) by Pb. Iron deficiency must be ruled out first since it can increase ALAD activity and mask Pb-induced reduction in ALAD activity.
    - Blood Pb levels:
      - Significantly elevated in acute exposure but may not be elevated in chronic exposure
      - Assessment for total body Pb accumulation is recommended for chronic exposure:
        - Calcium disodium edetate (EDTA) chelation test (given at 1 g IM × two doses 12 hours apart or 1 g IV × one dose to immobilize body stored Pb) followed by 24-hour urine collection to measure for Pb-EDTA. In patients with CKD, urine collection should be done over 3 to 6 days.
        - Radiographic fluoroscopy, a procedure whereby X-ray excitation of skeletal Pb atoms leads to fluorescence that can be detected and calculated.
  - Management: chelation therapy with EDTA

Organic Solvents

- Exposure to organic solvents (i.e., products or processes that contain solvents or petroleum products such as paint, printing ink, adhesives, degreasers, cleaning agents, aerosols, pesticides, gasoline, etc.) have been linked to various GN.
- Chronic organic solvent exposure has been linked to various glomerular diseases including RPGN with or without antiglomerular basement membrane antibodies, MGN, IgAN, and FSGS.
- Recent data suggest that organic solvent exposure may worsen the progression of existing GN rather than contributing to the development of the GN.

SPECIFIC DRUG ADVERSE EFFECTS OF INTEREST TO THE NEPHROLOGIST

- Drug metabolite accumulation of commonly used drugs leading to significant adverse effects in patients with reduced kidney function:
  - Allopurinol → oxypurinol (tubulointerstitial nephritis)
  - Glyburide → hydroxyglibenclamide (hypoglycemia)
  - Meperidine → normeperidine (seizures)
  - Morphine → morphine-t-glucuronide (altered mental status, seizures)
  - Nitroprusside → thiocyanate (cyanide toxicity)
  - Propoxyphene → norpropoxyphene (cardiac toxicity)

- Tramadol → O-desmethyltramadol (altered mental status, seizures)
- Venlafaxine → O-desmethylvenlafaxine (altered mental status). Other adverse effects: HTN (may be accelerated), orthostatic hypotension
- Notes regarding pain control in CKD:
  - Mild to moderate chronic pain: tramadol is acceptable at adjusted dose. However, although tramadol is primarily hepatically metabolized, the metabolites are eliminated by the kidneys. Approximately 30% of the dose is excreted in the urine as unchanged drug and 60% as metabolites. The use of tramadol in severe CKD is not recommended. Avoid codeine and dihydrocodeine due to risks for severe hypotension, respiratory arrest, narcolepsy.
  - Severe chronic pain: oxycodone, fentanyl (black box warning of respiratory arrest, particularly in opioid naïve patients), methadone
  - Fentanyl is primarily (more than 90%) eliminated by biotransformation to N-dealkylated and hydroxylated inactive metabolites. Less than 7% of the administered dose is excreted unchanged in the urine. While it is recommended that Fentanyl are titrated to clinical effect for all patients, special care should be taken in patients with severe hepatic or renal disease.
  - Neuropathic pain: Gabapentin is excreted unaltered in urine. Dose adjustment in CKD is required. Accumulation and toxicity can lead to reduced consciousness, confusion, ataxia, myoclonus, tremulousness, and asterixis.
- Neuromuscular-blocking agents are renally excreted and have increased t½ in ESRD patients.
- Immunosuppressive therapy (also see Transplantation):
  - Induction therapy:
    - Antithymocyte globulin (polyclonal antibodies that induces T-cell depletion): Cytokine release syndrome with flu-like symptoms and myelosuppression with leukopenia and thrombocytopenia. Premedications are needed.
    - Basiliximab and daclizumab (IL-2R antagonists): well-tolerated; no known drug interaction; no dose adjustment necessary for renal impairment
  - Maintenance therapy:
    - CNI (inhibit dephosphorylation of the nuclear factor of activated T-cell [N-FAT] molecules and resultant reduced IL-2 synthesis):
      - CsA, derived from the fungus *Tolypocladium inflatum*:
        - Plasma concentration at 2 hour postadministration better correlates with the area under the curve (AUC) compared with that of 12-hour trough levels.
        - GI absorption varies depending on food fat content, gastrointestinal motility (diabetic gastroparesis), diarrhea. Microemulsion formulation (Neoral) improved pharmacokinetic properties but not proven graft survival. Oral to IV conversion is one-third of oral dose.
        - CsA is predominantly metabolized by cytochrome P450 3A4. NOTE: St. John wort induces cytochrome P450 3A4 and can lead subtherapeutic CsA level and rejection, while grapefruit juice does the opposite and can cause CsA toxicity.
        - No dose adjustment necessary for renal impairment or dialysis
        - Side effects: hypertension, nephrotoxicity, fluid retention, hyperchloremic metabolic acidosis, hyperkalemia, hyperuricemia, hypomagnesemia
        - Hirsutism and gingival hyperplasia are common with CsA, but not with Tac. Gingival hyperplasia may be treated with azithromycin.
        - Rare adverse effects: thrombotic microangiopathic hemolytic anemia
        - Histopathology findings: afferent arteriolopathy, "striped" tubulointerstitial atrophy, and fibrosis

- Tacrolimus (Tac, FK-506), derived from the fungus *Streptomyces tsukubaensis*:
  - Oral bioavailability is only 20% to 25%.
  - Tac is highly bound to albumin, α-1 acid glycoprotein, and erythrocytes.
  - Levels should be measured from whole blood, not plasma.
  - Oral to intravenous conversion is 20% to 25% of total oral dose.
  - Metabolism is via cytochrome P450 3A4. Similar drug interactions as CsA.
  - Common adverse effects: nephrotoxicity (similar to CsA: striped interstitial fibrosis, arteriolar hyalinosis), new-onset diabetes mellitus after transplant (NODAT), hair loss, neurotoxicity, hyperkalemia, hyperuricemia, hypomagnesemia
  - Hypertension and hyperlipidemia are also common side effects with Tac, but both seem to be less severe compared with CsA.

> **NOTE** Enterocolitis/diarrhea can significantly increase tacrolimus levels due to reduced drug efflux into the gut via P-glycoproteins.

- Antiproliferative agents:
  - Azathioprine: imidazole analogue of 6-mercaptopurine that inhibits both de novo and salvage pathways for T and B lymphocyte proliferation.
    - Oral bioavailability is 50% to 60%
    - Major side effects: bone marrow suppression, venoocclusive disease, pancreatitis

> **NOTE** Avoid or reduce dose (i.e., 0.5 mg/kg/d) of azathioprine in patients on allopurinol. Allopurinol interferes with the metabolism of azathioprine which leads to a significant increase in 6-mercaptopurine levels and resultant severe bone marrow suppression (pancytopenia).

  - Mycophenolic acid (MPA): inhibits de novo purine biosynthesis in both B and T cells via noncompetitive inhibition of inosine monophosphate dehydrogenase
    - Formulated as mycophenolate mofetil (MMF) (CellCept or generic formulation) or mycophenolate sodium (Myfortic). Both undergo hepatic conversion to MPA, the active form. Mycophenolate sodium is thought to reduce GI intolerance due to its delayed absorption which occurs in the lower GI tract versus gastric absorption with MMF.
    - Used as adjunctive immunosuppressive therapy to improve long-term allograft survival as well as reducing acute rejection in kidney transplantation.
    - Major side effects: GI intolerance, anemia, leukopenia
    - Level monitoring of mycophenolate is not necessary since plasma concentration does not seem to correlate with incidence of acute rejection or side effects.
- Mammalian target of rapamycin (mTOR) inhibitors: mTOR inhibition leads to cell-cycle arrest at G1 and inhibition of T-cell proliferation.
  - Sirolimus and everolimus
  - Used in combination with low-dose CNIs or CNI-avoidance protocols
  - Adverse effects: myelosuppression (thrombocytopenia), delayed wound healing, hyperlipidemia, proteinuria (FSGS)
- Pregnancy and immunosuppression therapy:
  - Drugs with limited risk for congenital anomalies: prednisone, CsA, tacrolimus, azathioprine.
  - Contraindicated immunosuppressive therapy in pregnancy: mycophenolate, sirolimus, everolimus. See Kidney Transplantation chapter for more details.

Anticoagulants

- Low-molecular-weight heparin:
  - Half-life increases with eGFR < 30 mL/min/1.73 m^2.
  - Drug accumulation may cause excessive bleeding, not easily reversed.
  - If used, anti-factor Xa levels must be monitored and dose frequency reduced as needed.
- Warfarin: $>90\%$ protein bound (poor dialyzability), long t½ (40 hours), $>90\%$ renal elimination
- Novel oral anticoagulants:
  - Oral anticoagulants:
    - Rivaroxaban (avoid use in Cockroft-Gault CrCl < 30 mL/min):
      - Inhibits coagulation factor Xa
      - $>90\%$ protein bound, primary albumin, (poor dialyzability)
      - Shortest t½ (5 to 9 hours), compared to others; 60% to 70% renal elimination
    - Apixaban (safety data lacking for Cockroft-Gault CrCl < 25 mL/min):
      - Inhibits coagulation factor Xa
      - 85% to 90% protein bound (poor dialyzability), 25% to 30% renal elimination
  - Dabigatran:
    - Inhibits coagulation factor IIa
    - Used for atrial fibrillation and stroke prophylaxis
    - 35% protein bound, 80% renal elimination
    - For creatinine clearance 15 to 30: dose at 75 mg b.i.d.; no data for more advanced CKD
    - Dialyzable
  - For advanced CKD or ESRD, warfarin remains the anticoagulant of choice due to the lack of safety data for novel oral anticoagulants in this subpopulation.
    - Novel oral anticoagulants are not approved for patients on dialysis.
    - Unlike warfarin, there is no antidote for reversal of anticoagulant effect.

Other Agents

- Colchicine: increased risk of myopathy and polyneuropathy
- Selective serotonin reuptake inhibitors (SSRIs): Most do *not* require dose adjustment, except paroxetine (Paxil). SSRIs have increased risk of hyponatremia and GI bleed when taken with NSAIDS.
- Lithium: Acute lithium toxicity may be exaggerated by concurrent use of thiazide diuretics, NSAIDS, and ACEI/ARB.
- Anticonvulsants:
  - Phenytoin: No dose reduction is generally required. However, monitoring free versus total phenytoin level is recommended due to reduced protein binding with uremia but higher plasma clearance by hepatic P450.
  - Most newer anticonvulsants require dose reduction: gabapentin, felbamate, levetiracetam, pregabalin, topiramate, zonisamide
  - Lamotrigine does not require dose reduction.
- Calcium channel blockers (CCB):
  - Mechanism of CCB-induced edema: CCB causes relaxation of the precapillary sphincter which transmits systemic hypertension into the venous bed. The increased intravenous pressure (hydraulic pressure) favors net fluid filtration into the interstitium.
  - CCB are inhibitors of CYP34A and P-glycoprotein. Strongest inhibitors: diltiazem, verapamil

- Methyldopa, α-blockers, clonidine, and minoxidil are renally cleared. NOTE: Clonidine accumulates in advanced CKD and can lead to severe bradycardia or even asystole if used in high dose and in combination with β-blockers.

DRUG INTERACTIONS/ADVERSE EFFECTS (OTHER THAN NEPHROTOXICITY)

- Proton pump inhibitors can reduce GI absorption of MMF due to reduced acid-dependent dissolution of MMF (Cellcept) prior to absorption, but not enteric coated mycophenolate sodium (Myfortic), which is absorbed at neutral pH in the small intestines.
- CsA may inhibit recirculation of MMF and reduce MPA plasma levels. Tac does not. CsA switch to Tac may increase MPA levels and associated side effects.
- CsA can increase plasma hepatic hydroxymethyl glutaryl-CoA reductase (HMG-CoA) inhibitor (statin) and increase risk of rhabdomyolysis. Unlike CsA, Tac has limited effect on HMGCoA inhibitors. Rhabdomyolysis associated with TAC and HMGCoA inhibitors is only generally seen with concurrent use of diltiazem.
- Use of amphotericin B, AG, foscarnet, cidofovir, and NSAIDS can potentiate CNI toxicity.
- Use of ganciclovir, valganciclovir, and co-trimoxazole in combination with MMF and azathioprine can increase myelosuppression risk.
- St. John wort reduces while grapefruit juice increases CNI levels.
- Amlodipine increases simvastatin blood levels, hence risk of rhabdomyolysis. Both amlodipine and simvastatin are metabolized by P450 3A4.
- Barbiturate coma therapy (BCT) with thiopentone: Hypokalemia, a potentially life-threatening complication, has been recently reported to occur in 85% of patients, with severe hypokalemia occurring in up to 25%. Hypokalemia is thought to be due to increased cellular uptake. The severe rebound hyperkalemia following discontinuation of thiopentone is due to reshifting of intracellular into the extracellular space and high doses of potassium supplement during the hypokalemic phase. Gradual tapering of thiopentone has been suggested to reduce the risk for rebound hyperkalemia.

DIALYSIS AND OTHER TREATMENT OF POISONINGS

Pharmacokinetics of toxin removal by various dialytic methods are similar as those outlined for drug dialyzability. In addition, there are a few other extra considerations:
- Electrolytes: Electrolyte and acid–base disturbances are not necessarily similar to those seen with ESRD. Dialysate composition (i.e., K^+, HCO_3^-, Ca^{2+} dialysate concentrations) should therefore reflect patients' specific needs. Intravenous Mg^{2+} and PO_4^{2-} supplements may be necessary.
- Specialized dialysis systems to improve albumin-bound toxin removal:
  - Hemoperfusion: This is a form of dialysis where a cartridge containing an adsorbent material such as activated charcoal or resin is added to the circuit to compete for binding and removal of albumin-bound toxins from circulation. Not widely available
    - Hemoperfusion may be needed for amanita mushroom, barbiturate, carbamazepine, valproic acid, phenytoin, meprobamate, theophylline, dapsone, methotrexate. (Urinary alkalinization also facilitates renal elimination of barbiturate.)

- Hemoperfusion-related complications: hypocalcemia, charcoal embolization, leukopenia, thrombocytopenia, coagulopathy due to adsorption of co-agulation factors
  - High-flux dialysis may improve solute removal, thus less need for hemoperfusion.
- Molecular adsorbent recirculating system (MARS): This form of dialysis has an added albumin circuit to improve removal of albumin-bound toxins. Not widely available
- Hemofiltration alone may be considered for AG, desferrioxamine, sodium edetate, and theophylline.
- Drugs removable by HD: salicylates, lithium, methanol, ethylene glycol, isopropyl alcohol, theophylline, valproic acid, methotrexate, phenobarbital, metformin
- Plasma exchange:
  - 1-2 plasma volume exchanges may be considered for rapid removal of toxins that exist predominantly in the plasma (Vd < 1 L/kg).
  - Agents removable by plasma exchange: amanita mushroom, digoxin, snake envenomation, cisplatin, natalizumab (used for treatment of multiple sclerosis)

Common Poisonings That May Require Extracorporeal Removal

- Alcohols:
  - Ethylene glycol, methanol:
    - Significant ingestion of either alcohol can give rise to high anion gap metabolic acidosis and high osmolal gap > 10 mOsm/kg.
    - Fomepizole should be given to inhibit hepatic alcohol dehydrogenase in patients with blood levels of either alcohol above 20 mg/dL and serum osmolal gap > 20 mOsm/kg. Fomepizole should be continued until alcohol level is below 20 mg/dL or below 10 mg/dL in presence of end-organ damage.
    - Alkalinize blood to keep pH above 7.35
    - If fomepizole is not available, infuse 10% ethanol until blood ethylene glycol or methanol level is undetectable.
    - HD if the alcohol level is above 50 mg/dL in the setting of severe metabolic acidosis or end-organ damage (e.g., AKI or visual disturbances). Note that fomepizole and ethanol are dialyzable and their doses must be adjusted. Large surface area dialyzers (>1.5 m^2) should be used along with blood flow rate greater than 300 mL/min. Ethylene glycol and methanol levels should be monitored 2 hours postdialysis to assess for rebound. HD may be discontinued once the alcohol level is below 25 mg/dL.
    - In malnourished patients with ethylene glycol poisoning, add thiamine 100 mg and pyridoxine 50 mg IV to increase the metabolism of glyoxylate.
    - In methanol poisoning, add folinic acid 50 mg IV q6h to increase metabolism of formic acid to CO_2 and H_2O.
  - Isopropyl alcohol (a.k.a., isopropanol, rubbing alcohol): Both isopropanol and its metabolite acetone can cause CNS suppression, nausea/vomiting.
    - Since isopropanol is metabolized to acetone (not an acid) by alcohol dehydrogenase, isopropanol ingestion does *not* cause an anion gap metabolic acidosis. However, the acetone can be measured as positive "ketones" in either serum or urine. Low or absent serum ketones by the nitroprusside test after 2 hours from time of ingestion in the absence of alcohol dehydrogenase inhibition (e.g., concurrent ethanol ingestion or use of fomepizole) essentially rules out significant isopropanol ingestion.
    - Increased serum osmolal gap reflects the presence of exogenous isopropanol molecules.

- Isopropranol intoxication is not as toxic as ethylene glycol or methanol and rarely fatal. Fomepizole or ethanol infusion are thus not necessary.
- Management typically only requires routine supportive care including IV fluid support and, airway protection. For refractory and severe hemodynamic instability in association with very high levels > 500 mg/dL and osmolal gap > 100 mOsm/kg, HD may be considered.
- β-blockers:
  - Activated charcoal should be administered to all patients presenting within 2 hours of β-blocker overdose.
  - Supportive care with IV fluids for hypotension, atropine for severe bradycardia, β-agonists for bronchospasm, glucose for hypoglycemia
  - Dialyzable β-blockers (hydrophilic, low protein-binding): atenolol, metoprolol, acebutolol, nadolol
  - Nondialyzable β-blockers: carvedilol, labetalol, propranolol, timolol

> **NOTE**   There is evidence to suggest increased cardiovascular death in dialysis patients using dialyzable β-blockers compared to nondialyzable β-blockers.

- Lithium:
  - Patients may present with hemodynamic instability, altered mental status, prolonged QT interval, arrhythmias, renal insufficiency.
  - Signs and symptoms of lithium toxicity do not correlate well with lithium levels.
  - Lithium is highly dialyzable due to its low molecular weight and protein-binding.
  - Indications for dialysis:
    - Lithium level above 4 mEq/L, or
    - 2.5 to 4.0 mEq/L with CNS manifestations (altered mental status, seizures, coma), impaired renal excretion, or hemodynamic instability, or
    - Less than 2.5 mEq/L in ESRD patients or with increasing levels
  - NOTE: Rebound is a common problem; thus, prolonged or continuous dialysis is recommended. Close postdialysis level monitoring (e.g., q6h) is necessary.

> **NOTE**   Regarding metformin dosing in patients with CKD: KDIGO suggests that metformin should be continued in patients with GFR ≥ 45 mL/min/1.73 m^2, "reviewed" in patients with GFR 30 to 44 mL/min/1.73 m^2, and discontinued in those with GFR < 30 mL/min/1.73 m^2.

- Metformin induced lactic acidosis:
  - Routine supportive therapy and alkalinization with sodium bicarbonate
  - HD support if unresponsive to medical therapy or presence of kidney failure
- Digitalis toxicity:
  - Clinical manifestations: CNS symptoms ranging from drowsiness, lethargy to hallucinations seizures, visual disturbances with classic yellow halos around lights, nonspecific GI symptoms, cardiac arrhythmias. Electrolytes: hyperkalemia in acute toxicity, hypokalemia, and hypomagnesemia in chronic toxicity
  - Toxicity risks: advanced age, hypothyroidism, renal insufficiency, hypo- or hyperthyroidism, alkalosis or acidosis, myocardial disease, ischemia, or infarction, hypoxemia, electrolyte abnormalities (hypo- or hyperkalemia, hypercalcemia, hypomagnesemia, hypernatremia)
  - Management:
    - Routine supportive care, fluids, airway protection, drug discontinuation
    - Activated charcoal in acute overdose or accidental ingestion

- Cholestyramine may bind enterohepatically recycled digoxin in acute overdose.
- Hyperkalemia: insulin plus glucose, sodium bicarbonate if metabolic acidosis
- Concurrent hypokalemia and hypomagnesemia: supplement as needed
- Indications for digoxin immune Fab (digibind): life-threatening dysrhythmias, acute ingestion dose > 10 mg, steady-state serum digoxin level > 10 ng/mL in acute ingestions or >6 ng/mL in chronic ingestion, hyperkalemia > 5 mEq/L, altered mental status, rapid clinical deterioration
- Digoxin is not dialyzable. However, dialysis is indicated for hyperkalemia and kidney failure. Digibind is also not or minimally dialyzable.
- If digibind is not available or contraindicated, hemoperfusion should be considered.
- Salicylates
  - Initial presentation may be respiratory alkalosis alone due to activation of respiratory center, followed by high anion gap metabolic acidosis due to accumulation of lactic acids and ketoacids. Other characteristic manifestations: fevers, tinnitus, vertigo, blurry vision
  - Gastric lavage should be considered within 12 hours of ingestion if airway is protected.
  - Urinary alkalinization to keep urine pH > 7.5 in nonoliguric patients to increase levels of ionized salicylates (NaHCO$_3$ 1 to 2 mEq/kg bolus followed by infusion (100 to 150 mL/h) of 100 to 150 mEq mixed in 1 L of 5% dextrose). Ionized salicylates are more easily renally excreted and less likely to penetrate and accumulate in tissue than the nonionized form. NOTE: Acidemia increases salicylate CNS toxicity.
  - Glucose supplementation to avoid CNS hypoglycemia which may occur despite serum normoglycemia
  - Indications for HD: serum levels > 100 mg/dL or lower if presence of AKI, pulmonary edema, or altered mental status
- Theophylline
  - Theophylline is highly dialyzable due to its low Vd and protein binding.
  - High-efficiency HD is more effective than hemoperfusion in theophylline removal.
  - HD indications for acute intoxication: serum level > 80 mg/L or >60 mg/L in patients older than 65 years or history of seizures, ischemic heart disease, or liver or cardiac failure.
  - HD indications for chronic intoxication: theophylline level > 40 mg/L in patients older than 65 years or any patient with a history of seizures or any arrhythmias.

Access the eBook for self-assessment questions.

Acute Kidney Injury/ICU Nephrology

Phuong-Chi T. Pham, Cynthia C. Nast, Phuong-Anh T. Pham, and Son V. Pham

ACUTE KIDNEY INJURY

Clinical Impact of Acute Kidney Injury

- Acute kidney injury (AKI) increases the risk of de novo chronic kidney disease (CKD), accelerated CKD progression in those with underlying CKD, and mortality.
- Even non–dialysis-requiring AKI is associated with increased risks for poor long-term outcomes and increased mortality.

Classification of Acute Kidney Injury

- Purpose for classification system:
  - Early identification and management of AKI
  - Standardized AKI definitions for AKI-related research
- The diagnosis of AKI may be made based on specific criteria defined by various organizations: RIFLE (risk, injury, failure, loss of kidney function, end-stage renal disease [ESRD]), acute kidney injury network (AKIN), KDIGO (Table 10.1).
- KDIGO combines AKIN and RIFLE criteria and defines AKI as:
  - Increase in SCr by ≥ 0.3 mg/dL within 48 hours or increase in SCr by >1.5 times baseline SCr within prior 7 days, or
  - Urine volume < 0.5 mL/kg/h for ≥ 6 hours
- Worse stages of AKI based on RIFLE and AKIN are associated with increased mortality.
- An ideal biomarker (other than serum creatinine [SCr]) for the early identification of AKI would have the following characteristics:
  - Level of the biomarker is increased in urine or blood within minutes to hours after a renal insult
  - Level remains elevated as long as the injury is present
  - Level correlates quantitatively with the extent of injury
  - Level decreases with renal recovery
  - Notable biomarkers for the early detection of AKI:
    - Kidney injury molecule 1 (KIM-1): transmembrane glycoprotein; undetectable in normal kidney tissue or urine, but is expressed at high levels in dedifferentiated proximal tubular cells after ischemic or toxic injury and in renal cell carcinoma
    - Neutrophil gelatinase-associated lipocalin (NGAL): NGAL is predominantly detected in proliferating nuclear antigen-positive proximal tubular cells.

| Table 10.1 | Classification of acute kidney injury |

RIFLE (2002, by the Acute Dialysis Quality Initiative Group ADQI): SCr Criteria		AKIN (2005, Acute Kidney Injury Network): SCr Criteria		RIFLE and AKIN: Urine Output Criteria
SCr/eGFR (MDRD) criteria compared to baseline. If baseline not available, assume 75 mL/min/1.73 m²		SCr criteria: Change in SCr within 48 h following fluid resuscitation		
Risk	↑SCr × 1.5 or ↓eGFR > 25%	Stage 1	↑SCr ≥ 0.3 mg/dL or ↑SCr > 1.5–2 times baseline SCr	<0.5 mL/kg/h for >6 h
Injury	↑SCr × 2.0 or ↓eGFR > 50%	Stage 2	↑SCr > 2–3 times baseline SCr	<0.5 mL/kg/h for >12 h
Failure	↑SCr × 3.0 or ↓eGFR > 75% or if baseline SCr ≥ 4 mg/dL, ↑SCr ≥ 0.5 mg/dL	Stage 3	↑SCr > 3 times baseline SCr or acute RRT	<0.3 mL/kg/h for ≥24 h or anuria ≥ 12 h
Loss of kidney function	Complete loss of kidney function > 4 wk	NOTE: *KDIGO* criteria for AKI: 1. SCr criteria: either RIFLE "Risk" *or* AKIN "Stage 1" *or* 2. Urine output criteria: <0.5 mL/kg/h (>6 h)		
End-stage renal disease	Complete loss of kidney function > 3 mo			
Clinical studies: RIFLE improves detection rate of AKI during the first 48 h of ICU stay. Limitations: • Assumes baseline GFR of 75 mL/min/1.73 m² if baseline GFR is not available • Does not consider etiology of AKI (i.e., does not first rule out obstruction and volume depletion) • Does not include requirement of RRT, thus compromise accuracy in predicting mortality in patients requiring RRT		Advantages of AKIN over RIFLE: • Excludes volume depletion and urinary obstruction as cause of AKI • Does not rely on GFR • Does not need baseline SCr Limitations: • Does not identify AKI occurring in a time frame > 48 h • Stage 3 includes RRT requiring patients. Criteria for initiation/discontinuation of RRT vary widely among physicians and institutions. May affect accuracy in prediction of outcomes/mortality.		Commonalities between RIFLE and AKIN: • AKI was associated with increased hospital mortality, longer lengths of stay, and higher likelihood to be discharged to an extended care facility. • The use of UO criteria adds the number of AKI cases with lower mortality than those defined by SCr changes alone.

eGFR, estimated glomerular filtration; RIFLE, Risk, Injury, Failure, Loss of kidney function, End-stage renal disease classification; RRT, renal replacement therapy; SCr, serum creatinine; UO, urine output.

• Tissue insulin-like growth factor binding protein 7 and tissue inhibitor of metalloproteinase 2 (IGFBP7 and TIMP-2): IGFBP7 and TIMP-2 function as both autocrine and paracrine signals to arrest cell-cycle and shut down cell function with early kidney injury. IGFBP7 and TIMP-2 levels are increased in early kidney injury.

Routine Diagnostic Tools for the Diagnosis of AKI

• Microscopic examination of urinary sediment: The use of a scoring system based on the number of granular casts (muddy brown casts) and renal tubular epithelial cells has been shown to improve the differential diagnostic and prognostic evaluation of AKI.

- Evaluation of cells, cellular casts:
  - Hyaline casts: reduced renal perfusion (e.g., volume depletion, hypotension, acute cardiopulmonary event, drug-induced reduction in glomerular filtration, abdominal compartment syndrome)
  - Red blood cell casts:
    - Acute glomerulonephritis until proven otherwise
    - May be seen in acute tubulointerstitial nephritis, but must rule out acute glomerulonephritis
  - White blood cell casts: pyelonephritis or tubulointerstitial nephritis
  - Granular casts: nonspecific, indicates presence of cells that have degenerated
  - Muddy brown casts: acute tubular necrosis
  - Waxy casts: degraded cellular casts seen in CKD with poor urine flow
- Urine volume:
  - Anuria is more likely seen with complete urinary obstruction, vascular catastrophe, severe acute tubular necrosis (ATN), or severe rapidly progressive glomerulonephritis.
  - Oliguric AKI, defined as having urine output < 500 mL/d may also be seen in patients with early prerenal AKI or acute tubulointerstitial nephritis (ATIN).
  - Oliguric AKI is associated with worse outcome than nonoliguric AKI.
- Fractional excretion of sodium (FeNa) and fractional excretion of urea (FeUrea):
  - In nonoliguric AKI, FeNa < 1% or FeUrea < 35% generally indicates prerenal AKI as opposed to ATN.

> **NOTE** • Exceptions:
> - FeNa may be <1% *despite the presence of ATN* in patients with sepsis, hemoglobinuria, myoglobinuria, radiocontrast exposure, heart failure, and advanced cirrhosis presumably due to severe vasoconstriction.
> - In cirrhosis, FeNa < 0.1 may be consistent with hepatorenal syndrome (HRS), FeNa > 0.3 ATN, and FeNa 0.1 to 0.3 prerenal AKI.

- FeUrea versus FeNa rationale: urea reabsorption occurs primarily in the proximal tubules, and is less affected by loop and thiazide diuretics, whereas Na^+ excretion; hence, FeNa can be affected by diuretics.

HEMODYNAMIC (PRERENAL ACUTE KIDNEY INJURY)

Etiologies of Prerenal AKI

- Rapid fall in baseline blood pressure (BP) (e.g., overly rapid treatment of hypertension [HTN], acute volume loss)
- Volume depletion:
  - True volume depletion: bodily fluid loss, no access to adequate fluid intake
  - Reduced effective circulating volume: heart failure, cirrhosis
- "Third-spacing" (e.g. sepsis, acute pancreatitis, muscle trauma)
- Acute cardiopulmonary event (e.g., acute pulmonary embolism, myocardial infarction, valvular rupture, rapid (re)-accumulation of pericardial effusion, acute obstruction of renal artery (e.g., with aortic dissection extending into renal artery, use of angiotensin-converting-enzyme inhibitor/angiotensin-receptor blocker [ACEI/ARB] in severe bilateral renal artery stenosis)
- Intraglomerular hemodynamic compromise:
  - Predominant afferent vasoconstrictors: nonsteroidal anti-inflammatory drugs (NSAIDS), calcineurin inhibitors, amphotericin, contrast agents

- Predominant efferent vasodilators in patients with suboptimal baseline glomerular filtration: ACEI/ARB
- Hyperoncotic AKI:
  - This is seen with the rapid infusion of large quantities of osmotically active substances such as mannitol, dextran
  - Glomerular oncotic pressure far exceeds glomerular hydrostatic pressure, resulting in *net* reduction in glomerular filtration, hence oliguric/anuric AKI
- Intra-abdominal hypertension (IAH) leading to abdominal compartment syndrome (ACS): Updated consensus definitions and practice guidelines from the World Society of the ACS
  - IAH is defined as having sustained intra-abdominal pressure (IAP) $\geq$ 12 mm Hg. IAP is measured at end-expiration in supine position after ensuring absence of abdominal muscle contractions, with transducer zeroed at level of midaxillary line.
  - ACS is defined as having a sustained IAP $\geq$ 20 mm Hg ($\pm$ abdominal perfusion pressure (APP) < 60 mm Hg) that is associated with new-organ dysfunction/failure.
  - APP = mean arterial pressure (MAP) $-$ IAP
  - Risks for IAH/CAS:
    - Diminished abdominal wall compliance: abdominal surgery, major trauma/burns, prone positioning
    - Increased intraluminal contents: gastroparesis/gastric distention/ileus, colonic pseudo-obstruction, volvulus
    - Increased intra-abdominal contents: acute pancreatitis, distended abdomen, hemo-/pneumoperitoneum or intraperitoneal fluid collections, intra-abdominal or retroperitoneal tumors, laparoscopy with excessive insufflation pressures, liver dysfunction/cirrhosis with ascites, peritoneal dialysis
    - Capillary leak/fluid resuscitation: acidosis, hypothermia, massive fluid resuscitation or positive fluid balance, polytransfusion
    - Others: age, bacteremia, coagulopathy, increased head of bed angle, massive incisional hernia repair, mechanical ventilation, obesity, positive end–expiratory pressure (PEEP) > 10 mm Hg, peritonitis, pneumonia, sepsis, shock, or hypotension
  - Management of IAH/ACS: If IAP $\geq$ 12 mm Hg, begin medical therapy to reduce IAP:
    - Measure IAP $\geq$ every 4 to 6 hours. Titrate therapy to maintain IAP $\leq$ 15 mm Hg
    - Therapeutic measures to reduce IAP:
      - Evacuate intraluminal contents: nasogastric and/or rectal tube, initiate gastro-/colo-prokinetic agents, minimize or discontinue enteral nutrition, lower bowel decompression with enemas, or even colonoscopy as needed.
      - Evacuate intra-abdominal space occupying lesions or fluids as applicable (e.g., large volume paracentesis if safely tolerated)
      - Improve abdominal wall compliance: ensure adequate sedation and analgesia: remove constrictive dressings, consider reverse Trendelenburg position +/− neuromuscular blockade.
      - Minimize fluid administration, remove excess fluids with use of diuretics or even ultrafiltration (UF), consider hypertonic fluids, colloids.
      - Optimize systemic/regional perfusion: goal-directed fluid resuscitation with hemodynamic monitoring to guide resuscitation
      - If IAP > 20 mm Hg and new-organ dysfunction/failure occurs despite maximal medical intervention, consider surgical abdominal decompression.
    - Clinical manifestations of IAH/ACS:
      - Increased IAP with typically tense abdomen

- Increased peak inspiratory pressure, decreased tidal volume (due to abdominal compartment encroaching into thoracic cavity)
      - Reduced venous return
      - Increased central venous pressure (CVP), pulmonary arterial wedge pressure
      - Reduced cardiac index (blood pumped against high-pressured abdominal cavity)
      - Oliguria (reduced blood flow in renal vein and direct cortical pressure)
- Poor effective circulating volume: HRS and congestive heart failure
- HRS: functional kidney failure associated with liver failure characterized by:
  - Increased intrahepatic resistance leading to:
    - Portal HTN with compensatory increased production of vasodilators, nitric oxide leading to:
    - Splanchnic vasodilation and splanchnic blood pooling
    - Reduced peripheral vascular resistance (PVR), systemic arterial hypotension leading to:
      - Compensatory systemic activation of vasoconstrictor systems (RAAS, SNS) and hyperdynamic cardiac function, leading to:
      - HRS, cirrhotic cardiomyopathy, hepatic encephalopathy (severe cerebral vasoconstriction is thought to contribute to hepatic encephalopathy)
  - Criteria for the diagnosis of HRS:
    - Diagnosis of cirrhosis with ascites, and
    - AKI defined per AKIN/KDOQI as
      - Increase in SCr by $\geq$0.3 mg/dL from stable baseline in less than 48 hours, *or*
      - $\geq$50% increase in stable baseline SCr within the prior 3 months
    - No improvement of serum Cr (decrease to a level of $\leq$1.5 mg/dL) after $\geq$2 days with diuretic withdrawal and volume expansion with albumin (recommended dose: 1 g/kg of body weight per day up to 100 g/d), and
    - Absence of shock, and
    - No current or recent nephrotoxic drugs, and
    - Absence of parenchymal kidney disease as indicated by proteinuria > 500 mg/d, microhematuria > 50 RBC/HPF, and/or abnormal renal ultrasound
  - Subtypes of HRS:
    - Type 1: $\geq$doubling of initial SCr to >2.5 mg/dL or a 50% reduction of the initial creatinine clearance (glomerular filtration rate [GFR]) to <20 mL/min within 2 weeks; type I may occur spontaneously, but frequently occurs in close relationship with a precipitating factor: severe bacterial infection (spontaneous bacterial peritonitis [SBP]), GI hemorrhage, major surgical procedure, or acute hepatitis superimposed on cirrhosis.
    - Type 2: a moderate and stable reduction in GFR. Renal failure does not have a rapidly progressive course; type 2 is thought to represent the extreme expression of renovasoconstriction; dominant clinical feature of type 2: severe ascites with poor or no response to diuretics
  - Management of HRS:
    - Prevention of HRS precipitating factors:
      - SBP: intravenous infusion of albumin at 1.5 g/kg at time of SBP diagnosis and 1 g/kg IV 48 hours later
      - SBP prophylaxis:
        - Prolonged therapy (quinolone or double-strength trimethoprim–sulfamethoxazole daily):
          - $\geq$1 SBP

- Patients with cirrhosis and low ascitic fluid total protein < 1 g/dL with poor liver/kidney function (Child–Pugh score > 9, serum bilirubin > 3 mg/dL, SCr > 1.2 mg/dL or BUN > 20 mg/dL) or $S[Na^+]$ < 130 mEq/L
  - Short-term therapy:
    - Patients hospitalized for gastrointestinal bleed (ceftriaxone 1 g daily); transition to oral quinolone or trimethoprim–sulfamethoxazole b.i.d. $\times$ 7 days after stabilization
    - Patients hospitalized for other reasons with ascitic total protein < 1 g/dL
- Severe acute alcoholic hepatitis: administer pentoxifylline 400 mg t.i.d. (tumor necrosis factor inhibitor)
- Dietary sodium $\pm$ water restriction, the latter if hyponatremic, diuretics (loop + aldosterone antagonist)
- Transjugular intrahepatic portosystemic shunt (TIPS):
  - Diverts portal blood flow to hepatic vein
  - Redistributes splanchnic/portal blood to central volume
  - Improves variceal bleed
  - Improves renal perfusion
  - Improves central venous return, cardiac output
  - Complications: bleeding, infections, hepatic encephalopathy, renal failure
  - Limitations: poorly tolerated in advanced, end-stage liver patients
- Vasopressors:
  - Improves short-term mortality (i.e., 15 days), but not beyond
  - Europe: European Association for the Study of the Liver:
    - Terlipressin (a synthetic analogue of vasopressin with reduced anti-aquaretic effect used to raise peripheral vascular resistance (PVR) and BP and reduce portal venous blood flow and hepatic venous pressure gradient - [not available in the United States; terlipressin use is contraindicated in ischemic cardiovascular disease]) *plus* albumin, or
    - Combination of (1) norepinephrine (NE), vasopressin, or combination midodrine plus octreotide and (2) albumin (1 g/kg/d up to 100 g/d on day 1, followed by 20 to 40 g/d)
    - Maximum treatment duration: 14 days

> **NOTE**
> - Terlipressin + albumin: Start 0.5 mg over 4 to 6 hours infusion, increase to maximum of 2 mg over 4 to 6 hours if SCr decreases by $<25\%$ at day 3. Treatment is maintained until SCr has decreased <1.5 mg/dL, *or*
> - NE + albumin: Start 0.5 mg/h infusion, increase dose by 0.25 to 0.5 mg/h every 3 hours up to a maximum of 3 mg/h to achieve a MAP increase of ≥ 10 mm Hg, *or*
> - Vasopressin + albumin: Start 0.01 units/min, increase dose to a maximum of 0.8 U/min to achieve increase in MAP > 10 mm Hg
> - Efficacy of terlipressin in HRS reversal is comparable to NE.

- USA: American Association for the Study of Liver Disease:
  - Midodrine (~7.5 mg p.o. t.i.d., titrate up to 12.5 to 15.0 mg p.o. t.i.d. to increase MAP by ≥ 15 mm Hg as tolerated) *plus* octreotide (splanchnic vasoconstrictor, start at 100 μg subcutaneously t.i.d., titrate up to 200 μg as

needed for response) *and* albumin (~20 to 40 g/d: 40 g/d if CVP < 12 mm Hg or failure to reduce plasma renin activity level to <50% of baseline after 3 days of treatment). Duration of treatment is undefined.
- If failure to midodrine + octreotide + albumin above (i.e., no response within 3 days), change to NE + albumin outlined above.
- There are no data comparing the efficacy of midodrine/octreotide versus NE in HRS reversal.
  - Predictors of response:
    - Baseline serum bilirubin level < 10 mg/dL and increase in mean arterial BP ≥ 5 mm Hg
    - If positive response, effect is generally seen within 3 days.
- Molecular adsorbent recycling system (MARS) and fractionated plasma separation and adsorption (FSPA): systems designed to clear protein bound toxins not metabolized by the diseased liver.
  - Current data suggest improvement in kidney function, bilirubin, prothrombin time, grade of encephalopathy, MAP, systemic vascular resistance (SVR), and cardiac output.
  - May be considered for HRS type 1, patients with severe hepatic encephalopathy, or Child–Pugh score ≥ 12, but more data are needed.
- Liver transplantation is only cure. Nonetheless, the incidence of ESRD following liver transplantation in patients with HRS is 7% versus 2% in those without HRS.
- Cardiorenal syndrome (CRS):
- Pathologic disorder of the heart and kidneys whereby acute or chronic dysfunction of one organ induces acute or chronic dysfunction of the other.
  - CRS type 1: (acute cardiorenal syndrome): abrupt worsening of cardiac function → AKI
  - CRS type 2: (chronic cardiorenal syndrome): chronic abnormalities in cardiac function → progressive CKD
  - CRS type 3: (acute renocardiac syndrome): abrupt worsening of renal function → acute cardiac dysfunction.
  - CRS type 4: (chronic renocardiac syndrome): CKD → decreased cardiac function, cardiac hypertrophy and/or increased risk of adverse cardiovascular events.
  - CRS type 5: (secondary CRS): systemic condition → both cardiac and renal dysfunction.
- Incidence of CKD in heart failure: 20% to 70%
- Risk factors: older age, female gender, baseline CKD, Caucasian American race, diastolic heart failure, history of CHF, diabetes mellitus, SBP > 160 mm Hg
- Pathophysiology of CRS:
  - Heart failure → reduced cardiac output → arterial underfilling
  - Increased synthesis and release of antidiuretic hormone (ADH)
  - Activation of sympathetic nervous system
  - Activation of renin angiotensin aldosterone system (RAAS)
  - Reduced renal perfusion and increased renal Na^+ and H_2O reabsorption
- Management of heart failure:
  - Decongesting therapeutic options: diuretics, UF, aquaretics
  - Diuretic optimization strategies evaluation in acute heart failure (DOSE trial):
    - There was no statistically significant difference in global symptom relief or change in renal function at 72 hours for either bolus or continuous infusion of loop diuretics → intravenous bolus of diuretic = continuous infusion.

- High intensification (double home dose of loop diuretics given intravenously) was associated with trends toward faster diuresis, greater symptomatic relief, and greater reduction in NT-proBNP only.
  - Ultrafiltration:
    - UF versus IV diuretics for Patients Hospitalized for Acute Decompensated Congestive Heart Failure ADHF (UNLOAD trial):

Early UF results in greater weight and fluid loss without adverse effect on kidney function. UF arm had reduced rehospitalization and number of hospital days, emergency room visits, and unscheduled office visits at 90-day follow-up.

    - UF in patients with decompensated heart failure (HF) and CRS, Cardiorenal Rescue Study in Acute Decompensated Heart Failure (CARRESS-HF) trial: effect of UF versus guided "stepped pharmacologic" therapy: "Stepped pharmacologic" based on target urine output (UO) 3 to 5 L/d:
      - IV loop diuretic → If not at UO goal:
      - Add thiazide (metolazone up to 5 mg b.i.d.) → If not at UO goal:
      - Add dopamine or dobutamine at 2 µg/kg/h if SBP < 110 mm Hg and EF < 40% or right ventricular systolic dysfunction *or* add nitroglycerin or nesiritide if SBP > 120 mm Hg (any ejection fraction) and severe symptoms → If not at UO goal:
      - Add left ventricular assist device (LVAD) → If not at UO goal:
      - Dialysis or UF crossover

Conclusions: The use of a stepped pharmacologic therapy algorithm was superior to a strategy of UF for the preservation of renal function at 96 hours, with a similar amount of weight loss. UF group had higher rate of adverse events.

Class IIa recommendation from the ACC/AHA: Ultrafiltration is reasonable for patients with refractory congestion not responding to medical therapy. (Level of evidence: B)
  - Aquaretics (vasopressin V2 receptor antagonist, vaptans): tolvaptan
    - Approved for treating hyponatremia
    - Improves free water excretion, reduces furosemide use and body weight
    - Early benefit in dyspnea and edema/weight, but no benefit on heart failure, hospitalization, or mortality (Efficacy of Vasopressin Antagonism in Heart Failure Outcome Study With Tolvaptan (EVEREST) trial)
    - Vaptans are currently *not* indicated in the treatment of CRS.
  - Others:
    - Natriuretic hormones: nesiritide (synthetic atrial natriuretic hormone)
      - Potent arterial and venous vasodilator
      - Potentially ↓cardiac filling pressures and inhibits neurohormonal systems
      - Acute Study of Clinical Effectiveness of Nesiritide in Decompensated Heart Failure (ASCEND-HF):
        - Nesiritide did not reduce the rate of recurrent heart failure hospitalization or death at 30 days.
        - Nesiritide reduced dyspnea to a modest degree, consistent with previous findings but did not meet prespecified protocol criteria for statistical significance at 6 and 24 hours.
        - Nesiritide did not affect 30-day all-cause mortality nor did it worsen renal function as had been suggested by prior meta-analyses of smaller studies.
    - Vasodilators: nitroglyceride, nipride, ACEI/ARB
    - Inotropes: dobutamine, milrinone, dopamine, digoxin, levosimendan (novel agent in United States, approved in Europe)

- A1-adenosine antagonists:
  - Adenosine levels are increased in heart failure.
  - A1 receptor activation → ↓GFR → glomerular arteriolar vasoconstriction → ↑Na^+ reabsorption in proximal and distal tubules (tubuloglomerular feedback) → ↓renin secretion
  - A2 receptor activation (renally beneficial) → vasodilation → ↑renal medullary blood flow
  - Clinical data: Placebo-Controlled Randomized Study of the Selective Adenosine A1 Receptor Antagonist Rolofylline for Patients Hospitalized with Acute Decompensated Heart Failure and Volume Overload to Assess Treatment Effect on Congestion and Renal Function (PROTECT): no clinical benefit
- Erythropoiesis-stimulating agents:
  - Reduction of Events by Darbepoetin Alfa in Heart Failure (RED-HF): no benefit from raising hemoglobin from as low as 9.0 to target of 13.0 g/dL
  - Recommendation: follow same guideline regarding routine anemia management in CKD.
- Hypertonic saline solution (HSS) with diuretics:
  - Theory:
    - Offsets the counterproductive neurohormonal upregulation and transiently improves hemodynamics
    - Promotes renal Na^+ extraction with accompanied net water loss and preservation of renal function
    - CAUTION: HSS is contraindicated in oliguric patients.
  - Proposed therapy: infusion of furosemide plus HSS (150 mL of 1.4% to 4.6% NaCl — tonicity depends of current serum sodium, i.e., 4.6% for SNa < 125 mEq/L, 1.4% to 2.1% for SNa > 135 mEq/L) twice daily for a period of 6 to 12 days
  - Early results: more rapid achievement of dry weight, improved renal function without adverse cardiac effects, shorter length of stay, faster decline in BNP, and better survival at 48 months (55 vs. 13%)
  - United States and Brazil with ongoing large studies. *Not yet* routinely recommended. Confirmatory data are needed.

AKI Prevention in Surgical Setting

- Cardiac surgery, coronary artery bypass grafting (CABG):
  - Causative factors for AKI: hypoperfusion, inflammatory response induced by cardiopulmonary bypass pump (CPB), intraoperative anemia/hemolysis, and hemoglobinuric nephrotoxicity
  - Risk factors for AKI: age > 70 years, females, large body surface area (>2.1 m^2), (insulin requiring) diabetes mellitus, congestive heart failure, ejection fraction < 35%, atrial fibrillation, chronic obstructive pulmonary disease, urgent surgery, CPB duration, preoperative intra-aortic balloon pump, underlying CKD, use of aprotinin (anti-fibrinolytic agent used to reduce bleeding)
  - Off-pump versus On-pump CABG:
    - Potential benefits of off-pump: reduced AKI, neurologic complications (strokes), ICU and hospital stays, and mortality
    - Potential risks: hemodynamic instability; risks may be minimized with surgeons/anesthesiologists' experience
    - Data for preferential use of on- versus off-CPB pump CABG are lacking.

- Sodium bicarbonate infusion during cardiac surgery requiring CPB:
  - Benefits thought to be due to reduced hemoglobinuria-induced nephrotoxicity via urinary alkalinization and/or reduced generation of CPB-induced oxygen-free radicals produced by ischemia–reperfusion and inflammation
  - Incidence of AKI has been shown to decrease with the use of sodium bicarbonate compared to normal saline in a double-blind randomized control pilot trial involving 100 cardiac surgical patients at risk for postoperative AKI (32% vs. 52%, $p = 0.043$).
- Perioperative use of RAAS inhibitors:
  - Inadequate data to suggest routine discontinuation prior to surgery
  - Discontinuation should be considered in patients with hypotension, hyperkalemia, and/or requirement for vasopressors.
- Remote ischemic preconditioning in cardiac surgery: recently shown (2015) to reduce incidence of AKI within 72 hours and need for RRT
- Natriuretic peptide (nesiritide): AKI preventive use following cardiac surgery
  - Current data suggest that the prophylactic use of perioperative human ANP (hANP) in patients who have left ventricular dysfunction and undergo CABG may confer reno- and cardioprotective effects and reduce postoperative complications.
  - However, both all-cause mortality and in-hospital mortality are not significantly reduced.
  - hANP reduces incidence and severity of AKI after cardiac surgery.
  - Further studies still necessary
- Avoid NSAIDS, nephrotoxins, hyperglycemia.
- Management of high-risk surgical patients:
  - Protocolized use of inotropes to optimize oxygen delivery in late critical illness has not been shown to reduce incidence of AKI or improve outcomes.
  - Key beneficial interventions: hemodynamic monitoring and optimization, avoidance of hypotension and hypoperfusion
- Abdominal aortic aneurysm surgery:
  - Endovascular aortic aneurysm repair (EVAR) versus open laparotomy:
    - EVAR avoids aortic cross-clamp, but still requires general anesthesia and aortic manipulation with associated atheroembolic complications.
    - Potential problem with EVAR: radiocontrast use, contrast-induced AKI
  - Current data are inadequate to suggest that EVAR is better than open repair in terms of AKI

Mechanisms of AKI

- Ischemia-related ATN:
  - Proximal and distal tubules may be affected in a patchy distribution: irregular vacuolization, loss of proximal cell brush border, disruption and sloughing of epithelial cells lining the tubule, intratubular epithelial cell casts
  - Necrosis of tubular cells
  - Apoptosis of proximal tubular cells
  - Functional changes:
    - Loss of tubular cell polarization (loss of differentiation between the apical and basolateral sides, resulting in reabsorption of intraluminal urine, known as "urine back-leak")
    - Microvascular injury, vascular congestion

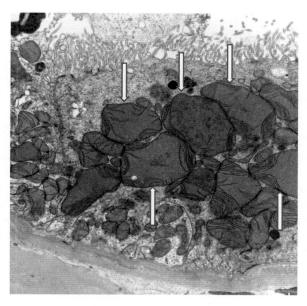

FIGURE 10.1 Electron micrograph of abnormal proximal tubular cell mitochondria due to exposure to tenofovir (nucleotide reverse transcriptase inhibitor). The affected mitochondria (*arrows*) are enlarged with atypical shapes and broken or absent cristae. Note that not all mitochondria are enlarged (×10,000).

- Nephrotoxin-related AKI:
  - Aminoglycosides, radiocontrast agents, cisplatin, cyclosporine, tacrolimus, tenofovir, amphotericin B, methotrexate, foscarnet, pentamidine, organic solvents, heavy metals, sucrose-based immunoglobulins infusion (IVIG).
  - Nephrotoxin induced AKI typically involves proximal tubules. Radiocontrast agents, cyclosporine, tacrolimus, and sucrose-based IVIG can lead to the formation of tubular cell cytoplasmic small uniform (isometric) vacuoles. Tenofovir injures mitochondrial DNA with large atypical tubular cell mitochondria (Fig. 10.1). Heavy metals such as gold and lead cause intracytoplasmic and intranuclear inclusions, respectively. With medications such as gentamycin, electron microscopy may reveal proximal tubular cell "myeloid bodies" which are multilamellar lysosomes filled with undigested drug–phospholipid complexes or drug-bound cytoplasmic structures.
- Sepsis-related AKI a.k.a. "hyperemic" AKI: Glomeruli have increased renal blood flow due to dilatation of both afferent and efferent arterioles, thus "hyperemia." However, GFR is reduced because there is greater efferent vasodilation compared to afferent vasodilation which results in reduced glomerular filtration pressure.

PARENCHYMAL (INTRINSIC) ACUTE KIDNEY INJURY

Vascular Causes of AKI

- Acute intrinsic diseases:
  - Microangiopathy and hemolytic anemia (MAHA), thrombotic thrombocytopenic purpura–hemolytic uremic syndrome (TTP/HUS), scleroderma, malignant HTN
  - Renal vasculitides

- Large vessel involvement:
  - Aortic dissection extending into renal artery, renal artery aneurysm
  - Systemic thromboembolism (atheroemboli, spontaneous bacterial endocarditis)
- Atheroembolic disease:
  - May occur with any invasive arterial procedure, arteriography, vascular surgery, or thrombolytic therapy and may occur up to months following inciting event
  - Diagnosis: clinical history *plus* classic triad of livedo reticularis, AKI, and eosinophilia with or without hypocomplementemia
    - Fundoscopic examination may reveal cholesterol emboli a.k.a. Hollenhorst plaque.
    - Laboratory findings: leukocytosis, eosinophilia, anemia, thrombocytopenia, elevated blood urea nitrogen, SCr, liver function tests, creatine phosphokinase (CPK), and amylase, hematuria, positive inflammatory markers: hypocomplementemia; elevated rheumatoid factor, antinuclear antibodies, C-reactive protein, and sedimentation rate
    - Histopathology: as cholesterol dissolves during tissue processing, cholesterol crystal embolization is seen as clear needle-shaped structures within vascular lumens or walls, sometimes with surrounding multinucleated giant cells. They may be in large or small arteries, arterioles, or capillaries (Fig. 10.2).
    - Presentation: unexplained fevers, weight loss, myalgias, anorexia, end-organ infarction/injury occurring weeks to months following inciting event (e.g., stroke, myocardial/bowel/renal infarction, pancreatitis, adrenal failure, muscle infarction)
    - Management:
      - Supportive, nutritional support given high catabolic state in these patients
      - Avoid further invasive procedures if possible.
      - Do not use anticoagulants or thrombolytics
- Renal vein or even artery: thrombosis associated with severe nephrotic syndrome

Glomerular Diseases

Many glomerular and vascular diseases may also present with a rapidly progressive course and AKI. See Glomerular/Vascular Diseases chapter.

Tubulointerstitial Diseases

In addition to the following conditions, also see Tubular, Interstitial, and Cystic Diseases chapter for other conditions that may present as AKI.

- Heme-pigment induced AKI (hemoglobin, myoglobin):
  - Hemolysis:
    - Causes: ABO-incompatible blood transfusions, G6PD deficiency, poisoning, snake/insect envenomation, drugs (cephalosporins, paroxysmal nocturnal hemoglobinuria, malaria)
    - Laboratory findings: reduced haptoglobin, increased lactate dehydrogenase and bilirubin, increased reticulocytes and spherocytes, hyperkalemia
  - Rhabdomyolysis:
    - Causes: trauma, immobilization (particularly overweight patients), prolonged vascular/orthopedic surgery, extreme exertion (exacerbated by heat, underlying metabolic/inflammatory myopathies), seizures, neuroleptic malignant syndrome, alcoholism (particularly if concurrent electrolyte abnormalities, e.g., hypophosphatemia, hypomagnesemia), drugs/toxins

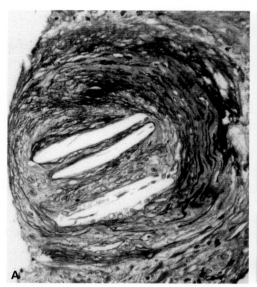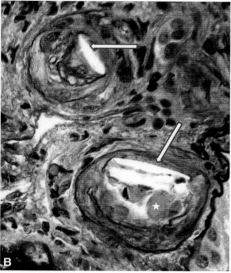

FIGURE 10.2 Cholesterol crystal embolization. Cholesterol emboli (atheroembolic). **A.** Artery with clear needle-shaped cholesterol crystals in the fibrotic lumen. (Periodic acid methenamine silver, ×325) **B.** Arterioles with cholesterol crystals (*arrows*) in the lumina with associated swollen endothelial cells and fibrin deposition (*asterisk*) (Periodic acid methenamine silver, ×400).

- Diagnosis:
  - Myalgias
  - Elevated CPK
    - Levels < 5,000 to 10,000 units/L: AKI uncommon
    - Levels > 40,000 units/L may be associated with moderate to severe AKI.
  - Reddish brown urine due to myoglobinuria
  - NOTE: Reddish brown urine can be due to hematuria, myo- or hemoglobinuria, or agents with reddish brown coloring effect (beet, phenazopyridine, porphyria).
    - Centrifuge urine:
      - Red sediment → hematuria
      - Red supernatant → myoglobinuria *or* hemoglobinuria *or* agents with coloring effect (see earlier examples)
    - Heme dipstick (presence of "blood" on urine dipstick):
      - Positive myoglobinuria or hemoglobinuria
      - Negative (agents with coloring effect)
  - Plasma color:
    - Clear: myoglobinuria (due to its low molecular weight, myoglobinuria is easily filtered and does not remain/accumulate in plasma)
    - Red/pink: hemoglobinuria (high molecular weight, binds to haptoglobin, not easily filtered, remains in plasma as red/pink color). Hemoglobinuria suggests high plasma concentration.
- Pathogenesis of AKI associated with heme-pigment-induced AKI:
  - Tubular obstruction, with or without association with uric acid crystals
  - Direct proximal tubular cell injury
  - Vasoconstriction (explains why FeNa may be <1% even in the presence of ATN)

- AKI risks: volume depletion, low urine pH
- Complications of rhabdomyolysis:
    - Electrolyte abnormalities: hyperkalemia (potassium levels may increase at >1 mEq/L/day versus ~0.3 mEq/L/d in other nonhypercatabolic AKI), hyperphosphatemia (release from injured muscle cells), hypocalcemia (due to calcium phosphate deposition into injured muscles, reduced bone sensitivity to parathyroid hormone), hyperuricemia, and metabolic acidosis
    - Transaminitis (elevated aspartate aminotransferase [AST]) and aldolase
    - AKI
- Management:
    - Early and aggressive volume administration:
        - Start normal saline at 100 to 200 mL/h. If good diuresis, aim for goal urine output 200 to 300 mL/h. Monitor volume status.
        - Theoretical benefits of alkalinization with $NaHCO_3$ over normal saline:
            - Urine pH > 6.5 may reduce heme-induced renal toxicity and pigment cast formation.
            - $NaHCO_3$ may reduce the release of free iron from myoglobin
            - There is no clear evidence of benefits of $NaHCO_3$ over NaCl except possibly in severe rhadomyolysis.
            - NOTE: Alkalinization should be avoided in patients with hypocalcemia, hypokalemia, existing CO_2 retention (chronic respiratory acidosis in chronic obstructive pulmonary disorder), or high calcium × phosphorus product (i.e., >70).
    - Benefits of mannitol remain undefined and not routinely recommended.
    - Loop diuretics do not change outcome in AKI. Use in volume overload only.
    - Benefit of dialysis to remove myoglogin, hemoglobin, or uric acid has not been shown.
- Hyperbilirubinemia: severe hyperbilirubin (serum bilirubin levels > 20 mg/dL) has been reported to be associated with ATN with bile granules in tubular epithelial cells and bile thrombi in tubules. Kidneys appear green on autopsies.
- Radiocontrast-induced AKI (CI-AKI):
    - Pathogenic mechanisms:
        - Medullary hypoxia (radiocontrast induces vasoconstriction of both afferent and efferent arterioles, but greater effect in afferent arterioles)
        - Direct cytotoxicity
        - Generation of reactive oxygen species
    - Histopathology: proximal tubular cell with small uniform (isometric) vacuoles
    - Prevention is *key*:
        - Use of nonionic low or iso-osmolal agents:
            - Low-osmolal nonionic agent: iohexol, ioxaglate
            - Iso-osmolal (~290 mOsm/kg) nonionic agent: iodixanol
            - Controversy: iso-osmolal iodixanol may be better than low-osmolal iohexol among patients with DM and CKD, but not better than other low-osmolal agents.
            - Iohexol has specific adverse effect on kidneys and not necessarily the "low-osmolal" effect.
            - KDIGO recommends the use of low-osmolal or iso-osmolal rather than high-osmolal contrast agents. Current evidence is not reliable to preferentially recommend one agent over the other.
        - Avoid concurrent use of nephrotoxins.

- Use of magnetic resonance imaging with gadolinium:
  - Concerns for the development of nephrogenic systemic fibrosis
  - Possible nephrotoxicity has been reported
- Hydration:
  - Normal saline or isotonic sodium bicarbonate: 3 mL/kg over 1 to 2 hours prior to contrast study, followed by 1 mL/kg/h × 6 to 12 hours postcontrast—assuming patient can tolerate volume expansion.
  - POSEIDON trial: left ventricular end diastolic pressure guided fluid administration among patients undergoing cardiac catheterization lowered risk of CI-AKI.
  - Rationale for bicarbonate over normal saline hydration: added protection against free radical injury. Meta-analysis only revealed trend for better outcome.
    - KDIGO does *not* preferentially recommend one agent over the other.
  - Isotonic is preferred over one-half isotonic saline.
  - Outpatient oral hydration: salt-containing fluid is likely more renoprotective than free water.
  - No or undefined benefit and potentially harmful agents/therapy and *not* recommended: diuretics, mannitol, dopamine, atrial natriuretic peptide (ANP)
- Hemofiltration, hemodialysis for the sole indication of CI-AKI prevention:
  - In patients on established dialysis: benefit of immediate dialysis (i.e., within 24 hours of contrast exposure) versus waiting for next regularly scheduled dialysis treatment is unclear.
  - In pre-ESRD patients, dialysis initiation for the sole indication of CI-AKI is not recommended.
- In patients with congestive heart failure: Optimize cardiac function. If volume overload, continue diuretics to improve cardiac contractility, hence cardiac output and renal perfusion.
- Ongoing use of ACEI/ARB in *stable* patient: discontinuation may be beneficial.
- Acetylcysteine (mucomyst):
  - Has antioxidant and vasodilatory properties
  - Benefits unproven, but given low cost, tolerability, and potential benefits, 2012 KDIGO suggests administration (1,200 mg orally b.i.d. day prior and day of contrast study) to high-risk patients in addition to hydration and selection of low-risk contrast agents. American College of Cardiology/American Heart Association, however, does not recommend its use.
  - Inhibition of renal vasoconstriction:
    - Theophylline—little or no effect.
    - Iloprost—prostacyclin analog; less CI-AKI than placebo in small trial, but severe hypotension. More data needed for both efficacy and safety.
    - Fenoldopam—no benefit; unclear if benefit would be evident if administered intrarenally
    - (Nonselective) endothelin receptor antagonist—worse CI-AKI
  - Remote ischemic preconditioning:
    - Deliberate induction of transient nonlethal ischemia to an organ (e.g., inflating BP cuff to 50 mm Hg above patient's SBP × 4 cycles of 30 second on/off duration) to activate systemic vasodilatory response/release of vasodilators such as nitric oxide to protect other ischemic organs (e.g., kidneys exposed to radiocontrast).

- Two small studies in patients undergoing elective coronary angiography and PCI suggested benefits in reducing risk of CI-AKI as well as short-term rehospitalization and death.
  - Atrial natriuretic peptide (ANP):
    - Available data suggest *no* benefit compared to placebo. It is possible that negative result was due to short duration of treatment (30 minutes pre and 30 minutes post).
    - A larger prospective, controlled, randomized trial of 254 patients with SCr $\geq$ 1.3 mg/dL receiving either ANP (0.042 mg/kg/min vs. Ringer solution alone) for 4 to 6 hours prior to angiography and continued for 48 hours revealed a reduction in the incidence of CI-AKI (defined as $\geq$25% or $\geq$0.5 mg/dL increase in SCr within 48 hours) in the treatment group compared with placebo (3.2 vs. 11.7%). Confirmatory studies are still needed.
  - Statins:
    - Rationale: statins have anti-inflammatory and antioxidant properties. Statins also improve endothelial function and reduce endothelin-induced arterial vasoconstriction.
    - Recent meta-analysis (2015) of short-term, high-dose statin revealed benefit in prevention of CI-AKI in patients undergoing cardiac angiography.
    - Recommendation: reasonable to start statins in patients who will need statins, but not everyone
  - Ascorbic acid: insufficient data to support use
  - Forced diuresis: likely increases risk of CI-AKI and is not recommended
  - Avoid NSAIDs
- Tumor lysis syndrome (TLS):
  - Associated with high cellular turnover following chemotherapy for large tumor burdens
  - May be spontaneous due to high cellular proliferation and rapid cellular turnover (non-Hodgkin lymphoma, particularly Burkitt lymphoma) and other hematologic malignancies.
  - Criteria for laboratory TLS: $\geq$2 of the following:
    - Hyperuricemia: uric acid $\geq$ 8 mg/dL or $\geq$25% increase from baseline
    - Hyperkalemia: potassium $\geq$ 6 mEq/L, or $\geq$25% increase from baseline
    - Hyperphosphatemia: phosphorus > 6.5 mg/dL, or $\geq$25% increase from baseline
    - Hypocalcemia: calcium < 7 mg/dL, or $\geq$25% decrease from baseline
  - Criteria for clinical TLS:
    - Meeting laboratory criteria above *plus*
    - One or more of associated complications involving AKI, cardiac arrhythmias, seizures, or death
  - Etiologies of AKI associated with TLS:
    - Hyperuricemia:
      - Tubular obstruction from uric acid crystals
      - Uric acid induced inflammatory response, tubular interstitial nephritis
      - Uric acid-induced renal vasoconstriction
    - Hyperphosphatemia: tubular obstruction from calcium oxalate crystals
  - Treatment of TLS:
    - Prevention is *key*:
      - Volume expansion with crystalloid solutions
      - NOTE: Urinary alkalinization to increase uric acid solubility is *no longer* routinely recommended due to

- Inability to increase xanthine solubility (purine metabolite that may also precipitate and cause tubular obstruction) and
  - Increased risk for metabolic alkalosis and calcium phosphate precipitation
- Dietary potassium and phosphorus restriction
- Renal replacement therapy as needed
- Management of hyperuricemia:
  - Purine metabolites of nucleic acids are converted to uric acid via a multistep process requiring the enzyme xanthine oxidase (XO):

  Purine metabolites → hypoxanthine + XO → xanthine + XO →
  uric acid + urate oxidase → allantoin

  - Allopurinol is converted to oxypurinol, a competitive inhibitor of XO to decrease downstream uric acid formation. Allopurinol is therefore *not* effective in reducing *preexisting* hyperuricemia.
  - Febuxostat, a nonpurine XO inhibitor, approved for treatment of hyperuricemia in patients with gout, has not been used in TLS.
  - Rasburicase: recombinant form of urate oxidase, converts uric acid to the more soluble metabolite, allantoin, which can be renally excreted.
    - NOTE: Rasburicase is contraindicated in patients with glucose-6-phosphate dehydrogenase and catalase deficiencies due to the development of hemolytic anemia and methemoglobinemia.
    - Rasburicase is associated with hypersensitivity (including anaphylaxis) in 1% of patients.
    - Rasburicase effectively reduces hyperuricemia, but not shown to reduce incidence of clinical TLS.
- Hematopoeitic stem cell transplant (HSCT)-associated AKI:
  - Associated complication: veno-occlusive disease involving liver, hepatic failure, and HRS
  - Higher risk in association with myeloablative compared with nonmyeloablative therapy
  - Management: supportive care
- AKI in pregnancy:
  - Early: before 20 weeks gestational age: volume depletion due to hyperemesis gravidarum and poor oral intake, septic abortion, medication-induced AKI
  - After 20 weeks to postpartum: obstruction, bleeding (e.g., placenta abruption), acute fatty liver of pregnancy (AFLP), pregnancy-associated atypical HUS (aHUS), HELLP (hemolysis, elevated liver enzymes, low platelets), renal cortical necrosis, drug induced
    - Obstruction:
      - Late pregnancy: Large uterus compressing on ureters, right-sided involvement is more common, resolves with delivery. Advise positional changes with sleeping.
      - Postpartum: consider injury of soft tissues surrounding urethra or urethra itself with marked inflammation and resultant obstruction of urine flow.
    - AFLP:
      - Clinical manifestations: anorexia, nausea, vomiting, marked transaminitis, coagulopathy, AKI. No hemolytic anemia
      - Supportive therapy
    - Pregnancy associated aHUS:
      - Patient typically develops symptoms postpartum: hemolytic anemia, thrombocytopenia, AKI, CNS symptoms

- Etiology thought to be due to the loss of placental regulatory proteins that compensate for increased complement activation from maternal mutations of complement genes
  - HELLP:
    - Clinical manifestations: HTN, headaches, chest pain, right upper quadrant abdominal pain, laboratory findings of both AFLP and aHUS (transaminitis and hemolytic anemia respectively), AKI
    - Similar pathogenesis as preeclampsia/eclampsia. See Hypertension chapter.
  - Renal cortical necrosis:
    - May be associated with obstetrical complications such as placenta abruption, sepsis, amniotic emboli, retained product of conception
    - Patient may present with persistent anuria postpartum.
    - Diagnostic imaging: pericortical rim due to infarction may be seen on CT.
- Others:
  - Hantavirus infection (most commonly subtype Puumala) is associated with flu-like symptoms and acute kidney failure: biopsy findings include tubulointerstitial nephritis, hemorrhage into medullary tissues, interstitial edema, and tubular cell necrosis. Podocyte effacement in association with glomerular proteinuria has been described.
  - H1N1 influenza A: AKI is common and predominantly associated with ATN +/− rhabdomyolysis. The latter is typically mild. AKI requiring renal replacement therapy has been reported to be ~20%.

POSTRENAL ACUTE KIDNEY INJURY

Definitions

- Obstructive uropathy refers to structural or functional changes in the urinary tract that adversely affect urine flow. Obstruction may be complete or partial and may involve upper or lower collecting system and unilateral or bilateral systems.
- Obstructive nephropathy refers to kidney injury due to impaired urine flow.

Etiologies of Postrenal AKI

- Intrinsic causes:
  - Stones/calculi (kidney or bladder), transitional cell carcinoma, blood clots, sloughed papillae from papillary necrosis (e.g., excessive NSAIDS, sickle cell disease, diabetics, renal tuberculosis), fungus balls, intratubular obstruction from drug crystallizations (e.g., acyclovir, sulfonamides, sulfadiazine, ethylene glycol, methotrexate, indinavir), calcium phosphate precipitation (e.g., from high phosphate-containing enemas), oxalate crystals, light chain precipitations (cast nephropathy), debris.
  - Warfarin-related kidney injury: Mechanisms thought to be related to RBC casts causing renal tubular obstruction. Risks: older age, diabetes mellitus, HTN, cardiovascular disease, over-anticoagulation, for example, INR > 3 (See Figure 7.16).
- Extrinsic causes:
  - Malignancy (particularly female pelvic malignancies, GI malignancies, retroperitoneal fibrosis), benign prostate hypertrophy (BPH) or malignancy, pregnancy (may begin in first trimester, typically right-sided obstruction and resolves within 2 to 3 weeks postpartum)

- Retroperitoneal fibrosis:
  - Thought to arise from exaggerated local inflammatory response to aortic atherosclerosis, tissue injury, or autoimmune disease
  - Etiologies: idiopathic, drug induced (e.g., ergot derivatives, methysergide, bromocriptine, β-blockers, methyldopa, hydralazine, analgesics), infections, malignancies, prior surgeries or retroperitoneal hemorrhage, radiation therapy, smoking, asbestos exposure
  - Clinical manifestations: back pain, abdominal pain, or lower flank pain that may radiate to inguinal area (testicular pain), nonspecific constitutional symptoms of malaise, weight loss, fevers, nausea/vomiting, constipation, symptoms associated with mesenteric ischemia, obstructive uropathy, upper leg claudication, lower extremity phlebitis or deep vein thrombosis (DVT), new-onset HTN, elevated erythrocyte sedimentation rate or C-reactive protein levels
  - Diagnosis: computed tomography scan (may be seen as mass encasing anterior and lateral sides of aorta, often also encasing and compressing inferior vena cava [IVC], thus tendency for DVT), tissue biopsy (particularly to rule out underlying infections/malignancy)
  - Management: relief of obstruction (e.g., ureteral stenting, anti-inflammatory medical therapies such as glucocorticoids)
- Collecting system malformations or strictures: phimosis, meatal stenosis, urethral or ureteral strictures from recurrent infections, manipulations
- Functional obstruction:
  - Diabetic neurogenic bladder
  - Large output urine volume that overwhelms the patient's ability to void (severe diabetes insipidus)
  - Drugs that can lead to neurogenic bladder:
    - Anticholinergics (tricyclic antidepressants, diphenhydramine): reduce bladder detrusor muscle contraction
    - NSAIDS: inhibit prostaglandin-mediated detrusor muscle contraction
    - Sympathomimetics: α-adrenergic agents increase tone in prostate and bladder neck
- Transplant setting:
  - Ureteral strictures due to trauma, ischemia, or BK virus infection
  - External compression by lymphoceles
  - Bladder dysfunction

Pathogenesis of Obstructive Kidney Injury

- Obstruction leads to increased intratubular pressure, which in turn leads to reduced glomerular filtration (tubular luminal hydraulic pressure exceeds glomerular filtration pressure). The reduced filtration pressure leads to local renal vasoconstriction, a process mediated by increased release of angiotensin II and thromboxanes.
- Influx of inflammatory cells, synthesis of transforming growth factor-β, other inflammatory cytokines, proteases, and oxygen-free radicals
- Histopathology may reveal tubulointerstitial fibrosis, tubular atrophy, and glomerulosclerosis.

Clinical Manifestations of Obstructive Uropathy

- Reduced urine output, partial reduction in urine output to anuria:
  - Anuria: consider lower tract obstruction (bladder neck or urethral obstruction), clotted foley catheter, bilateral ureteral (papillary necrosis, large tumors)

> **NOTE** A "good" urine output does not necessarily imply absence of obstruction. Patient may still have a partial obstruction.

- Pain (depends on level of obstruction—see Kidney Stones in Calcium, Phosphorus, Magnesium, and Kidney Stones chapter)
- Hematuria
- Urinary symptoms: sensation of incomplete voiding, frequency, nocturia, overflow incontinence
- Suprapubic tenderness, fullness, sometimes mass-like effect from distended bladder
- HTN

Laboratory Findings of Obstructive Kidney Injury

- Elevated SCr unless unilateral obstruction in the setting of normal kidney function in contralateral kidney
- Hyperkalemia, metabolic acidosis out of proportion to the degree of kidney injury. This is essentially a form of distal renal tubular acidosis that arises from urinary stasis (see Renal Tubular Acidosis in Acid-Base/Potassium chapter).
- Elevated blood urea nitrogen to creatinine ratio may be seen due to tubular reabsorption of urea with urinary stasis

Diagnostic Imaging Studies of Obstructive Uropathy

- Ultrasound: inexpensive, readily available
  - False-positive in up to 25% of cases as hydronephrosis can occur in the absence of obstruction (e.g., high urine production in diabetes insipidus)
  - False-negative: severe volume depletion, oliguric state, retroperitoneal fibrosis
- CT urogram:
  - Avoid in childbearing age women due to radiation exposure
  - Consider study if suspicious for obstructing kidney stones or stones in patients with polycystic kidney disease.
- Magnetic resonance imaging:
  - No radiation exposure
  - Poor visibility for stones
- Findings:
  - Parenchymal (cortical thickness): thinning implies long-standing obstruction, hence poor recovery potential
  - Ureteral obstruction with an empty bladder indicates obstruction at the ureteral orifice or more proximal segments.
  - Hydronephrosis in patients with a ureteral stent in the presence of a full bladder does not necessarily imply obstruction since the pressure from the full bladder can be transmitted up to the kidneys via the ureteral stent.
  - Doppler imaging showing "ureteral jets" typically implies ureteral patency. Absence of ureteral jets, however, does not rule in obstruction.

Management of Obstructive Kidney Injury

- Relief of obstruction:
  - Removal of source of obstruction if possible
  - Foley insertion for bladder neck obstruction; ureteral stenting for ureteral obstruction; nephrostomy placement for obstruction proximal to proximal ureters.

- Removal of extrinsic compression (e.g., treatment of malignancy, evacuation of compressing lymphocele or mass)
- Correction of functional obstruction:
  - Discontinue responsible medications
  - Use of α-adrenergic blockers in diabetic neurogenic bladder or BPH
  - Treat diabetes insipidus if etiologic (see Polyuria in Sodium/Water chapter)
- Monitor and replace fluid and electrolytes as needed for postobstructive diuresis:
  - Causes of postobstructive diuresis:
    - Excessive fluid administration
    - Appropriate diuresis of accumulated sodium/water retention during kidney failure
    - Osmotic diuresis from accumulated urea, other toxins/solutes during kidney failure
    - Obstruction-induced tubular dysfunction and nephrogenic diabetes insipidus (may be transient or chronic)
    - Increased ANP
    - Delayed tubular recovery of reabsorptive function relative to recovery of glomerular filtrating function
  - Typical fluid replacement: 0.5 mL of fluid for every mL of urine output above 100 mL/h with 0.5 normal saline; Adjust as clinically indicated.
  - Monitor serum potassium and magnesium levels and replete as needed during postobstructive diuresis phase

Prognosis of Obstructive Kidney Injury

- Depends on duration, severity, preexisting CKD, and kidney mass affected (i.e., one or two kidneys involved)
- Functional recovery typically occurs by 7 to 10 days following relief of obstruction. Recovery may take longer in more severe and prolonged cases.

TREATMENT OF AKI

Pharmacologic Options

- Erythropoietin (EPO): no benefit
  - Experimental models: effective if used within 6 hours of ischemia–reperfusion injury
  - Clinical studies: no definitive renoprotective effect shown thus far
- ANP: possible benefit with low dose — more data needed
  - Initial studies did not show benefits in mortality or need for RRT. Low-dose ANP, however, was associated with a significant reduction in RRT requirement.
  - More recent AKI-prevention trials indicate possible benefits.
  - More studies needed, particularly, regarding the use of low-dose hANP (<0.1 μg/kg/min) for the prevention of AKI in high-risk patients with cardiovascular disease

Renal Replacement Therapy

- Timing of RRT: Current data are not adequate to recommend optimal timing of initiation of RRT in AKI.
  - Consider isovolumic "furosemide stress test": nonresponders predict progression to more severe AKI and likely indicate prompt need for RRT initiation

- Early initiation of RRT is not associated with benefit, but delayed initiation is associated with higher mortality and increased hospital/ICU lengths of stay.
- Large ongoing trials pending
- NOTE: Fluid overload at the time of RRT initiation in critically ill patients with AKI may be associated with adverse outcomes.
- Intermittent versus continuous RRT (IRRT vs. CRRT):
  - Good direct comparative data are lacking for various reasons: lack of CRRT in some centers, preferential use of CRRT in hemodynamically unstable patients.
  - Current data suggest *no definitive mortality benefit* between IRRT and CRRT.
  - CRRT has been suggested to be associated with a *higher rate of renal recovery* compared with IRRT in critically ill patients.
  - IRRT or prolonged IRRT provide faster solute removal than CRRT and is preferred for hyperkalemia, severe metabolic acidosis, and poisoning.
  - IRRT and CRRT or hybrid modalities (using both IRRT and CRRT on the same patient) should be considered complementary, not competing, techniques.
  - Use of sustained low-efficiency daily dialysis (SLEDD):
    - Slow dialysis ≥ 6 hours per session every other day
    - Provides similar degree of hemodynamic stability as CRRT
    - Drug dosing may be problematic (particularly for antibiotics)
- Intensity (dose) of RRT:
  - Recent data from large trials do not show improved outcomes with high-intensity RRT. However, higher dose may be considered for patients with high catabolic rates or sepsis.
  - Possible problem with head-to-head comparison between low and high dialysis dosing groups: actual delivery dose may be lower than that prescribed (may be due to delay in therapy initiation and/or technical issues during the dialysis procedure).
  - KDIGO AKI guidelines recommend minimal RRT dose:
    - CRRT: effluent volume of 20 to 25 mL/kg/h (actual delivery dose)
    - Intermittent, conventional hemodialysis: Kt/V (urea) of 3.9 per week or equivalent of 1.2 to 1.4 three times per week
  - Measurement of solute clearance should be measured routinely to assure adequate dose delivery.
- Continuous renal replacement therapy:
  - Indications:
    - Hemodynamic instability (e.g., patients with liver failure awaiting transplant, sepsis, systemic inflammatory response syndrome [SIRS])
    - Increased intracranial pressure (ICP):
      - CRRT is associated with lower increase in ICP compared with IRRT.
      - CRRT is associated with less hypotension, thus reduced cerebral hypoperfusion risk.
      - Use of bicarbonate buffers can increase CO_2 production which can cause cerebral vasodilation and increased ICP.
      - Use of citrate has also been suggested to be neuroprotective via attenuation of hypoxic neuronal injury.
    - Acute respiratory distress syndrome
    - Severe burns, post-trauma, rhabdomyolysis, or tumor lysis (high catabolic state)
    - Postcardiovascular surgery
    - Organ transplants

- Vascular access:
  - Arteriovenous system requires arterial line and adequate patient's BP.
  - Venovenous system requires double lumen venovenous hemodialysis catheter and blood pump
  - Suggested length of catheter based on site of insertion:
    - Most preferred: right internal jugular (IJ), 15 cm
    - Femoral: 25 cm
    - Left IJ: 20 cm: *note* greater rate of catheter dysfunction with left than right IJ or femoral
- Types of CRRT:
  - Slow continuous ultrafiltration (SCUF): large fluid removal via UF without need for dialysate or replacement solution (up to 2 L/h)
  - Hemofiltration:
    - Continuous venovenous (or arteriovenous) hemofiltration (CVVH)
    - Provides convective solute clearance of middle/large molecules and UF
    - Corrects electrolytes, acid/base disturbance
  - Hemodialysis:
    - Continuous venovenous (or arteriovenous) hemodialysis (CVVHD)
    - Provides diffusive solute clearance of small molecules and UF
    - Corrects electrolytes, acid/base disturbances
  - Hemodiafiltration
    - Continuous venovenous (or arteriovenous) hemodiafiltration (CVVHDF)
    - Provides diffusive and convective solute clearance of small, middle, large molecules and UF
    - Corrects electrolytes, acid/base disturbances
- CRRT selection:
  - If primary goal is UF: SCUF, CAVH, CVVH
  - If primary goal is solute removal: CAVHD, CVVHD
  - Both UF and solute removal are necessary: CAVHDF, CVVHDF
- Fluid management:
  - Prescribed net fluid removal rate (UF rate) + input (IV fluids, total parenteral nutrition, medications) − output (urine, other fluid losses) = patient fluid removal rate (set in dialyzer)
  - Pre versus postdilution:
    - Predilution: lower efficiency; lower risk of filter clotting
    - Postdilution: better clearance, clearance is equal to effluent rate; higher membrane fouling and filter clotting
    - Decision to use pre- or post- is based on clinical experience.
- Anticoagulation:
  - Unfractionated heparin:
    - Used for patients with low bleeding risk
    - Bolus 30 IU/kg, followed by initial rate of 5 to 10 IU/kg/h
    - Activated partial thromboplastin time > 45 to 50 seconds may be associated with increased bleeding risk
    - Potential problems with heparin: heparin-induced thrombocytopenia (HIT), adverse effects on serum lipids, efficacy is dependent on antithrombin levels
  - Low-molecular-weight heparin (LMWH):
    - LMWH is dialyzable and requires continuous infusion to achieve systemic anti-factor Xa levels of 0.25 to 0.35 units/mL.
    - Lower incidence of HIT

- Regional citrate anticoagulation:
  - KDIGO suggests the use of regional citrate anticoagulation over heparin for all patients if there is no contraindication.
  - Regional citrate anticoagulation is used for patients with moderate to high bleeding risk
  - Citrate binds to Ca^{2+} thus inactivating Ca^{2+}-dependent procoagulants. Most of the citrate calcium complexes formed are removed in the effluent. The remaining calcium citrate is returned to circulation, where citrate undergoes hepatic conversion to bicarbonate at a 1:3 conversion ratio.
  - NOTE: *Extracorporeal* ionized Ca^{2+} concentrations must be below 0.35 mmol/L for adequate regional anticoagulation.
  - Calcium reinfusion into patient via a separate central line is required to reverse the anticoagulant effect.
  - Potential problems with regional citrate anticoagulation:

    > **NOTE** Citrate toxicity may occur if hepatic conversion to bicarbonate is reduced. This may be detected by having an increased total serum calcium to ionized calcium ratio > 2.5 (a.k.a. increased "Ca^{2+} gap")
    >
    > Calcium ratio = (total serum Ca^{2+} (mg/dL) $\times$ 0.25)/(systemic ionized Ca^{2+} (mmol/L))
    >
    > The 0.25 factor is only used to convert mg/dL to mmol/L.

  - Patients with liver failure or shock liver who cannot convert citrate to HCO_3^- should not receive regional citrate anticoagulation.
  - Citrate toxicity can result in the following:
    - Metabolic alkalosis in patients with good hepatic conversion to HCO_3^-
    - High anion gap metabolic acidosis in patients with no liver function
    - Hypercalcemia but with low ionized Ca^{2+}
    - Hypernatremia
  - Potential benefits of regional citrate anticoagulation:
    - Lower bleeding risk than heparin
    - Lower blood, antithrombin III, platelet transfusion rates
    - Potential anti-inflammatory benefits
    - Long-term outcome not known
- Other possible anticoagulant therapies alternative to heparin:
  - Hirudin: need to monitor PTT, Ecarin clotting time; no reversal agent
  - Danaparoid: monitor PTT, antifactor Xa; no reversal agent
  - Argatroban: monitor PTT, *reduce* dose if hepatic dysfunction; no reversal agent
- No anticoagulation option: consider in patients active with bleed or in those with liver failure and high bleeding risk who cannot receive either citrate or heparin
- CRRT-specific complications:
  - Fluid volume deficit due to excessive UF with inadequate fluid replacement
  - Electrolyte abnormalities: hypophosphatemia, hypomagnesemia, hypokalemia. Close monitoring and replacement as needed.
  - Hypothermia due to blood exposure to room temperature and large volume replacement with room temperature fluids: use warming blankets, blood warmer
  - Air embolus due to line leakage or faulty connections

- Filter clotting:
  - Predominantly due to accumulation of proteins, a process called "concentration polarization"
  - Preventive measures: maximize blood flow; keep UF-to-plasma flow ratio (filtration fraction percentage) < 20% for postdilution; use anticoagulation
- Discontinuation of CRRT may be considered when:
  - Urine output > 400 mL/d or
  - Patient's own creatinine clearance > 20 mL/min or decrease in SCr while on CRRT when urine output exceeds 30 mL/h
- Calculations for CRRT:
  - Solute clearance: recall clearance = UV/P. In CRRT, U is the solute concentration in the effluent (E[solute]), V is the effluent rate, and P is the plasma concentration of the solute (P[solute]). As the effluent rate is much lower compared to blood flow, full equilibrium can be assumed to occur, allowing the concentration of the solute in the effluent to be the same as that in the blood.

$$\text{Clearance} = (E[\text{solute}] \times \text{effluent rate})/P[\text{solute}] = \text{effluent rate},$$
$$\text{denoted as } Q_E$$

  - Sieving coefficient of solute = E[solute]/P[solute], a ratio of 1 indicates free passage of fluid across the membrane
  - Solute clearance with predilutional fluid:

$$\text{Clearance} = Q_E \times \text{dilutional factor of } [Q_B/(Q_B + Q_R)], \text{ where } Q_B \text{ is the blood}$$
$$\text{flow, } Q_R \text{ is the rate of predilutional fluid administration}$$

  - Filtration fraction = UF rate/*plasma* flow rate

Example: Whole blood flow rate = 200 mL/min = 12,000 mL/h, hematocrit of 30%, and UF rate is 1,500 mL/h. Plasma flow would be $(12,000 \times (1 - 0.3)) = 8,400$ mL/h. Filtration fraction would be 1,500/8,400 = 18%

ICU NEPHROLOGY

Management of Acute Lung Injury/Acute Respiratory Distress Syndrome (ALI/ARDS):

- Berlin definition for acute respiratory distress syndrome (ARDS):
  - PaO_2/FiO_2 ratio ≤ 300 when using PEEP at 5 cm H_2O minimum (Example of calculation: a patient with PaO_2 of 100 mm Hg and FiO_2 of 40% has a PaO_2/FiO_2 ratio of 100/0.4 = 250). PaO_2 = arterial partial pressure of oxygen, FiO_2 = fraction of inspired oxygen.
    - Mild: PaO_2/FiO_2 ratio 200 to 300 (previously denoted ALI)
    - Moderate: PaO_2/FiO_2 ratio 100 to 199
    - Severe: PaO_2/FiO_2 ratio < 100
  - Onset within 1 week of a known clinical insult or new or worsening respiratory symptoms
  - Chest imaging revealing bilateral opacities not fully explained by effusions, lobar collapse, or nodules
  - Origin of edema not fully explained by cardiac failure or fluid overload must be objectively evaluated (e.g., echocardiography) if no clear predisposing factor for ARDS is present.

- Clinical impact of ARDS:
  - Patients with ARDS have mortality of 30% to 40%. The occurrence of AKI with ARDS may increase mortality up to 60%.
  - ARDS survivors have been shown to suffer long-term physical, psychological, and cognitive dysfunction.
- Management of ARDS:
  - Use of low tidal volumes (6 mL/kg of predicted body weight) to decrease plateau airway pressures
  - Maintenance of airway pressures < 30 cm H_2O to avoid alveolar overdistension
  - Use of PEEP:
    - Rationale:
      - Improve oxygenation by recruiting collapsed alveoli
      - Reduce ventilator-induced lung injury by preventing repetitive alveolar collapse and reexpansion
    - Concerns:
      - Circulatory depression due to increased intrathoracic pressure
      - Lung overdistension
    - Recent meta-analysis:
      - Patients with higher PEEP 15 ± 3 cm H_2O compared with PEEP of 9 ± 3 cm H_2O on day 1:
        - Higher PEEP had better oxygenation (lower Fio_2 requirement)
        - No difference in in-hospital mortality, but ICU mortality rates were lower in those with higher PEEP.
        - In patients with ARDS at randomization who received higher PEEP:
          - Both ICU and hospital mortality rates were lower (30.3 vs. 36.6%, $p = 0.001$).
          - Shorter time to unassisted breathing
          - Required less rescue therapies for refractory hypoxemia
        - In patients without ARDS at randomization who received higher PEEP:
          - Tendency toward harm (risk of hypotension or barotrauma)
          - Nonsignificant increase in in-hospital mortality rates (27.2 vs. 19.4%).
      - Bottom line: High PEEP strategy is relatively safe and may be considered in severe ARDS. *However*, PEEP > 10 cm H_2O may adversely affect kidney hemodynamics and the renin−angiotensin−aldosterone axis, especially in patients not yet adequately volume resuscitated.
- The link between ARDS and AKI:
  - AKI increases production and reduces clearance of inflammatory cytokines which can lead to increased pulmonary neutrophil chemotaxis and capillary permeability.
  - AKI downregulates ion and water transport channels involved in the removal of solute and water from injured alveoli in animal models.
- Fluid management in ARDS:
  - The Fluids and Catheters Treatment Trial (FACCT):
    - Patients with ARDS and without shock (i.e., no end-organ hypoperfusion), conservative fluid management (goal CVP < 4 vs. CVP of 10 to 14 cm H_2O) with fluid restriction and/or diuresis improves lung function and shortens duration of mechanical ventilation. Of note, at 7-day, there was a net zero fluid balance in the conservative group and 7 L positive in the liberal fluid group.
    - Conservative fluid management did not predispose patients to AKI, but was associated with a trend toward decreased RRT requirement.

- There was no survival benefit with the conservative fluid strategy.
- The Sepsis Occurrence in Acutely Ill Patients (SOAP):
  - Positive cumulative balance within the first 72 hours was associated with an increased risk of mortality in sepsis.
  - Early fluid resuscitation (e.g., fluid bolus, vasopressors as needed to reach hemodynamic stability within 6 hours of presentation in septic patients) and conservative late fluid management (maintaining even or negative fluid balance following hemodynamic stability) likely improve outcomes and survival rates.

Fluid Management in ICU Patients with AKI

- In general, volume overload is thought to delay diagnosis of AKI and has been shown to be associated with worse outcomes.
- Program to Improve Care in Acute Renal Disease (PICARD) trial:
  - Fluid overload, defined as an increase in >10% of admission weight, was associated with an increase in mortality at 60 days following study enrollment.
  - Fluid overload at the time of AKI diagnosis was *not* associated with recovery of kidney function.
  - Patients with fluid overload at their peak SCr were less likely to recover kidney function.
- Finland AKI (FINNAKI) trial: Patients with fluid overload at RRT initiation had an increased risk of 90-day morality after adjusting for disease severity, time of RRT initiation, modality, and sepsis compared to those without.
- Use of diuretics in AKI:
  - KDIGO: recommends not using furosemide to prevent or treat AKI, except for the management of volume overload.
  - There is no clear benefit with the use of diuretics on kidney function recovery.

Transfusion in Non-hemorrhagic Critically Ill Patients

- Red blood cells (RBC):
  - Stored RBCs may develop membrane injury, potassium leakage, altered oxygen affinity and delivery, and increased adhesions to endothelial cells.
  - Safety of aged versus fresh blood transfusions study is ongoing.
  - Recommended indications:
    - Hemoglobin < 7 g/dL for patients without cardiac disease
    - Hemoglobin < 7 to 8 g/dL in patients with coronary artery disease
    - Hemoglobin < 8 g/dL or when symptomatic in patients with acute coronary syndrome
    - Transfusions for higher Hb if symptomatic in isovolemic patients (e.g., cardiac chest pain, congestive heart failure, unexplained tachycardia, or hypotension not responsive to fluid replacement)
- Platelet transfusion:
  - Most bleeding occurred at a platelet count < 7,000/μL.
  - Transfuse for platelets < 10,000/μL
  - Prophylactic transfusion for invasive procedures: poor data; current expert opinion suggests transfusion for platelets < 50,000/μL
  - For CNS injury, multisystem trauma, neurosurgery: transfuse for platelets < 100,000/μL

- In patients requiring massive blood transfusion for exsanguinating hemorrhage, e.g., >10 units of PRBCs within 24 hours, transfuse 1:1:1 ratio for RBCs, plasma, and single-donor platelets.
- Plasma transfusion, fresh-frozen plasma (FFP):
  - Contains albumin, coagulation factors, fibrinolytic proteins, and immunoglobulins
  - May be given for patients with coagulopathy and active or anticipated bleeding
  - FFP may not correct INR of 1.85 or less.
  - Plasma transfusion is associated with an increased risk for lung injury and trend toward increased mortality. FFP should not be used for the sole purpose of a plasma expander.
- Complications associated with transfusions of blood products:
  - Volume overload, transfusion-related dyspnea and allergic reaction
  - Transfusion-related acute lung injury (TRALI):
    - TRALI: new-onset acute lung injury within 6 hours of receiving a plasma-containing blood component in the absence of other causes of ALI
    - Incidence: up to 1 in 20 patients
    - Risks:
      - Recipient factors: high IL-8 levels, high peak airway pressures (e.g., >30 cm H_2O), shock, tobacco and alcohol abuse, positive fluid balance
      - Blood product factors: plasma-rich products, increased antihuman leukocyte antigen class II antibodies and antihuman neutrophil antibodies, blood from female donors
  - Transfusion-related immunomodulation (TRIM): a transient transfusion related immunosuppressive effect that has been suggested to increase the risk of malignancy recurrence and hospital acquired infections. TRIM remains a debatable transfusion complication.

Vasopressors

- Indications for vasopressors: end-organ dysfunction due to hypoperfusion (i.e., MAP < 60 mm Hg or fall in SBP by >30 mm Hg from baseline with associated end-organ dysfunction [e.g. reduced urine output, altered mental status])
- Types of vasoactive agents:
  - α-1 adrenergic receptor stimulation → vasoconstriction
  - β-1 receptor stimulation → increase cardiac inotropy plus chronotropy
  - β-2 receptor stimulation → vasodilation
  - Dopamine: clinical effects are dose-dependent
    - Low dose (1 to 2 µg/kg/min): predominantly vasodilates cerebral, coronary, renal, and mesenteric vascular beds via dopamine-1 receptors
    - Intermediate dose (2 to 5 µg/kg/min): mix of vasodilation + increased stroke volume + some degree of α-adrenergic receptor activation; overall net effect may be seen as increased MAP
    - High dose (5 to 10 µg/kg/min): increases stroke volume, cardiac output; variable chronotropic effect
    - Very high dose > 10 µg/kg/min: predominantly vasoconstrictive via α-adrenergic receptors
    - Caution: dysrhythmias with doses > 2 µg/kg/min
- Special considerations regarding the use of vasoactive agents:
  - Optimize fluid status *prior* to the use of vasopressors (e.g., pulmonary capillary wedge pressures of 18 to 24 mm Hg for cardiogenic shock, and 12 to 14 mm Hg for septic or hypovolemic shock)

- Avoid excessive increase in systemic vascular resistance (SVR), hence cardiac work load, in patients with poor cardiac function (e.g., keep SVR 700 to 1,000 dynes $\times$ s/cm^5)
- Absorption of subcutaneous medications (e.g., heparin, insulin) may be reduced due to peripheral vasoconstriction
- Special uses of vasoconstrictors:
  - Hyperdynamic septic shock:
    - First line: NE (levophed) activates both α-1 and α-2 receptors. Activation of α-1 increases vasoconstriction and cardiac contractility/output, both of which lead to reflexive bradycardia. Activation of α-2 provides a mild positive chronotropic effect which opposes any α-1-induced bradycardia.
    - Alternative: epinephrine (neo-synephrine, acts on α-1 receptor to cause vasoconstriction, thus increasing MAP via increasing SVR, without altering cardiac inotropy or chonotropy).
      - Useful in hypotensive patients (e.g., hyperdynamic sepsis, neurologic or anesthesia related hemodynamic instability, with SVR < 700 dynes $\times$ s/cm^5)
      - NOTE: Phenylephrine may reduce stroke volume and should be last resort option.
      - Contraindicated if SVR > 1,200 dynes $\times$ s/cm^5
    - For patients with tachyarrhythmias or failed other therapies: phenylephrine
    - Add vasopressin if inadequate vasopressor effect with above agents
  - Hypodynamic shock (e.g., neurologic or anesthesia-related): first line: NE
  - Anaphylactic shock, hypotension following CABG:
    - Epinephrine (adrenalin: potent β-1 adrenergic receptor activity and moderate β-2 and α-1 adrenergic receptor effects; at high dose, predominant effects include increased cardiac output and SVR).
    - Epinephrine may be considered as second-line agent for patients with septic shock (who failed NE).
    - Considerations: dysrhythmias and splanchnic vasoconstriction
  - Cardiogenic shock:
    - First line: NE
    - *Once adequate perfusion pressure has been achieved*, dobutamine may be added as safely tolerated. Dobutamine acts predominantly on β-1 adrenergic receptor, thus leading to increased inotropy and chronotropy to reduce left ventricular filling pressure and improved cardiac output. NOTE: There may be an overall slight reduction in BP as a reflex response to the increased cardiac output.

> **NOTE** Dobutamine is contraindicated in patients with idiopathic hypertrophic subaortic stenosis.

- Others:
  - Vasopressin 0.3 IU/min:
    - Used as second-line or add-on vasopressor in refractory vasodilatory shock, for example, septic shock or anaphylaxis.
    - Potential adverse effects: coronary and mesenteric ischemia, skin necrosis, pulmonary vasoconstriction, hyponatremia

> **NOTE** Rebound with drug discontinuation: dose tapering is recommended.

- Isoproterenol (Isuprel):
  - Acts on β-1 adrenergic receptors resulting in prominent chronotropic effect as well as β-2 receptor to cause vasodilation and decrease in MAP.
  - Only indication: bradycardia-induced hypotension
- Complications of vasopressor therapy:
  - Hypoperfusion (e.g., blue distal extremities, skin necrosis, bowel ischemia, reduced kidney perfusion, myocardial ischemia). For skin necrosis due to IV infiltration, consider local subcutaneous injection with phenolamine (5 to 10 mg in 10 mL normal saline).
  - Dysrhythmias (e.g., tachycardia, atrial fibrillation, reentrant atrioventricular node tachycardia, or ventricular tachyarrhythmias; seen with agents with potent chronotropic effects via β-1 receptor stimulation)
  - Hyperglycemia (particularly with NE and epinephrine)
  - Electrolyte disturbances: hyponatremia with vasopressin, hypokalemia with agents with potent β2-receptor agonist effects such as dobutamine and isoproterenol, hyperkalemia with agents with strong α-adrenergic activity such as phenylephrine and NE in at-risk patients.

Fluid and Diuretics in AKI

- Colloids versus crystalloids:
  - Theoretical benefit: colloids remain intravascularly better than crystalloids, hence lower requirement for high volume resuscitation and less complications with pulmonary and peripheral edema.
  - 2011 Cochrane Collaboration group review: Colloids are *not* superior to isotonic crystalloids in terms of mortality when used for intravascular volume repletion in patients with trauma, burns, or after surgery.
  - KDIGO: suggests that isotonic crystalloids be used ahead of synthetic and nonsynthetic colloids for intravascular volume expansion in patients at risk or presenting with AKI in the absence of hemorrhagic shock.
  - Special considerations regarding colloids: albumin and synthetic colloids (hydroxyethylstarch [HES], gelatin, dextran):
    - Colloids (particularly hyperoncotic colloids including hyperoncotic albumin): increased AKI risk
    - Risks of albumin:
      - Virus transmission, Creutzfeldt–Jakob disease
      - 4% albumin infusion in patients with traumatic brain injury may be associated with higher mortality.
  - Albumin (4%) may be considered in other clinical scenarios including severe sepsis.
  - Hyperoncotic albumin (20% to 25%) appears to be renoprotective in cirrhotic patients, but should probably be avoided in other patients due to the lack of data.
- Calcium-free balanced crystalloid solution (i.e., plasma-lyte) on the day of a major surgery may be associated with fewer complications compared with normal saline, including infections and AKI requiring RRT. Confirmatory studies are needed.

Sepsis:

- Definitions:
  - SIRS: can arise from noninfectious insult

- Sepsis: systemic inflammation arising from infection
- Sepsis + organ dysfunction (including circulatory dysfunction): severe sepsis
- Septic shock: circulatory dysfunction (hypotension refractory to volume resuscitation or evidence of end-organ hypoperfusion, lactic acidosis)
- Early recognition:
  - Markers such as C-reactive proteins and serum procalcitonin are not useful.
  - Early recognition relies on routine clinical history and laboratory and imaging studies.
- Early resuscitation:
  - Hemodynamics and tissue oxygenation goals:
    - Maintain CVP of 8 to 12 mm Hg.
    - MAP > 65 mm Hg, but must individualized (higher in patients with chronic HTN; lower in end-stage liver disease may be acceptable).
    - Central venous oxygen saturation ($SCvo_2$) > 70% or lactate clearance > 10%.
  - Fluid resuscitation:
    - No consensus on type (0.9% normal saline, 4% albumin) and amount of fluid used for resuscitation of septic patients
    - Albumin:
      - Possible harm in patients with traumatic brain injury
      - Trend for benefit in patients with sepsis
    - Hydroxyl ethyl starch and pentastarch:
      - Associated with higher rates of AKI and death risk
      - Not recommended
- Antibiotics:
  - Goal: appropriate antibiotic initiation within the first hour of documented hypotension
  - Identification of infectious source within 24 hours
- Vasopressors for patients with septic shock:
  - NE is the preferred initial agent (5 μg/min).
  - Current data do not demonstrate survival difference between patients with shock treated with either dopamine or NE.
  - Dopamine may be associated with increased adverse events.
  - For patients with impaired cardiac contractility who require inotropic support:
    - Add dobutamine to NE, *or*
    - Use epinephrine as both vasopressor and inotropic agent
- Steroids:
  - Hydrocortisone 50 mg every 6 hours × 5 days followed by taper regimen
  - If given within 8 hours of septic shock onset, improved mortality in patients who cannot increase serum cortisol level following 250 μg ACTH stimulation test ("nonresponders") compared with "responders."
  - May reverse shock more promptly
- Glycemic control:
  - Control to <180 mg/dL leads to similar outcomes compared with tighter control of 80 to 100 mg/dL and avoids hypoglycemic episodes.
- AKI:
  - Low-dose dopamine does not reduce the incidence of AKI or its associated mortality.
  - Loop diuretics do not reduce the need for RRT, duration on RRT, or mortality.
  - RRT support as indicated

- Others:
  - Recombinant activated protein C (rhAPC): PROWESS-SHOCK trial (randomized controlled trial comparing rhAPC treatment vs. placebo in vasopressor-dependent septic shock patients) revealed no mortality benefit.
  - Intravenous immunoglobulin:
    - Conflicting data; no benefit shown in high-quality trials
    - Routine use in septic patients not recommended
  - Extracorporeal blood purification:
    - Rationale: improve removal of inflammatory mediators.
    - No benefit found with higher intensity RRT (i.e., CRRT with UF rates > 20 to 25 mL/kg/h) in septic patients with AKI.
    - High-volume hemofiltration with rates (HVHF) > 60 mL/kg/h → small trials indicate improvement in hemodynamics and other physiological parameters.
    - The safety and efficacy of hemoperfusion (removes endotoxins with use of polymyxin-bound fibers) in patients with septic shock are not known pending ongoing EUPHRATES trial.
    - Ongoing trials on HVHF and hemoperfusion in sepsis

HEMODYNAMIC MONITORING

Static Testing for Fluid Responsiveness

- Static testing parameters:
  - CVP via central line (internal jugular or subclavian vein): estimates right atrial pressure, and in effect, right ventricular end diastolic volume, blood volume and right ventricular preload
  - Pulmonary arterial occlusion pressure (PAoP) via pulmonary artery (PA) catheter: estimates left atrial pressure, and in effect, left ventricular diastolic volume
  - Left ventricular end diastolic area (LVEAD) via transthoracic or transesophageal echocardiography: Theoretically, an increase in LVEDA corresponds to greater ventricular myocardial stretch, thus presumed greater cardiac output.
- Limitations to static testing:
  - CVP, PAoP, and LVEAD lack accuracy and precision.
  - CVP: invasive, falsely high readings with pulmonary HTN, right ventricular dysfunction, or high PEEP
  - PAoP: invasive, falsely high readings with ARDS due to misleadingly high cardiac filling pressure
  - LVEAD: cannot predict where in the Frank–Starling curve the myocardial stretch is to accurately determine actual cardiac output

Dynamic Testing for Fluid Responsiveness

- Pulse pressure variation (PPV) and stroke volume variation (SVV):
  - This should be measured with PEEP 8 to 10 cm H_2O and tidal volume of 8 to 10 mL/kg to be consistent with studies that document the usefulness of PPV/SVV.

- Technique is based on the principle of pulsus paradoxus, which is the variation of stroke volume and BP with respiration. Positive pressure ventilation causes decreased venous return and increased right ventricular afterload, hence reduced stroke volume or pulse pressure. Volume depletion exaggerates SVV and PVV.
  - PPV = [PP(highest value) − PP(lowest value)]/PP(lowest value). Variation > 12% suggests greater likelihood for fluid responsiveness.
  - SVV= [SV(highest value) − SV(lowest value)]/SV(lowest value). Variation > 12% suggests greater likelihood for fluid responsiveness.
- Inferior vena cava (IVC) diameter:
  - Subcostal measurement of IVC diameter (below junction with right atrium) changes during respiration by echocardiography.
  - A change of >10% to 18% in IVC diameter between inspiration and expiration (expiration is considered as "baseline") predicts fluid responsiveness with sensitivity 50% to 100% and specificity 53% to 100%. This test may be used for both ventilated and spontaneously breathing patients.
- Passive leg raising:
  - Measures changes in various hemodynamic parameters between semirecumbent position (head-of-bed elevation at 45°) and both leg raise to 45°.
  - Measures changes in cardiac output, pulse pressure/stroke volume, MAP, or PAoP. Improvement in hemodynamic parameters with leg raising suggests fluid responsiveness. This test is limited to patients who can lie flat.

Hemodynamic Methods for Measuring Cardiac Output and Body Volume Status

- Thermodilution: Requires a PA catheter, where a small volume of cold solution (injectate) is injected into the PA catheter. The change in blood temperature following blood mixing with the injectate can be used to calculate cardiac output.
- Transpulmonary thermodiluation: Similar theory as above. Injectate is injected through a standard central venous catheter and a thermistor which is inserted into the femoral artery. This method is thought to be less invasive compared to the thermodilution technique above.
- Esophageal Doppler:
  - Doppler is positioned in the esophagus to measure aortic diameter and velocity of blood flow through the aorta, where cardiac output is estimated by the equation: velocity = flow/cross-sectional area. Flow (blood flow) reflects cardiac output.
  - Limitations: Measurements may be affected by flow turbulence (e.g., from aneurysm, atherosclerotic disease) and by upward flow from the aortic arch (blood volume that does not reach aortic area of interest leads to falsely low cardiac output).
  - Good correlation with thermodilution method
- Thoracic electrical bioimpedance (TEB):
  - Technique is based on Ohm's law: voltage = current × resistance
  - Measures electrical resistance on an applied current, where the resistance is affected by the relative water content in the descending aorta, which is the amount of blood flow through the aorta. A volume-repleted patient will theoretically

have a low TEB (i.e., low resistance) compared with that of a volume depleted patient.

- Pulse contour analysis: Measures/calculates cardiac performance based on variations in arterial line tracings with bedside computers/programs
- Pulse oximetry waveform variation: The pulse oximetry curve represents the amount of infrared light absorbed by circulating hemoglobin during a cardiac cycle. Variation in the amplitude of this curve relates to the amount of blood in the capillary bed/volume status.

Access the eBook for self-assessment questions.

Core Resources and Selected Readings

CORE TEXTBOOKS

Danovitch G, ed. *Handbook of Kidney Transplantation*. 5th ed. Philadelphia, PA: Lippincott Williams & Wilkins; 2010.

Daugirdas JT, Blake PG, Ing TS, eds. *Handbook of Dialysis*. 4th ed. Philadelphia, PA: Lippincott Williams & Wilkins; 2007.

Johnson RJ, Feehally J, Floege J, eds. *Comprehensive Clinical Nephrology*. 5th ed. Philadelphia, PA: Elsevier; 2015.

Kurtz I, ed. *Acid-Base Case Studies*. Victoria, Canada: Trafford; 2004.

Nissenson AR, Fine RN, eds. *Dialysis Therapy*. 3rd ed. Philadelphia, PA: Hanley & Belfus, Inc.; 2007.

Ronco C, Bellomo R, Kellum JA, eds. *Critical Care Nephrology*. 3rd ed. Philadelphia, PA: Saunders Elsevier; 2009.

Rose B, ed. *Clinical Physiology of Acid-Base and Electrolyte Disorders*. 5th ed. New York, NY: McGraw-Hill Companies, Inc.; 2001.

ONLINE RESOURCES

Aasld.org
Asn-online.org//education/brcu
Kdigo.org/home/guidelines
Medscape.com
UptoDate.com

SELF-ASSESSMENT SERIES

Nephrology Self-Assessment Program (NephSAP), American Society of Nephrology

CHAPTER-SPECIFIC SELECTED READINGS

Chapter 1
Sodium/Water

Berl T. Vasopressin antagonists. *N Engl J Med*. 2015;372(23):2207–2216.

Crowly RK, Sherlock M, Agha A, et al. Clinical insights into adipsic diabetes insipidus: a large case series. *Clin Endocrinol (Oxf)*. 2007;66(4):475–482.

Fenske W, Allolio B. Current state and future perspectives in the diagnosis of diabetes insipidus: a clinical review. *J Clin Endocrinol Metab*. 2012;97(10):3426–3437.

Liamis G, Milionis H, Elisaf M. A review of drug-induced hyponatremia. *Am J Kidney Dis*. 2008;52(1):144–153.

Pham PM, Pham PA, Pham PT, et al. Correction of hyponatremia and osmotic demyelinating syndrome: have we neglected to think intracellularly? *Clin Exp Nephrol*. 2014;19(3):489–495.

Robertson GL. Diabetes insipidus. *Endocrinol Metab Clin North Am*. 1995;24(3):549–572.

Sam R, Feizi I. Understanding hypernatremia. *Am J Nephrol*. 2012;36(1):97–104.

Schrier RW, Gross P, Gheorghiade M, et al. Tolvaptan, a selective oral vasopressin V2-receptor antagonist, for hyponatremia. *N Engl J Med*. 2006;355(20):2099–2112.

Sterns RH. Disorders of plasma sodium – causes, consequences, and correction. *N Engl J Med*. 2015;372(1):55–65.

Verbalis JG, Goldsmith SR, Greenberg A, et al. Diagnosis, evaluation, and treatment of hyponatremia: expert panel recommendations. *Am J Med*. 2013;126(10 Suppl 1):S1–S42.

Chapter 2
Acid-Base/Potassium

Batlle D, Haque SK. Genetic causes and mechanisms of distal renal tubular acidosis. *Nephrol Dial Transpl.* 2012;27(10):3691–3704.

Berend K, de Vries APJ, Gans ROB. Physiological approach to assessment of acid-base disturbances. *N Engl J Med.* 2014;371(15):1434–1445.

Fenves AZ, Kirkpatrick HM 3rd, Patel VV, et al. Increased anion gap metabolic acidosis as a result of 5-oxoproline (pyroglutamic acid): a role for acetaminophen. *Clin J Am Soc Nephrol.* 2006;1(3):441–447.

Kraut JA, Madias NE. Lactic acidosis. *N Engl J Med.* 2014;371(24):2309–2319.

Naesens M, Steels P, Verberckmoes R, et al. Bartter's and Gitelman's syndromes: from gene to clinic. *Nephron Physiol.* 2004;96(3):65–78.

Palermo M, Quinkler M, Stewart PM. Apparent mineralocorticoid excess syndrome: an overview. *Arq Bras Endocrinol Metabol.* 2004;48(5):678–696.

Venance SL, Cannon SC, Fialho, et al. The primary periodic paralyses: diagnosis, pathogenesis and treatment. *Brain.* 2006;129(Pt 1):8–17.

Chapter 3
Calcium, Phosphorus, Magnesium, and Kidney Stones

Cunningham J, Locatelli F, Rodriguez M. Secondary hyperparathyroidism: pathogenesis, disease progression, and therapeutic options. *Clin J Am Soc Nephrol.* 2011;6(4):913–921.

Khashayar S, Maalouf NM, Sinnott B. Kidney stones 2012: pathogenesis, diagnosis, and management. *J Clin Endocrinol Metab.* 2012;97(6):1847–1860.

Kovesdy CP, Quarles LD. Fibroblast growth factor-23: what we know, what we don't know, and what we need to know. *Nephrol Dial Transplant.* 2013;28(9):2228–2236.

Martin KJ, Gonzalez EA. Long-term management of CKD-mineral and bone disorder. *Am J Kidney Dis.* 2012;60(2):308–315.

Pearle MS, Goldfarb DS, Assimos DG, et al. Medical management of kidney stones: AUA guideline. *J Urol.* 2014;192(2):316–324.

Pham PC, Pham PA, Pham SV, et al. Hypomagnesemia: a clinical perspective. *Int J Nephrol Renovasc Dis.* 2014;7:219–230.

Zoppellaro G, Faggin E, Puato M, et al. Fibroblast growth factor 23 and the bone-vascular axis: lessons learned from animal studies. *Am J Kidney Dis.* 2012;59(1):135–144.

Chapter 4
Chronic Kidney Disease

Cooper BA, Branley P, Bulfone L, et al. Randomized controlled trial of early versus late initiation of dialysis. *N Engl J Med.* 2010;363(7):609–619.

Coresh J, Byrd-Holt D, Astor BC, et al. Chronic kidney disease awareness, prevalence, and trends among US adults, 1999 to 2000. *J Am Soc Nephrol.* 2005;16(1):180–188.

Farnett L, Mulrow CD, Linn WD, et al. The J-curve phenomenon and the treatment of hypertension. Is there a point beyond which pressure reduction is dangerous? *JAMA.* 1991;265(4):489–495.

Galperin TA, Cronin AJ, Leslie KS. Cutaneous manifestations of ESRD. *Clin J Am Soc Nephrol.* 2014;9(1):201–218.

Levey AS, Stevens LA, Schmid CH, et al. A new equation to estimate glomerular filtration rate. *Ann Intern Med.* 2009;150(9):604–612.

Maisonneuve P, Agodoa L, Gellert R, et al. Cancer in patients on dialysis for end stage renal disease: an international collaborative study. *Lancet.* 1999;354(9173):93–99.

Manisco G, Poti M, Maggiuli G, et al. Pregnancy in end-stage renal disease patients on dialysis: how to achieve a successful delivery. *Clin Kidney J.* 2015;8(3):293–299.

McCormick BB, Sydor A, Akbari A, et al. The effect of pentoxifylline on proteinuria in diabetic kidney disease: a meta-analysis. *Am J Kidney Dis.* 2008;52(3):454–463.

Miller PD. Bone disease in CKD: a focus on osteoporosis diagnosis and management. *Am J Kidney Dis.* 2014;64(2):290–304.

Roberts JM, August PA, Bakris G, et al. Hypertension in pregnancy. Report of the American College of Obstetricians and Gynecologists' Task Force on hypertension in pregnancy. *Obstet Gyn.* 2013;122(5):1122–1131.

Sjostrom P, Tidman M, Jones I. Determination of the production rate and nonrenal clearance of cystatin C and estimation of the glomerular filtration rate from the serum concentration of cystatin C in humans. *Scand J Clin Lab Invest.* 2005;65(2):111–124.

Vaqar S, Murray B, Panesar M. The medical-legal responsibilities of the dialysis unite medical director. *Semin Dial.* 2014;27(5):472–476.

Wang H, Wei Y, Kong X, Xu D. Effects of urate-lowering therapy in hyperuricemia on slowing the progression of renal function: a meta-analysis. *J Ren Nutr.* 2013;23(5):389–396

Zhou XJ, Saxena R, Liu Z, et al. Renal senescence in 2008: progress and challenges. *Int Urol Nephrol.* 2008;40(3):823–839.

Chapter 5
Hypertension

Cline DM and Amin A. Drug treatment for hypertensive emergencies. *Emergency Medicine Medical Research and Education Group International Newsletter.* 2008;1:1–12.

Joint National Committe on Prevention, Detection, Evaluation, and Treatment of High Blood Pressure: Seventh and Eight Reports (JNC 7 and JNC 8).

Pathare G, Hoenderop JG, Bindels RJ, et al. A molecular update on pseudohypoaldosteronism type II. *Am J Physiol Renal Physiol.* 2013;305(11):F1513–F1520.

Marzano L, Coluss G, Sechi LA, et al. Adrenalectomy is comparable with medical treatment for reduction of left ventricular mass in primary aldosteronism: meta-analysis of long-term studies. *Am Hypertens.* 2015;28(3):312–318.

Reincke M, Fischer E, Gerum S, et al. Observational study mortality in treated primary aldosteronism: the German Conn's Registry. *Hypertension.* 2012;60(3):618–624.

Roberts JM, August PA, Bakris G, et al. Executive summary: hypertension in pregnancy. *Obstet Gyn.* 2013;122(5):1122–1131.

Rossi GP, Cesari M, Cuspidi C, et al. Long-term control of arterial hypertension and regression of left ventricular hypertrophy with treatment of primary aldosteronism. *Hypertension.* 2013;62(1):62–69.

Shanmugam VK, Steen VD. Renal disease in scleroderma: an update on evaluation, risk stratification, pathogenesis and management. *Curr Opin Rheumatol.* 2012;24(6):669–676.

SPRINT Research Group, Wright JT, Williamson JD, et al. A randomized trial of intensive versus standard blood pressure control. *N Engl J Med.* 2015;373(22):2103–2116.

Weiner ID. Endocrine and hypertensive disorders of potassium regulation: primary aldosteronism. *Semin Nephrol.* 2013;33(3):265–276.

Chapter 6
Tubular, Interstitial, and Cystic Disorders

Chapman AB, Devuyst O, Eckardt KU, et al. Autosomal-dominant polycystic kidney disease (ADPKD): executive summary from a kidney disease: improving global outcomes (KDIGO) controversies conference. *Kidney Int.* 2015;88(1):17–27.

Hall AM, Bass P, Unwin RJ. Drug-induced renal Fanconi syndrome. *QJM.* 2014;107(4):261–269.

Markowitz GS, Radhakrishnan J, Kambham N, et al. Lithium nephrotoxicity: a progressive combined glomerular and tubulointerstitial nephropathy. *J Am Soc Nephrol.* 2000;11(8):1439–1448.

Raissian Y, Nasr SH, Larsen CP, et al. Diagnosis of IgG4-related tubulointerstitial nephritis. *J Am Soc Nephrol.* 2011;22(7):1343–1352

Rossert J. Drug-induced acute interstitial nephritis. *Kidney Int.* 2001;60(2):804–817.

Yarlagadda SG, Perazella MA. Drug-induced crystal nephropathy: an update. *Expert Opin Drug Saf.* 2008;7(2):147–158.

Chapter 7
Glomerular/Vascular Diseases

Beck LH, Bonegio RGB, Lambeau G, et al. M-type phospholipase A2 receptor as target antigen in idiopathic membranous nephropathy. *N Engl J Med.* 2009;361(1):11–21.

D'Agati VD, Kaskel FJ, Falk RJ. Focal segmental glomerulosclerosis. *N Engl J Med.* 2011;365(25):2398–2411.

Fakhour F, Roumenina L, Provot F, et al. Pregnancy-associated hemolytic uremic syndrome revisited in the era of complement gene mutations. *J Am Soc Nephrol.* 2010;21(5):859–867.

George JN, Nester CM. Syndromes of thrombotic microangiopathy. *N Engl J Med.* 2014;371(7):654–666.

Goldschmidt H, Lannert H, Bommer J, et al. Multiple myeloma and renal failure. *Nephrol Dial Transpl.* 2000;15(3):301–304.

Hudson BG, Tryggvason K, Sundaramoorthy M, et al. Alport's syndrome, Goodpasture's syndrome, and type IV collagen. *N Engl J Med.* 2003;348(25):2543–2556.

Kallenberg CGM. Key advances in the clinical approach to ANCA-associated vasculitis. *Nat Rev Rheum.* 2014;10:484–493.

Korbet SM. Treatment of primary FSGS in adults. *J Am Soc Nephrol* 2012;23:1769–1776.

McCormick BB, Sydor A, Akbari A, et al. The effect of pentoxifylline on proteinuria in diabetic kidney disease: a meta-analysis. *Am J Kidney Dis.* 52(3):454–463.

Rovin BH, Prikh SV. Lupus nephritis: the evolving role of novel therapeutics. *Am J Kidney Dis.* 2014;63(4):677–690.

Sethi S, Fervenza F. Membranoproliferative glomerulonephritis – a new look at an old entity. *N Engl J Med*. 2012;366(12):1119–1131.

Stanhope TJ, White WM, Moder KG, et al. Obstetric nephrology: lupus and lupus nephritis in pregnancy. *Clin J Am Soc Nephrol*. 2012. 7(12):2089–2099.

Sterner RM, Hartono SP, Grande JP. The pathogenesis of lupus nephritis. *J Clin Cell Immunol*. 2014;5(2):PMC4131745.

Tomas NM, Beck LH, Meyer-Schwesinger C, et al. Thrombospondin type-1 domain-containing 7A in idiopathic membranous nephropathy. *N Engl J Med*. 2014;371(24):2277–2287.

Wyatt RJ, Julian BA. IgA nephropathy. *N Engl J Med*. 2013;368(25):2404–2414.

Chapter 8
Kidney Transplantation

Alberu J, Pascoe MD, Campistol JM, et al. Lower malignancy rates in renal allograft recipients converted to sirolimus-based, calcineurin inhibitor-free immunotherapy: 24-month results from the CONVERT trial. *Transplantation*. 2011;92(3):303–310.

Dols LF, Kok NF, Roodnat JI, et al. Living kidney donors: impact of age on long-term safety. *Am J Transplant*. 2011;11(4):737–742.

Euvrard S, Morelon E, Rostaing L, et al. Sirolimus and secondary skin-cancer prevention in kidney transplantation. *N Engl J Med*. 2012;367(4):329–339.

Fernandez-Ruiz M, Lopez-Medrano F, Varela-Pena P, et al. Monitoring of immunoglobulin levels identifies kidney transplant recipients at high risk of infection. *Am J Transplant*. 2012;12(10):2763–2773.

Florescu MC, Miles CD, Florescu DF. What do we know about adenovirus in renal transplantation? *Nephrol Dial Transplant*. 2013;28(8):2003–2010.

Garg AX, Muirhead N, Knoll G, et al. Proteinuria and reduced kidney function in living kidney donors: a systematic review, meta-analysis, and meta-regression. *Kidney Int*. 2006;70(10):1801–1810.

Garg AX, Nevis IF, McArthur E, et al. Gestational hypertension and preeclampsis in living kidney donors. *N Engl J Med*. 2015;372(2):124–133.

Glotz D, Chapman JR, Dharnidharka VR, et al. The Seville expert workshop for progress in posttransplant lymphoproliferative disorders. *Transplantation*. 2012;94(8):784–793.

Hurst FP, Belur P, Neer R, et al. Poor outcomes associated with neutropenia after kidney transplant: analysis of United States Renal Data system. *Transplantation*. 2011;92(1):36–40.

Kalanta-Zadeh K, Molnar MZ, Kovesdy CP, et al. Management of minerals and bone disorders after kidney transplantation. *Curr Opin Nephrol Hypertens*. 2012;21(4):389–403.

Kucirka LM, Sarathy H, Govindan P, et al. Risk of window period hepatitis C infection in high infectious risk donors: systematic review and meta-analysis. *Am J Transplant*. 2011;11(6):1188–2000.

Oriquen J, Fernadez-Ruiz M, Lumbreras C, et al. Potential role of post-transplant hypogammaglobulinemia in the risk of Clostridium difficile infection after kidney transplantation: a case-control study. *Infection*. 2015;43(4):413–422.

Chapter 9
Pharmacology

Bayliss G. Dialysis in the poisoned patient. *Hemodial Int*. 2010;14(2):158–167.

Bennett WM. Principles of drug therapy in patients with renal disease. *West J Med*. 1975;123(5):372-379.a

Coco TJ, Klasner AE. Drug-induced rhabdomyolysis. *Curr Opin Pediatr*. 2004;16(2):206–210.

Fissell WH. Antimicrobial dosing in acute renal replacement. *Adv Chronic Kidney Dis*. 2013;20(1):85–93.

Gabardi S, Munz K, Ulbricht C. A review of dietary supplement-induced renal dysfunction. *Clin J Am Soc Nephrol*. 2007;2(4):757–765.

Gao Y, Zhao MH. Review article: drug-induced anti-neutrophil cytoplasmic antibody-associated vasculitis. *Nephrology (Carlton)*. 2009;14(1):33–41.

Jha V. Herbal medicines and chronic kidney disease. *Nephrology (Carlton)*. 2010;15(suppl 2):10–17.

Johnson CA. 2010 Dialysis of Drugs. Verona, WI: CKD Insights, LLC; 2010.

Laniado-Laborin R, Cabrales-Vargas MN. Amphotericin B: side effects and toxicity. *Rev Iberoam Micol*. 2009;26(4):223–227.

Lo A, Burckart GJ. P-glycoprotein and drug therapy in organ transplantation. *J Clin Pharmacol*. 1999;39(10):995–1005.

Singh NP, Ganguli A, Prakash A. Drug-induced kidney diseases. *J Assoc Physicians India*. 2003;51:970–979.

Chapter 10
Acute Kidney Injury/ICU Nephrology

Haase M, Haase-Fielitz A, Bellomo R, et al. Sodium bicarbonate to prevent increases in serum creatinine after cardiac surgery: a pilot double-blind, randomized controlled trial. *Crit Care Med*. 2009;37(1):39–47.

Hollenberg SM. Hemodynamic monitoring. *Chest*. 2013;143(5):1480–1488.

Kirkpatrick AW, Roberts DJ, De Waele J, et al. Intra-abdominal hypertension and the abdominal compartment syndrome; updated consensus definitions and clinical practice guidelines from the World Society of the Abdominal Compartment Syndrome. *Intensive Care Med*. 2013;39(7):1190–1206.

Konstam MA, Gheorghiade M, Burnett JC, et al. Effects of oral tolvaptan in patients hospitalized for worsening heart failure: the EVEREST outcome trial. *JAMA*. 2007;297(12):1319–1331.

Lenz K, Buder R, Kapun L, et al. Treatment and management of ascites and hepatorenal syndrome: an update. *Therap Adv Gastroenterol*. 2015;8(2):83–100.

Liu KD, Matthay MA. Advances in critical care for the nephrologist: acute lung injury/ARDS. *Clin J Am Soc Nephrol*. 2008;3(2):578–586.

National Heart, Lung, and Blood Institute Acute Respiratory Distress Syndrome (ARDS) Clinical Trials Network, Wiedemann HP, Wheeler AP, et al. Comparison of two fluid-management strategies in acute lung injury. *N Engl J Med*. 2006;354(54):2564–2575.

Perazella MA, Coca SG, Hall IE, et al. Urine microscopy is associated with severity and worsening of acute kidney injury in hospitalized patients. *Clin J Am Soc Nephrol*. 2010;5(3):402–408.

Rafat C, Burbach M, Brocheriou I, et al. Bilirubin-associated acute tubular necrosis in a kidney transplant recipient. *Am J Kidney Dis*. 2013;61(5):782–785.

Ronco C, Haapio M, House AA, et al. Cardiorenal syndrome. *J Am Coll Cardiol*. 2008;52(19):1527–1539.

Ronco C, Ricci Z, De Backer D, et al. Renal replacement therapy in acute kidney injury: controversy and consensus. *Crit Care*. 2015;19:146–156.

Index

Page numbers followed by "*f*" indicate figures; page numbers followed by "*t*" indicate tables.